Health and Healing in the Igbo Society

European University Studies
Europäische Hochschulschriften
Publications Universitaires Européennes

Series XXIII
Theology

Reihe XXIII Série XXIII
Theologie
Théologie

Vol./Bd. 857

PETER LANG
Frankfurt am Main · Berlin · Bern · Bruxelles · New York · Oxford · Wien

Victor Nkemdilim Onyeador

Health and Healing in the Igbo Society

Basis and Challenges for an Inculturated Pastoral Care of the Sick

PETER LANG
Internationaler Verlag der Wissenschaften

Bibliographic Information published by the Deutsche Nationalbibliothek
The Deutsche Nationalbibliothek lists this publication in the Deutsche Nationalbibliografie; detailed bibliographic data is available in the internet at <http://www.d-nb.de>.

Zugl.: Vallendar, Philos.-Theol. Hochsch., Diss., 2007

ISSN 0721-3409
ISBN 978-3-631-57151-4

www.peterlang.de

To my Sister, Sr. Dr. med. Virgie M. Onyeador who is now resting in the Lord

And to all People of Goodwill

Forword

In the introduction to the Rite of Anointing of the Sick, published 1972 we read:

It is part of God's plan that we should combat all illness and should prudently seek the blessing of good health. We will thus be able to play our part in the secular society and in the Church. Arthur Schopenhauer, the astute German philosopher, puts it another way: 'The greatest mistake a man can make is to sacrifice health for any other advantage.'

This Work is first and foremost, a fruit of my immense experience as a Hospital Chaplain and a Pastor in one of the biggest Catholic Charismatic Renewal Parish in Enugu Diocese of Nigeria.

Health care of the sick in the Healing Ministry now occupies a strategic position in the activities of the Catholic Church world–wide, and this has also awakened my interest in this area of scientific study. Being a study "from within", I hope it will help whoever has interest in the Healing Ministry in accordance with the tradition and approval of the Catholic Church.

Health is a good companion of our lives, not to be taken advantage of. Occasionally it is like the timid student in school who raises his hand for help but finds the teacher too busy to notice, until a time comes when, like health, he loses his cool and refuses to stay silent any longer. His frustrations reach such a pitch that he scrams for attention.

Looking at Man as a complex being, this work endeavours to capture the various aspects of the suffering man giving no preference to one or the other; since each aspect is only but the part of a whole, to dislocate one part is to dislocate equally the unity of the whole. From my experience as Chaplain, most people are notoriously negligent when it comes to maintaining good health. Even when hospitalized, they are occupied with their businesses at home and other related matters.

In the words of Proverbs 17:22: A joyful heart is good medicine (the Hebrew says, '... causes good healing ...') but a broken spirit dries up the bones. Therefore good health is an essential requirement for effective evangelisation.

Acknowledgements

As Karl Jaspers puts it, “no matter how minute an individual is among the factors that make up history, he is a factor” Hence, for the success of this work, I heartily acknowledge the collaboration, sacrifices and encouragement of friends and colleagues, which would be impossible to mention all here but their names have been written in my heart.

My unalloyed gratitude goes first and foremost to my Moderator, Professor Dr. Ernst Leuninger, for his scholarly guidance and moderation of this Dissertation. Remembered in the same spirit is my second moderator: Professor Dr. P. Rheinbay and the Rector of the Philosophisch – Theologische Hochschule, Vallendar: Professor Dr. H. Niederschlag for the approval of this work.

I give special thanks to my former Bishop, Most Rev. Dr. M.U. Eneja, for granting me the permission to complete my theological studies. My thanks also to His Lordship, Most Rev. Dr.A.Gbuji, the present Bishop of Enugu. I am grateful to them for the enriching horizon they left at my disposal.

I would also like to acknowledge the overwhelming support and encouragement I received from my friends Frau Hildegard Höller, Herrn Karl–Josef Höller, Frau A. Gonschor and M. Lakenbrink to them I own special gratitude. I will ever remain grateful to Professor Dr. Ludwig Bertsch, who was a splendid mentor and he is now resting in the Lord. I commend them to God to reward them most abundantly.

Finally I should like to express my deepest thanks to my family for all they have been and meant for me all these years and above all to Almighty God for the health and inspiration to complete my work. Read on!

Table of Contents

0 General Introduction

0.1 Introduction

Throughout the history of Christianity the problem of Christian faith and human suffering has been a major focus of theological reflection. This problem is a serious and enduring challenge to Christian faith, making striking at the heart of traditional belief in God. Some theologians contend that evil makes theistic belief in an omnipotent, omniscient and perfectly good God problematic. According to Hans Küng, the problem is so severe that is has become "the rock of atheism." Through the centuries, many great thinkers have wrestled with this intellectual difficulty which arises equally for the three major theistic religions – Judaism, Christianity, and Islam.

A number of Western theologians have given it some attention from various perspectives for example, Michael J. Teylor, The Mystery of Suffering and Death (1973); John M. McDermott, The Bible on Human Suffering (1990); Hans Küng, On Being a Christian (1991); and Jurgen Moltmann, The Crucified God (1992); to mention but a few. All have respectively given detailed and theological reflection on the mystery of human sufferings and Death. Pope John Paul II, in his Apostolic Letter, Salvifici Doloris (1984), on the other gives a critical view on the Christian meaning of human suffering. Even some African theologians made their positive contributions regardless of their shortcomings.

The Catholic Church in Igboland of Nigeria which takes a lion share in this work is now over a hundred years old with her celebration of the centenary jubilee in 1985. Christianity has up to a point taken a deep step into permeating the life of the people. One will not hesitate therefore to observe that the mission of Jesus Christ to evangelise the world has reached the Igboland of Nigeria. Before Jesus left the world to go back to his father, he entrusted to his disciples the mission he received from his father and gave them the authority and power to heal the sick and preach the gospel.

> *He summoned his twelve disciples and gave them authority over unclean spirits with power to cast them out and cure all kinds of diseases and sickness. (Mt 10: 1–6; Lk 9: 1–2; Mk 6–7.)2*

Luke extended the commission further than Matthew and Mark by adding the commissioning of the seventy–two other disciples in his writing.

After this, the Lord appointed seventy–two others and sent them out ahead of him, in pairs, to all the towns and places he himself was to visit... Whenever you go into a town where they make you welcome, eat what is set before you. Cure those in it who are sick and say, 'The kingdom of God is very near to you. (Lk 10: 1–9)

The proclamation of the kingdom and the healing works of Jesus Christ were placed on the same plane by the evangelists. The healing works "authenticate the proclamation of the kingdom of God and stands as a sign of triumph over evil".[1] The first missionaries of this gospel landed at the bank of the River Niger in Onitsha in Igboland on December 5, 1885, with the Holy Ghost fathers as the pioneer missionaries. The fathers along with the preaching of the word "opened a dispensary as a vital point of contact with the people who came for treatment. The move was so successful that parents crowded the Catholic mission where Fr Lutz provided medication for their children's ailments".[2]

Since then the Church has continued with the establishment of healthcare institutions, as an avenue for the continuation of the healing mission entrusted to the Church by Jesus Christ.

The healing mission through prayer and faith/healing was not prominent in the Catholic Church in Igboland until very recently. According to G. Ikeobi., "Before the 10th of May 1973, no priest was fully involved in the healing ministry."[3] That is to say that this important aspect of the mission of Jesus

Christ has gone on rather slowly in the Church over years. The preaching of the word so to say suffocated the mission to heal. Today the situation is changing rapidly. The healing aspect of the mission of Jesus Christ has claimed an overwhelming prominence in the area.

According to C. Ejizu,

The practice of casting out evil spirits and prayer/faith healing is certainly one of the most outstanding features of popular religiosity in the contemporary Nigerian scene. It's record of achievement especially in the past thirty years or so appears quite spectacular.[4]

---

1 K. D. O'Rourke and P.Boyle, Medical Ethics: Sources of Catholic Teachings, C H A, St Loius, 1989, p.134

2 C. A. Obi, Background to the planting of the Catholic Christianity in the Lower Niger, in C.A. Obi, ed., "Hundred years of the Catholic Chruch in Eastern Nigeria", Onitsha, 1985, pp24 – 25

3 G. Ikeobi, "What I think God is doing and through me", paper presented at the National theological seminar on healing ministry, Enugu, Nigeria, 1992, p.33

4 C. Ejizu, Cosmoligical perspective on Exorcism and Prayer healing in Contemporary Nigeria, in C.U. Manus et al., eds, 'Healing and Exorcisms: The Nigerian Experience', Proceeings and Letures of the First Missiological Symposium on Healing and Exorcism, Snaap Press, Enugu, 1992. p11

Many priests, religious, and lay men and women especially members of the Catholic Charismatic Renewal engage in the healing ministry today. This has been a significant development for the still growing Church of Igboland. But the quest for healing and healing miracles is growing in a crazy proportion. This has invariably affected Christianity in particular and life in general. Prayer houses and healing centres of various types and proportions are germinating all over the place and people run helter–skelter from one healing centre to another in search of healing and security. They want instant wealth and health. People want by all means to have health and avoid suffering. This invariably seems to have increased the types of sickness and their dimensions which range from natural headache and fever to attacks from various demonic or evil forces, some of which sometimes defy solutions and cures except by some mystic inclinations.

Problems mostly reported by people in these centres include 'Amosu' (witchcraft), 'Ogbanje' or 'Ndi otu' (born to die), 'Muo mmili' (aquatic spirits), 'Nsi' (poisoning), 'Agwunsi or 'Muo mkpasasi'(type of malevolent spirits), to mention but a few. So many people today believe that their misfortune or illness is rooted in or caused out–rightly by one or more of the above. The young man who, has fever or cold believes he could not sleep in the night because he is being be–witched by 'amosu', while the young lady who is not yet married believes the Mermaid does not agree she should marry. And the young un–progressive trader is preoccupied with the 'Muo mgbasasi, which is believed to be responsible for his lack of success in the business world. We are not however, trying to show that these named forces or phenomena are non–existent. But, if they do, the gravity of the menace that they are believed to cause seems to be over–exaggerated.

> *This largely accounts for the kind of fanatical appeal and excitement which people who claim to possess the spiritual power to deliver others from demonic attacks and afflictions of one kind or the other generate in the society.*[5]

The frequency with which these prayer/healing centres and the acclaimed healing ministers spring up all over the place calls for a proper examination and re–appraisal.

The craze for miracles has also grown to question the authenticity of the pastoral life of the Church and the pastoral output of the ministers. The clergy man who has or claims to have the gift to heal or deliver people from ' these problems or give assurance to material upliftment and social security is considered the authentic pastor of the people, while the one who does not organise healing sessions is considered fake and unholy. Perhaps, this may account for one of the reasons

5 C.Ejizu, Cosmological perspective on Exorcism and Prayer healing in Contemporary Nigeria, in C. U. Manus, et. Al., eds, Healing and Exorcisms, p.11

why many priests are trying to identify themselves in the field. And so, it is therefore necessary to remark that,

> *Faith – healing as a charismata, like all other similar charismata, (as distinct from the prototypical gifts of personal sanctification, which the spirit of God will bestow on the stump of Jesse (Is 11:1–2), are not gifts, signs or fruits of personal sanctification or holiness, but gifts given, so that they can also be given out, served, and used to build up one body of Christ (1 Cor 14:12, Eph 4:12). As Paul amply described and even the Christ before him explained (1 Cor 12" 13,1 &14; Mtt 7:12ff), the Charismata are not signs of holiness or indications of acceptance by, or of one behaving in consonance with the desires of God; and moreover, they are easily abused and used contrary to their good purposes in the mind of God in first giving it to such people. The world experiences of these gifts in the modern world confirm these things from all denominational Christians as well as Catholic angles.*[6]

The attempt to identify in the field has a lot of pastoral questions. Some healing ministers have employed methods that have raised some serious questions and problems unfamiliar to the traditional Christian theology. Some are competing with the native doctors in some of their objectionable methods such as the performance of certain sacrifices at some joints in the village and the observations of a number of taboos. Some also make very sharp distinctions between what they call "Healing Masses" and perhaps "Non Healing Masses". The Catholic bishops of Igboland and of Nigeria are therefore concerned about the growing number of priests surging into the healing ministry. Hence at the National Theological / Pastoral Seminar held in Emene–Enugu in February 1992, the Nigerian Bishops strongly noted, "A good number of our priests are going in for the healing ministry. Care must be taken that our faith and practice are not compromised or put in jeopardy."[7] The bishops are really concerned and have called attention to that. The priests and some lay people have noticed the development and are also concerned and have called for a control of the situation. The development therefore, is a double dimensional one for the Church. It is a healthy development that the mandate of Christ is being carried out among the Ibos of Nigeria. Jesus himself commanded the Church to continue his healing mission, and stated that the healing power would be associated with the believers. (Mk 16: 17–18). The apostles worked many healing miracles, such that Luke in his second book puts it thus:

---

6 M.C. Asuzu, The Healing Apostolate of the Church, in the light of modem day faith–healing, "National/Theological Seminar", Emene, Enugu, 11th – 14th February 1992, pp.2–3

7 L. Madubuko, Healing and Liturgy, a paper presented at the National Theological/Pastoral Seminar, Emene, Enugu, 11th – 14th February 1992. p.1

So many signs and wonders were worked among the people at the hands of the apostles that the sick were even taken out into the streets and laid on beds and sleeping–mats in the hope that at least the shadow of Peter might fall across some of them as he went past. People came even crowding in from the towns around Jerusalem, bringing with them their sick and those tormented by unclean spirits, and all of them were cured. (Acts 5: 12–16)

Many of the Igbo priests and the lay faithful are becoming more disposed to the healing work by prayers, and many more are discovering their charisms in this area of the apostolate of the Church. The charismatic dimension of the Church is active and growing. On the other hand, it has to be followed with great care and caution as the bishops warned for fear of abuses and excesses that are already creeping in. The tension that already existed in the Church in the area seems to have emanated from the bestowal and administration of the gifts of the Holy Spirit, particularly the gift of healing. Our Lord has bestowed these gifts to His Church for the good and building up of the Community.

There is a variety of gifts but always the same Spirit; there are all sorts of service to be done, but always to the same Lord; working in all sorts of different ways in different people, it is the same God who is working in all of them. The particular way in which the spirit is given to each person is for a good purpose. ... All these are the work of one and the same Spirit, who distributes different gifts to different people just as he chooses (1 Cor 12: 4–11)

But it seems some priests and some of the lay faithful are improperly handling the application and use of these gifts, thus giving room for misunderstanding on the part of the hierarchy of the Church. There was therefore the danger of stifling the spirit blowing in the Church instead of discerning and controlling the spirit.

Those who have charge over the Church should judge the genuineness and proper use of these gifts, through their office not indeed to extinguish the spirit but to test all things and hold fast to what is good. (cf. Th. 5:12 & 19–21)[8]

This work therefore, among other things, makes an attempt to understudy the meaning of Charisms or gifts to help in avoiding the wrong interpretation and application of these gifts. This has to be addressed to give room for a healthy renewal and revival that this development is meant to bring.

8 Vatican Council 11, Lumen Gentium, No 12,21 November, 1964, p.364

0.2 Inspiration and Aim

The interest for the choice of this theme is not unconnected with some of the experiences on the current trend of affairs in the young and growing Church of Nigeria especially in this all important and embracing area of the healing ministry and culture. Shortly before 1 left home for further studies in Europe, 1 noticed that the issue of the healing ministry has not only generated fame and excitement for some people but it has also germinated one problem or the other for various people at various levels in the Church. There are some pastors who are at loggerhead with some members of their parishes especially the famous Charismatic renewal groups among whom are commonly found some of the lay healers. There are also some priests who are not in understanding with their Ordinaries because of the healing ministry. Some who engage in the healing ministry attract great attention and admiration of the society such that a few of them tend to lose sight of the authority of their local Ordinaries. Some priest–healers have been cautioned by their Ordinaries or in some cases suspended because of some of the practices found in the healing services that are considered unorthodox or unfamiliar with the traditional theology of the Church. Yet some of these healers do not understand why their attention should be called to those areas. This invariably raises further questions on the intentions and reasons for the ministry on the part of such healers. One is not sure anymore, whether many of the priests and lay members of the Church who are surging into the much elevated and loving ministry are doing it according to the mind of Christ and his Church. On the other hand, there are also unnecessary oppositions, over–reaction, hasty and unproductive criticisms against this loving ministry of the Church of Jesus Christ on earth.

Consequently, there is a need for a deep and comprehensive study into this area, for a better understanding of the loved ministry of Christ in the area. There is also a need to educate our Christians and protect them from the menaces of over indulgence to the attacks of evil spirits and other such forces or phenomena. They need to be informed and protected too from the menaces of dupes and nefarious antics that parade around as miracle workers. It is therefore on account of these developments that we have decided to study the health and healing in the Igbo society of Nigeria, vis a vis the basis and challenges for an inculturated pastoral care for the sick. This work is also intended to incite others into researching in this area.

0.3 The Scope of the Study

The culture and life of the Igbo people particularly their religion, which according to many writers was a fertile ground for the implantation of the Christian religion, has perhaps made some writers too, to trace the origin of the people to the Jewish descent. But the people did not migrate from anywhere. They are original to their position and culture. The Igbo has very much respect for life and community sense of living. Hence he cares very much for his health and that of his brother. The care he has for his health is very much holistic and he would approach his problems from the various dimensions of man – physical, spiritual, psychological emotional and social. This care he has for his life in its various aspects deeply affects the healing ministry of the Church. Hence this work covers a wide scope.

The work covers the study of the two major entities concerned, namely the healing ministry of the Church and the anthropological components of healthcare of the sick in Igbo community of Nigeria. To understand well the components of Igbo healthcare, the work explores the origin, location and language of the people. It also digs into the study of the life and culture of the people, in the original context of the people as a homogenous group without external influences. The examination of their religious and social life exposes the beautiful qualities of their life and culture such as their view of life, the sense of family and family unit, the extended family system, marriage and transmission of life, sense of community life and hospitality.

The Igbo's desire to preserve life can be seen in many aspects of his life particularly in his understanding of sickness and his care for the sick. Sickness for him is perceived as a big problem that comes from God, the devil or from the evil one and must have to be avoided or cured. The Igbo hardly believes that no sickness that attacks him is without an intervening cause. Hence he consults the "dibia" (medicine man) when he is sick. The medicine man prepares drugs for treatment of various ailments. Yet the Igbo believe that God is the ultimate healer. There are various types of medicine men as there are different types of sickness.

Healing as we discuss here is that notion of healing that is capable of generating some emotional and irrational reactions from the people but which could also serve as a source of evangelical power. It is that healing that includes the well-being of various dimensions of the personality of a man in his general relationships with both God and man – infact the healing that involves healing a whole person's world – body, soul and environment – social and economical. In treating the healing ministry of Jesus and the healing Tradition of the Church, the work exposes the main forms of healings of the Church, namely, Ordinary, Extra–

ordinary and Sacramental forms of healings. In this exposition lies the possibility for an understanding of a healing ministry much more clear and profound than today's Christianity in Igboland has recognised.

0.4 Sources

This research has as its primary source, the personal interest and experiences gathered after some years as a priest in the pastoral ministry of the Catholic Church in Nigeria. Various literatures in Igbo people, culture, and religion also form a major source of materials for this research. Source books like the Holy Scripture, the Christian Tradition and the Magisterium, dictionaries and encyclopaedias, books on healing and healthcare, biblical commentaries and different other forms of writings were used. Some libraries both private and public were consulted in Germany, Rome and in Nigeria. And since Igbo culture is a complex one, extensive oral interviews among the Igbo people of Nigeria were conducted for originality of the work. Responses from Questionnaires were also used.

0.5 Limitations and Problems

Looking at the title of this nature, any sound thinker knows that this work is bound to have its problems and limitations. The word healing generally speaking is acknowledged as an evocative word and to write on healing in today's world is to delve into a very complex area that generates a lot of reactions and problems. And to write on healing in the Nigerian Church, particularly in Igboland where almost more than ninety percent of the population are Christians, and where "the practice of traditional medicine has almost always been combined with some form of religious ministration"[9] is to dig into the minefield. Yet, theology and the theologians of the Church in Igbo Society today must adequately face the problems of the Church in the area. Our aim, therefore, is to attempt to better enlighten the people through a comprehensive and pastoral study of the healing ministry of Jesus Christ, taking into consideration the people's original understanding of health and healing. We therefore tried to avoid as much as possible the issues that will generate unnecessary and highly emotional reactions. But where it becomes impossible, all limitations accruing therein are hereby acknowledged.

---

9 M.C. Asuzu, The healing apostolate of the Church, Seminar paper, Op.Cit,. p.1

0.6 Methodology

The approach to this work is basically pastoral and generally theological. It is nonetheless also descriptive, expository, and synthetically analytical. It is expected to take cognisance of the two major entities in the study, examining the key concepts involved. Efforts were made to break down the concepts to the knowledge of the common man. A type of comparative study was made between the major areas of the healing Tradition of the Church and the Igbo traditional care of the sick.

0.6 The Sequence of the Study

This work is mainly divided into five major Chapters with a general introduction and conclusion. Chapter one of the work deals with the general background of the Igbo people, the anthropological components of healthcare of the sick and the qualities of the Igbo people of Nigeria. The second chapter shall examine the concept of 'Ndu' – (life), general notion of health, Sickness and healing with special reference to Igbo Myths on the Origin of Suffering and Death and care of the sick in Igbo society.

The third chapter of the work undertakes the study of Healthcare, popular notion of Healing and healing ministry in Igbo Church of Nigeria. It also takes an analysis of the Christian understanding of Suffering and Sickness in the light of European culture.

Chapter four looks at the healing ministry of Jesus Christ and the healing tradition of the Church. This chapter of our work makes an attempt to show that it was Jesus Christ who began the tradition of healing in the Church and that it is His own ministry that sets the pattern for Christian healers of all ages. His healing ministry ever since its inception, remains ever present and active in the Church never ceasing or remaining dormant at any time in the history of the Church. Jesus healed men and women in all their relationships with one another and with God. That is to say that his healing is holistic. Jesus also freely acknowledges that the father is the source of all powers and healings.

This chapter also exposes the fact that in the ministry of Jesus, preaching, healing and teaching all went together, each as an integral part of the message of Salvation. This part of the research also took care of the different dimensions of the healing works of Jesus, the methods of His healing works and the significance or aims of His healing ministry. Taking a special interest in the biblical injunction of Jesus to his Church to preach the gospel and heal the sick, the works traces the mission to our own age. In treating the major forms of healings of the Church, a little exposition was made of the term Charism, as a manifestation of the ordinary form of healing of the Church and thereby, bringing our service of Charity as the greatest of the healing gifts.

Chapter five examines and analyses the healing ministry and its pastoral contributions in Igbo society and possibly studies and evaluates some the pastoral challenges too. Attempts are made to unearth some positive and negative aspects of the healing ministry to the yet growing Church of Igboland. A fair study of this will very much help in understanding the type of healing ministry peculiar to the Igbo Church of Nigeria and probably shed some light to some misunderstanding and excesses currently immanent in the healing ministry among the Igbo Christians. Finally possible means for acculturating some of the practices current in the healing ministry in Igbo society into the Church's healing ministry shall be explored.

The conclusion makes a general analysis of the whole work, pointing out clearly what healing ministry should embrace and with caution and firmness amplifies the importance of the healing ministry in the Church.

1. Chapter One – The Igbos

1.1 The Basic Features of the Igbos

1.1.1 The Location and Whereabout of the People

Igboland is located on both banks of the River Niger south of its confluence with the River Benue. The greater part of the land and the majority of the people are found east of the Niger in Imo, Abia, Enugu, Anambra, and some parts of the River States of Nigeria: These are called the Eastern Igbo. The smaller group on the west bank of the Niger are called the Ika Igbo or Western Igbo in the Delta State. Thus, the Igbo people are native to six Nigerian states in the current state structure. (see Map). The Igbo number about fourteen million.[10] In 1972, Ekenem put the figure at twelve million.[11] The last official census in Nigeria was conducted in 1963, and it put the population at 8.3 million. If the growth is 2.5% annually, our estimated number should be a little higher without taking into account the live that were lost during the Nigeria and Biafra civil war. The recent census of 1992 was not conducted on ethnic or tribal lines.[12] That could have given a current estimation of the population of the Igbo. The majority of them are Christians and agriculturists. Before the "Colonial Era" (as we shall see later), they lived in segmentary independent socio–political groups called *Umunna.*

1.2 Whereabouts of the Ibos

It is not easy to ascertain the origin of the Igbo people since there are hardly any written records. The only records available are those based on oral Tradition, myth, and legends, all of which have been recorded in recent times. Nevertheless the Igbo people must have a historical origin. According to E. N. Njoku:

---

10 A conservative estimate.

11 Ekenem, I., The 1963 Nigerian Census: A Critical Appraisal (Benin City, SNNP Press, 1972, p.67

12 The provisional result of this census says that Nigeria has only 88.5 million people. "News watch Magazine," Ikeja, March 30, 1992

"If a race has no history/origin, if it has no worthwhile Tradition, it becomes a negligible factor on the thought of the world, and it stands in danger of being exterminated.[13]"

However, a number of hypotheses have been put forward by some historians backed up by archaeological evidence and other dating innovations in the sciences. Some of these have now been firmly established as additional credible sources of the development of the history of the Igbo people, thanks to extensive research work done in the past forty years by historians in Africa and elsewhere in the southern world. One of the hypotheses which is still current among Igbo scholars today is also based on linguistic kinship and environmental factors. According to one of these hypotheses, the Igbo people originally came from the Guinean zone of the middle belt region in the far north of Nigeria. From there they migrated southwards until they settled around what is known today as the Igbo heartland. In the words of A. E. Afigbo: "The Igbo after separating from their Kwa brothers somewhere around the Niger–Benue confluence, settled first on the Northern Plateau, where under the impact of agricultural and iron revolutions, they evolved their characteristic culture. Some however, under the pressure of population, left the Northern plateau for the plains and the upland where they developed their own lines of dialects while retaining the basic Igbo speech and culture."[14] The Igbo are people who share a common language known as "Igbo" and common culture known as *Omenala* custom. These two factors distinguish them from any other national group in Nigeria. They are people with a variety of traditions and culture.

1.2.1 Language of the People

One area where the Igbo people are homogeneous is in the aspect of language. The language helps to ascertain that the Igbos are indigenous to their land since the Igbo language "is not spoken as mother tongue anywhere else in Africa or in the world for that matter." The word Igbo did not even originally refer to the whole of the Igbo tribes as we know it today for there was no common name for the whole tribe. People were particular in identifying with the names of their towns.

---

13 Njoku, E., The Igbo of Nigeria (Ancestor, Rite Change and Survival), (New York, The Edwin Mellen Press, 1990), p.211

14 Afigbo, A.E., *Prolegomena to the Study of Culture*: History of the Igbo Speaking (Ibadan University Press, Nigeria, 1975), p.29

Until recently, people applied the word Igbo primarily to the language and secondarily to Igbo–speaking groups other than one's own. A person would refer to himself as 'Igbo' (or 'Ibo') only when speaking to a foreigner.[15]

One of the major characteristics of the language is that it is marked by a complex set of tones, which is primarily used to distinguish meaning and grammatical relationship. "This makes the language one step more difficult for the foreigner who has enough problems already mastering the various dialects."[16] For the Indigenous Igbos, without minding their dialects, "the tonality of the language signifies lexical economy as one lexical unit or morpheme can mean several things depending on the accents. For instance, the same lexical unit "igwe" can mean "sky", "multitude", "metal", or "to grind".[17] The Igbo language has however many dialects, the major and prominent ones being Onitsha and Owerri dialects.

1.2.1.1 Qualities of the Igbo People

Authors have given different characteristics peculiar to the Igbo people. Helen Chukwu, one of the Igbo anthropologists, has this to say of them: "What baffles us and probably may baffle any other student interested in Igbo culture is the two–fold opposing polarity in Igbo character. On the one hand, the Ibos are selfish and highly individualistic. On the other hand, they are generous, kind and humane especially to strangers." With this both Marioghae agrees:

Throughout the country, there are closely similar social traditions which remind us what people in Europe have lost. They welcome strangers with a glowing spirit of hospitality...and are heart–warming. It made us realise how the Igbos must respond to the cold reception they receive in Britain.[18]

15 Arinze, F.A., Sacrifice in Ibo Religion, Ibadan, 1978. p.2

16 Cf. Emenajo, E.N., "Slans and Colloquialism in Modern Igbo – A preliminary Socio–Linguistic study" in Ikenga vol. 4 no. 2 (1980), p.49) Igbo has many dialects, as many as twenty – Afigbo, Ropes of Sand ... Op. Cit., p.359, in L. Madubuko, Igbo World View, in Bigard Theological Studies, Op. Cit., p.27

17 Cf. Madubuko, L., Igbo World View, Op. Cit., p.27. By way of meeting the problems of Dialogue and tones in Igbo Language, the Seminar (referred to in note 71) made a number of recommendations including the following: The Seminar is of the opinion that tone marking is necessary in academic works, dictionaries and grammar books, But in works intended for more use, tones should be used only where necessary in order to avoid ambiguity. It is recognised that context is an important indicator of both the tone and meaning especially in literature and general works. Op. Cit., p.27

18 Marioghae, M., Nigeria Under the Cross (London, Geoffrey Chapman, 1965), p.4

Samuel Ottenberg, a British anthropologist, sees the Igbo as "one of the most unusual sets of Africans. They are both hated and admired by other Africans. They are moody people, quite irritable like every other normal son of nature."[19]

For me all these descriptions are labels, they represent no formula which exhausts the understanding of the Igbo people. I feel it is more realistic and objective to stress that among other qualities Igbos place a great emphasis on individual achievements and initiative. This individualism is rooted in group action, whereas traditional government is democratic in nature.

Within the realism of the Igbo's traditional individualism, greater emphasis is placed on communal co–operation and achievements. "The communal character of the Igbo peasant may be traced from the formative influences of traditional social patterns, and the influence of the nucleated residence pattern to the ideological urge to move ahead."[20]

The Igbos accepts changes easily and adapt to them. They readily embraced the Western type of education through the Christian philosophy of evangelization. The priesthood, farming, taking of titles, welfare, and trading are among the traditional avenues to status.[21] The nature of the exposure to different situations has made it possible for the Igbos to accept certain innovations, modify elements of their social, religious, economic, and political structures in order to accommodate the changes, and retain other basic patterns, such as achievement orientation, long–term goals, hatred of autocracy, and a strong community consciousness and solidarity in the family. The Igbos believes that the attainment of full human life consists in active participation in the life of the community. A community is a form of society in which people are more intimately bound by specific goals and natural force. Jean Vanier describes this type of community thus:

At one time, men lived in homogeneous groups composed of more or less the same family, with the same roots. In these groups, the tribe, the village, the people spoke the same language, lived by the same rites and traditions, had the same code of behaviour and accepted the same authority. There was solidarity among them. This solidarity came both from their flesh and blood and from the need to co–operate to meet material needs and to defend the group from enemy attack and natural dangers. There was a unity among people of the same group which etched itself deeply on their consciousness.[22]

---

19 Ottenberg, S., Leadership and Authority in an African Society (London, Heinemann, 1971), p.12

20 Ibid. p.5

21 Njoku, E., The Igbo of Nigeria (Ancestor, Rite Change and Survival), (new York, The Edwin Mellen Press, 1990), p.211.

22 Vanier, J., Community and Growth (London, Darton, Longmann and Todd, 1981), p.1

This is an apt description of Igbo community. The concept of community embraces four elements, namely: close personal relations with other persons that are sometimes called primarily "face to face" intimate relations; an emotional, sensitive involvement on the part of the individual in social functions and affairs of the group; moral dedication or commitment to the values that are considered high and significant by the group; and, a sense of solidarity with other members of the group.

This for the Igbo means first and foremost a moral, religious and affective quality of human relations in the sense that all the members of this community descend from a common ancestor. On this obvious fact Lazarus Esomonu, a moral theologian, affirms:

> *Every man is linked to his parents, on the natural level; he receives life from his parents and in their turn is bound to their grandparents, etc. This link which binds all members of the same family by propagation is broadened to include all the members of the community or clan, who are believed to be descendants of the same ancestor. Everyone thus considers himself a member of a definite community and as a part of the whole.*[23]

An Igbo is always conscious of belonging to a well–identified family within a well–known group. This idea is very clear in his head and mind. This quality of community consciousness and solidarity has been emphasised by different authorities in Igbo/African literature. This dimension of solidarity is closely linked with their religion. It is indeed through the worship of God and the veneration of their ancestors that people show that solidarity with the spiritual world. This is the link between their religion and life. Moreover, through this constant interplay between the community and individual each member is filled with a spirit of co–operation and responsibility in various areas of life. This explains the reason why they have a moral obligation to participate in the joys and sufferings of one another. The existence of the individual in corporate Igbo communal consciousness is underlined by a strong sense of solidarity, a feeling of being on board the same boat, and all have a responsibility to keep it afloat.

The Igbo people seem to say "I am because we are, and since we are therefore I am." It is through this relationship with others in the community that an Igbo defines himself, and his self–esteem depends more or less on those he values and those who value him in return. For a person to exist is to live in the group/community, to see things with the group, to do things with the group. Life is not an individual venture. This is what holds and strengthens them from hardship in life *Umunna buike or Igwe buike* (community or unity is strength) is an

23 Esomonu, L., Respect for Human life in Igbo Religion and Morality (Rome, C. Goodliff Neale, 1981), p.42

Igbo philosophical demonstration of community consciousness and spirit of solidarity, (see Diagram 1). This then will lead us to the Igbo sense of hospitality.

1.2.1.2 Culture of the People

The mention of the word culture often brings to the mind of many, the idea of the traditional aspects of the life of a group of people such as traditional dances, and dresses. But culture is much more than that. An English dictionary defines culture as a "state of manners, taste and intellectual development at a time or place"[24] The Concise Oxford Dictionary of Current English defines,

> *Culture is the arts and other manifestations of human intellectual achievement regarded collectively or the customs, civilisation and achievements of a particular time or people.*[25]

Hence Jacques Maguat sees culture as, "the totality of knowledge and behaviours, ideas and objects that constitute the common heritage of a society."[26] It can also be seen as, "the sum total of knowledge, belief, art, morality, customs and laws and other potentialities acquired by man as member of a society."[27] Culture could therefore be said to refer to the totality of the life of a society, embracing all aspects or needs of human life ranging from eating habits, housing, kinship system, marriage and family organisations, social class, religion and government to mention just a few. Similar responses to a number of these aspects of life make a people a homogenous community, homogeneity being an essential quality of a living culture. Culture gives a sense of identity to a group of persons.

Igbo people have a very great respect for their culture. A great interest is shown in marriage and family life. The sense of community and the extended family relations are very much encouraged. The Igbo believes that no man is an island and puts that in practice. For him, to exist is to live in groups and do things together.

Culture, however, exhibits a number of characteristics. Every culture often comes in contact with other cultures. The culture of the Igbo has therefore experienced great changes due to contact with modern scientific and technological

---

24 J.B. Foreman, (ed), Collins English Gem Dictionary, London, 1974, p.118

25 R.E. Allen, (ed), The Concise Oxford Dictionary of Current English, (eight edition), Oxford University Press, New York, 1990, p.282

26 J.Maguat, Africanity, p.4 as quoted in B.H. Kato., "African Cultural Revolution and the Christian Faith", Challenge publication, Jos, 1976, p.8

27 B.Taylor nel 1871: Cassics e la descrizione di cultura dall antropologo, in G. Orlandoni, "Culture e Communicazione" Rome, 1984, p.6

life. However a viable culture is known for its ability to admit changes. A culture that does not admit of changes is static and dead.

And culture, we know, is dynamic. Culture borrows from others and that makes it alive and dynamic. The Igbo culture is the pivotal point of the Igbo people's life and it is in a dynamic process of growth.

1.2.1.2.1 Religion of the People

The importance of the examination and the analysis of Igbo traditional religion in the context of our present work cannot be given enough credit. Scholars have ascertained that it is no longer possible to dissociate religion from the historical and geographical study of any group of people. This is very true as:

> *Religion originated as the response of the emotions and the dawning intelligence of man to the world around and within him, and as in the past, it served to satisfy certain human needs, so it has continued to do, sometimes widening, but at other times narrowing it's scope, in some instances deepening it's experience, in others becoming more and more superficial, occasionally it is stifled by convention and strangled by ritual, only to break away under the guidance of the reformer, the eternal conflict between the priest and the prophet. ...*[28]

The study and evaluation of Igbo traditional religion have over the years been influenced by many historical and geographical currents. The religion has undergone a wide range of misinterpretations and distortions. Some authors and ethnologists, including European, Asiatic and African writers, have pre–occupied themselves interpreting the religion as fetish, and paganish; some others interpret the religious beliefs in biological, psychological and sociological terms. But the designation of African religion and hence Igbo traditional religion as fetish is absurd and borders on ignorance and short – sightedness. Belief in the Supreme God "Chukwu" in Igbo religion or the veneration of ancestors cannot be described as fetish or paganish since the Igbo traditional believer does not worship inanimate object as God. He believes in the Supreme God who is worshipped in the other world religions. Some recent African authors in reaction to and in a bid to assert the truth and value in African Traditional Religion hold an extreme position, describing the traditional religious beliefs only in the Christian concepts and ideas. It is however, not our intention to go into semantics in this work or any examination of the currents going against African or Igbo traditional religion.

Our aim is to examine relevant topics in Igbo religious beliefs as a basis for anthropologically unearthing genuine traditional concepts and practices of Igbo

28 A.C. Hudson, Preface in A.G. Leonard, "The Lower Niger and it's tribes", London, 1968, p.8

concept of health and care of the sick and theologically evaluating the values therein with the proper equipments.

At this juncture, we have to prefix our discussion with the declaration of the Second Vatican Council, which strikes a note of hope for the non–Christian religions.

The Catholic Church rejects nothing of what is true and holy in these religions. She has a high regard for the manner of life and conduct, the precepts and doctrines which, although differing in many ways from her own teaching, nevertheless often reflect a ray of that truth which enlightens all men... The Church therefore urges her sons to enter with prudence and charity into discussion and collaboration with members of other religions. Let Christians while witnessing to their own faith and way of life, acknowledge, preserve and encourage the spiritual and moral truths found among non–Christians, and their social life and culture.[29]

The Igbo, like every other human being, is a religious being, "Homo religiosus". Religion permeates every aspect of his life. It occupies a central position in his social and cultural life such that we cannot get a clear idea of the life of the Igbo without referring to his religion. Writing on the Igbo tribes of the Lower Niger, Arthur Leonard says, "They are in the strict sense of the word a truly and deeply religious people of whom it can be said that they eat religiously, drink religiously, bath religiously and dress religiously."[30] Nwoga and Egudu writing of an Nri Chief express it thus:

The Igbo people are by nature religious. There is hardly any serious life activity in the society which is not very intimately punctuated by a religious exercise or expression. The entire life of the people follows a culturally rhythmical pattern making a cycle from birth to death, in which life begins and ends with religious sacrifices.[31]

In other to appreciate better the Igbo religious life, it is necessary to examine the structural elements of his belief namely – his beliefs in the Supreme Being, the spirits and the ancestors. Parinder in his book on West African Traditional

---

29 Vatican II, Nostra Aetate, (from hereafter, N.A.), AAS 58, 1966, no.2., p.739: We cannot truly pray to God the Father of all if we treat any people in other than brotherly fashion, for all men were created in God's image ... There is no basis therefore, either in theory or in practice for any discrimination between individual and individual, or between people and people arising either from human dignity or from the right which flow from it. Therefore, the Church reproves, as foreign to the mind of Christ, any discrimination against people or any harassment of them on the basis of their race, colour, condition in life or religion ... NA no. 5)

30 A. Leonard, Lower Niger and it's tribes, London, 1906, p.429

31 R.Egudu, and D. Nwoga, Igbo traditional verses, Op.Cit., p.10

Religion included "charms as the fourth element of the 1gbo religious belief."[32] In the strict sense of religion, charms are not elements of belief in Igbo religion. This brings to mind also another element medicine 'ogwu', considered by another author Ikenga Metuh as an element of belief in Igbo–World–View. According to him, "the Igbo recognises five categories of spiritual beings – Supreme Being (Chukwu), the Deities (Mmuo), the Spirits (Arusi), the Ancestors (Ndi ichie) and Medicine (ogwu).[33] But is medicine 'ogwu' actually an element of Igbo religious belief? However for the purpose of our work, we shall make a brief survey also on Charms and Medicines.

1.2.1.2.2 Belief in the Supreme Being

We have noted earlier that the religion of the African, including that of the Igbo has undergone a wide range of misinterpretations and distortions. This has been very clearly identified in his belief in the Supreme God. Some authors have concluded that the African God is a withdrawn God who has no temples or shrines and therefore has no prayers or sacrifices offered to him. Hence D. Westermann writes,

> *The High–God is as a rule, not the object of religious cult and is of small or almost no significance in practical religion. People acknowledge him but neither fear him nor love nor serve him ... The African God is a 'deus incertus' and a 'deus remotus', there is always an atmosphere of indefiniteness about him.*[34]

E. Smith held a more negative impression on African belief in the Supreme Being. He notoriously remarked, "How can the untutored Africa conceive God? ... How can this be? Deity is a philosophical concept which savages are incapable of framing."[35] The notion or thesis of the Igbo Supreme God or the African God as a withdrawn God 'Deus Remotus' or' deus incertus' who is said to have no temples or shrines and have no prayers or sacrifices offered to him is a misnomer.

---

32 Cf. G. Parinder, West African Traditional Religion, London, 1975, p.16

33 I.E. Metuh, God and Man in African Religion, London, 1981, in Metuh, "Comparative studies of African Traditional Religion" (A.T.R), Imico Publishers, Onitsha, 1987, p.58: Medicine "Ogwu" in Igbo traditional life and understanding has two meanings, namely, Medicine as drugs or mixture of herbs and roots used to cure diseases and illnesses, and Medicine as a type of Charms which is believed to have some mystical powers that can have influence on the life of man, positively as protective charms or negatively as dangerous charms. The Igbo believes in the existence and experience of the mystical powers of medicines and charms but not precisely as an object of religion.

34 D. Westermann, African and Christianity, London, Oxford, 1937, p.79

35 E. Smith, African ideas of God, London, 1961, p.1

And the remarks of Africans not having any conception or belief in the Supreme God borders on the realms of abstract ignorance tainted by pride and hatred.

The Igbo is a great lover of nature and he is imbued with the sense of wonder and mystery. His keen observation of the wonders and mysteries of nature such as birth and germination, growth of man and animals, enigma of sickness and death, the existence of seas and rivers and the general order of creation made him conclude there is a first and final cause of all these, an uncaused cause.

The Igbo has a very clear conception of and a strong belief in the existence of a Supreme Being called 'Chukwu' (the Great Spirit), or 'Chineke' (the spirit that creates) or 'Osebuluwa' (the Lord who upholds the world). This Supreme Being is all powerful and is believed by every Igbo "as the creator of all things, the almighty, all knowing, the giver of life and breath and the final judge of all men"[36] That is to say that the idea of the creator is central to Igbo theology. He is the author of life, the creator of heaven and earth. His presence looms round and permeates the entire life and culture of the Igbo such that all aspects of his life have a religious undertone. His name is often on his lips, especially in times of uncertainties and excitement, in times of grief and sorrows, also in times of enjoyment and festivities. God is not approached only as a last resort. The name is very often directly called in prayers, often used in proverbs and generally given in names. Hence the Igbos often have names like 'Chukwuemeka' (God is generous), 'Ikechukwu' (The power of God), 'Uchenna' (God's wish), and 'Chidiebele' (God is merciful). There are also phrases like 'Oge chukwu ka nma' (God's time is the best), 'ife dili chukwu' (Let God take control), 'Okwu Chukwu' (God's word). These three phrases are also used as Igbo names. In fact, Igbo belief in God is so established that one German missionary who worked among the people in 1841 had this to say.

The Igbos were in their own way religious people. The word "Tschukwu" God is continually heard. Tschukwu is supposed to do everything.... Their notions of the Attributes of the Supreme Being are in many respects correct, and their, manner of expressing them striking. "God made both White and Black" is continually on their lips. Some of their parables are descriptive of the perfections of God.[37]

So for the Igbo, the idea of 'Chukwu' as the Supreme God who is believed to be the creator and controller of all things is fundamental. Like other Africans,

---

36 E.G. Parrinder, West African Traditional Religion, London, SPCK, 1962, p.34

37 E. Isichei, History of the Igbo people, pp.24–25. Drawn from the "Journals of Rev. James Schon and Mrs. S. Crowther in 1841", London, pp.50–51

there are no atheists in the traditional life of the Igbo people and no traditional Igbo may be referred to as a pagan. Any wonder I. Igwegbe notes,

In traditional life of the African, there are no atheists. Only a doubly foolish person would doubt or negate the existence of God and refuse to worship him. And if the existence of such a 'strange fellow' is ascertained, it is a matter of urgent and serious concern for the entire community.[38]

V.C. Uchendu affirms this fact as he says that, "the Igbo believes in a Supreme God, a high God, who is all God."[39] The Supreme God is seen as a father of all who is interested in the affairs of men and can be always approached personally, directly and even without intermediaries, though the Igbos believe that this great God has intermediaries through the spirits who act between them and their God. With this we can go on to discuss the place of the Spirits in Igbo religious belief.

1.2.1.2.3 Belief in the Spirits or deities

The Igbo has a very strong believe in the existence of the spirits who are seen as "common spiritual beings beneath the status of divinities and above the status of men."[40]

In many respects they share some aspects of the nature and some of the Attributes of the Supreme Being. Some are said to live with the Supernatural being, in the heavenly realm and to act as his counsellors and collaborators. Others are associated with some natural phenomenon like the sky, the earth, thunder, rivers, forests, mountains over which they exercise a measure of control. They are personal, spiritual and powerful beings and exercise immense power over human life and destiny. They have powers to kill or save, reward or punish, bring fortunes or cause misfortunes to man.[41]

The spirits are believed to manifest God's providence and will for man. They are in fact messengers of God who have some influence on man and God seems to have given them much liberty of action. The Igbos prays and offer sacrifices to God through them as intermediaries; sometimes they ask the spirits expressly to intercede for them before God.

---

38 I. Igwegbe, Newman's Sacramental Theological Thinking: it's relevance to the Africans, Rome, 1994, p.31

39 V.C. Uchendu, The Igbo of South – Eastern Nigeria, Holt Rinehart and Winston, 1965, p.94.

40 J.S. Mbiti, African Religions and Philosophy, London, Edinburgh, 1977, p.22

41 E.I. Metuh, Comparative studies of African traditional religions, Jos, 1987

The spirits are all created by God and none of them claims equality with the Supreme Being. The spirits act as intermediaries between God and man. The origin of the spirit is not clear to the Igbo and he is not generally interested in finding out. The origin of these spirits is said to be wrapped up in mysteries. The Igbo thinks more of the powers and what the spirits can do. The Igbo believes that these spirits are invisible and ubiquitous. Hence the famous Igbo saying which asks, 'Onye fulu muo di'? (Who can see the spirits and live?). Yet in spite of this belief, people are said to experience their activities, and many folk stories describing the spirits in human form, activities, and personalities are told. There are therefore, many writers who say that, these spirits are personifications of natural phenomena.

There are spirits of rivers, hills, farms, and lightening. There is no part of the world, no object or creature, which does not have a spirit of its own or which is not inhabited by the apparitional entity known as spirit, whose goodwill men seek by appropriate offerings.[42]

"The four days of the Ibo week are also personified. Then there are spirits of destiny, of the household and of fertility"[43]

These spirits are many and are generally called 'ndi muo', 'alusi', or 'agbara'. These words mean spirit, according to different Igbo dialects.

> *Those spirits whose names are known have their cults; each has his or her shrine, priests and feast days. Many have sacred animals. Most spirits are regarded as male but some are regarded as female. The statuses of the spirits are called 'nkwu'.*[44]

Some of these spirits believed by the Igbo as influencing his life deserve to be mentioned here. They are 'Ani' (The earth spirit), 'Igwe' (The sky spirit), 'Anyanwu' (The sun spirit), 'Amadioha' (The spirit of Thunder and lighting), 'Udo', 'Idemili' and others.

1.2.1.2.3 Ani (The Earth Spirit)

Ani is the earth spirit, generally believed in all over Igboland. In some places it is called 'Ala' or 'Ana'. Ani is a Great Spirit, the most important spirit after Chukwu, the Supreme God. She is regarded as the "great mother" of the earth, having universal influence over the land. According to F. Arinze, "She is the Great Mother Spirit, the queen of the underworld, the 'owner' of men and custo-

---

42 G. Parrinder, West African Traditional Religion, London, SPCK, 1962, p.26

43 J. Whelan, The true and the false in Paganism, in Pagan Mission, 18, 1945, p.15; C. Meek., "The Religions of Nigerians in Africa", 14, 1943, p.113

44 F.A. Arinze, Sacrifice in Ibo religion, Op. Cit., p.13

dian of public morality in conjunction with the ancestors."[45] What a great belief the Igbos has on the Ani Spirit. Parents often name their children after this earth spirit. Hence 'Anichebe' (May Ani protect), 'Anidike' (Ani is strong), 'Anikamadu' (Ani is greater than man), 'Anikweobi' (May Ani allow to inhabit) are very common household names.

Ani spirit is believed to increase the fertility of man and the productivity of the land. Hence before and after every planting season, sacrifices are offered to the Ani spirit for good yield and protection during the season. The first of these rites is the 'sacred week' or 'week of peace'. This week precedes the planting of new seeds in the farm and it was a time when "no war or battle sound was heard the world around, the idle spear and shield were high up hung."[46] The second rite to Ani, the Harvest festival, takes its name from the stable food of the Igbo called 'ji' (yam). The feast has different names in various areas of the Igboland, such as 'lfejioku' festival, 'Iwaji', 'Ajoku' and 'Ahiaolu' festivals. It is a thanksgiving ceremony happily celebrated by the whole community,

> *Each community holds the rite on its market day, when elaborate preparations for it are made. Women prepare food and oil beans, children fetch water and wood, and everyone else works to clear the village paths and the market places.*[47]

The festival is widespread in Igboland. As a fertility deity to man, Ani is believed to give children to people and every family group had a cult of Ani.

> *Ala helps the Igbo family with many things. They ask her for children, for prosperity in trade and increase in livestock. As the source of strength, she must be notified before her children go to war. It is a great privilege to be a priest of Ala.*[48]

As the custodian of public morality, Ani acts as a true messenger of the Supreme God. According to Mozia, her role is to preserve unity and solidarity in the Igbo community by guiding the people towards the observance of the moral laws... She sometimes punishes the members of the community. But she is a merciful mother who intercedes for her children with God and other spirits.[49]

Some of the offences against Ani are adultery, homicide, stealing of yams, poisoning of another person, giving birth to twins. These sins or offences are called 'Nso ani' (abomination).

---

45 F.A. Arinze, Sacrifice in Ibo religion, p.15

46 P.A. Talbot, The tribes of the lower Niger, London, p.96

47 L. Esomonu, Respect for Human Life in Igbo Religion and Morality, Rome, 1981, p.81

48 Ibid. p.80

49 M.I. Mozia, Solidarity in the Church and Solidarity among the Igbos of Nigeria, Rome, 19, p.180

1.2.2 Igwe (The Sky Spirit)

Igwe is another spirit that has wide influence in Igboland. He is regarded as the son of God, sometimes called the husband of Ani the earth spirit. He is believed to fertilize her (the earth), with regular rains and thus make it possible for the earth to yield abundant harvests for the use of man. For without her harvests, "life would be impossible for the Igbos who attaches much sentiment to land."[50]

Igwe is believed to be much larger than the earth such that in the places where the cult is popular, it is celebrated with such praise name as 'Igwe ka Ala' (The sky that is greater than the earth). "Not much worship[51] is offered to Igwe as he is often better known through his 'wife', the earth spirit who happens to be the most important of the spirits of the Igbo religion and life."[52] He is the Sky spirit, who helps to maintain order and harmony among the heavenly bodies.

1.2.3 Amadioha (Spirit of Thunder and Lightening)

The Igbo believes that Igwe, the Sky spirit expresses his power and anger in thunderbolts and lightening. This is such that when it is raining or about to rain, and the sky is threatened with the signal of the oncoming thunder and lightening, the Igbo normally says 'ona asu ya' meaning that the sky is annoyed. Amadioha is the spirit of thunder and lightening and he is popularly called the "god of thunder".

He is popularly revered and widely acknowledged in Igboland. "He is regarded as an agent of Chineke against undetected criminals.[53] Igbos believes that thunder does not strike in vain.[54] It is accepted that it strikes as a direct vengeance for an evil committed by the man who is struck. Those who are struck by thunder or lightening are said to be killed by Amadioha as a penalty for the atrocities they might have committed. They are not mourned by the society. "Their corpses are not carried into the house and sacrifices must be offered at the

50 Ibid. p.179

51 The Igbos does not worship the spirits. Instead they venerate the spirits.

52 L.E. Esomonu, Respect for Human life in Igbo religion and morality, Op. Cit., p.78

53 V.C. Uchendu, The Igbo of Southern Nigeria, New York, 1965, p.97

54 "Thunder does not strike in vain" Recently in January 2006, thunder struck at Ogbete Market in Enugu in Enugu State of Nigeria, and killed one woman who sells in the sight of the onslaught. The rumour went about the city and environs, that charms were buried at the sight of the thunder hazard by woman hoteliers. It was believed that the acclaimed charms were buried to help the owner make good and quick sales.

fatal Spot."[55] This is how Chioma Madume, a priestess of Amadioha expresses the role of Amadioha,

Amadioha, like Ala and the Arochukwu Juju is against all those who act contrary to custom. The thunder god sends down his bolt to strike such sinners, so when a man is killed by lightening, people always know that he has done some bad thing. Witches and Wizards specially dread his power and never dare to go out during a storm.[56]

1.2.4 Anyanwu (the Sun Spirit)

Some spirits are called sons of 'Chukwu'. 'Anyanwu' (the sun) is one of such spirits. "Anyanwu is sometimes confused or even Market very near Onitsha town in Anambra State of Nigeria, and killed one woman who sells in the sight of the onslaught. The rumour went about the city and environs that charms were buried at the sight of the thunder hazard by women hoteliers. It was believed that the acclaimed charms were buried to help the owner make good and quick sales identified with Chukwu, the high God."[57] He is among the great sky deities that surround the Supreme Being above, just as the heavenly bodies decorate the sky. Anyanwu the 'sun spirit' has the duty to collaborate with the Supreme God to give sun and heat to the world. This collaboration is sometimes mistaken that the sun spirit is in some places "worshipped and addressed in prayers as if he were the same as Chukwu.... A popular way of offering prayers to the sun spirit is by addressing him as the companion of the kings of the heavens (Anyanwu na Eze – elu). This is prominent in Nsukka division of the Northern Igbo sub–cultural area.[58]

1.2.5 Idemili

Idemili is one of the water spirits popularly known and worshipped around the towns in what we today called Idemili local government area of Anambra State of Nigeria. Idemili is a water spirit. Rivers and lakes are believed to have guardian spirits and have particular laws concerning them. "Modern pagans believe that

---

55 F.A. Arinze, Sacrifice in Ibo religion, p.16

56 P.A.Talbolt, Some Nigeria Fertility Cults, London, Oxford University Press, 1929, p.57

57 C.K. Meek, Law and Authority in a Nigeria Tribe, London, 1937, p.21

58 L.E. Esomonu, Respect for human life in Igbo religion and Morality, Op. Cit., p.77–78

'mammy water' (a sort of nymph) dwells at the beds of big rivers."[59] Today, it is not only the modern pagans that believe this. Some modern Christians also believe that too. They are believed to cause sickness in various ways, sometimes, "a strange unknown sickness."[60]

1.2.6 Evil Spirit

Igbo religious traditions are generally concerned with the quest for the good much more as with the effort to ward off evil. Generally, evil are of two types – physical and moral evil. Physical evil is conceived as any misfortune, which befalls an individual or a community. While the moral evil is any voluntary infringement of the decrees of God, the deities and the ancestors. Evil spirits in the traditional belief are the beings that cause physical evils to individuals or communities. For the Igbos, "those spirits that come in contact with man whose names are known and who have priests and shrines are generally regarded as benevolent or neutral or as severe to those who disobey their laws."[61]

> *Among those spirits who have shrines and priests however, are some that do so little good and so great harm that they are called "wicked". Such are Udo, widespread in Iboland, Omaliko at Abatete, Okpimodu at Umunachi, and lyi–Oji at Nkwelle near Onitsha, to name only a few. No sane man wants to deal with them. Every one is afraid of swearing falsely on them. They delight in inflicting suffering almost capriciously and at the least provocation.*[62]

There are however a host of unknown non–human spirits who are regarded as malevolent says Basden. According to him, "The name 'Ekwensu' did not come with Christianity.[63] Ekwensu is not to be identified with the Christian concept of the Devil as some writers have in fact described it and as some Christians of today see it.

"Some see Ekwensu as the supreme author of evil and an arch–enemy of God whose purpose is to frustrate the goodness of God and disseminate evil."[64]

Ekwensu is an evil spirit in the Igbo traditional world–view, but some occasions refer to him as a good spirit.

---

59 F.A. Arinze, sacrifice in Ibo Religion, p.14

60 L.N. Odinkemelu, Mammy Water in the Society: Her influence in Igbo Culture, Ihiala, 1986, p.12

61 P.A. Talbot, The tribes of the lower Niger, London, 1932, p.63

62 F.A. Arinze, Sacrifice in Ibo religion, p.14

63 G.T. Basden, Niger Ibos, London, 1966, pp.36–37

64 G.T. Basden, Niger Ibos, p.36

Ekwensu is a deity of violence believed to incite people to do violent deeds. A person given to violence is said to be possessed by the Ekwensu, since he spells disaster for the community during peace time. But at war time, his activities are propitious and he is invoked as a good spirit. Warriors set up shrines where they make sacrifices to Ekwensu.[65]

This identification of Ekwensu as a good spirit is well explained by the Igbo proverb, 'Gbue Dike gbue Dike, mbosi ogu achoba Dike', (Kill the warrior, kill the warrior, during war he will be sought for). In Ukpor in Nnewi South Local Government of Anambra State, there is a hill that up till today bears the name 'Ugwu Ekwensu' (the Hill of Ekwensu). The name is not obviously connected with evil.

In Igboland, there are many other spirits who are believed to do so great harm to individuals and communities that they are said to be inherently evil. A great number of them are believed to be the spirits of the dead who are sometimes believed to work in groups. The Igbos classify the evil spirits of the dead into three age–groups, namely, "the 'Umu aro' (evil spirits of dead children), the 'Ogbunuke' (evil spirits of dead young men), and the 'Akalogeli' (evil spirits of adults who died without offsprings).[66] These groups of evil spirits are feared in Igboland. The groups of evil spirits most feared by young mothers and which disturb the society a lot are the famous 'Ogbanje' or born to die children. Lucas describes them as,

> *A confraternity of spirits who visit the world in incarnate form for short periods, the length of each being prearranged. The spirits are born into babies who will die in infancy or boyhood.*[67]

These Ogbanje spirits are regarded as one of the most devilish agents of misfortunes. However, it is good to note that many people in Igboland do not hold the belief in the Ogbanje phenomenon.

1.2.6.1 Veneration of the Ancestors

Belief in the continued existence and influence of the late members of the Igbo families has a special place in the religious life of the Igbo people. There is a general belief among the Igbos that communion and communication are possible between those who are alive and those who are dead. All those who have died

---

65 E.I.Metuh, God and Man in African Religion, Chapman, London, 1981, p.76
66 Ibid. P.156
67 J.O. Lucas, Religion in West Africa and Ancient Egypt, National Press, Lagos, 1970, p.168

and can communicate with the living; we call the living–dead. It is observed that various terms have been used for them such as ancestors or Ghosts or the ancestral spirits. But these terms are lacking in their contents if we are to include all the dead that still communicate with the living in our work. The term living–dead includes all categories of the dead children, men and women, in fact all members of the family who have died and are believed to interact in the world of the living. We are however more interested in those who are regarded as ancestors of the living. We shall therefore give special attention to those living–dead qualified to be ancestors to differentiate them from the other living dead and particularly for the place they occupy in Igbo religious life.

The ancestors are among the group of spiritual beings who were one–time human beings and later disincarnated and revered in Igbo traditional religion. F. Oborji says,

they are people who have made it to the Spirit–land and are being venerated by their descendants. They are regarded as the elder members of the family. As spirits, they have enhanced powers, which they are believed to use mainly to protect the interest of their families, or clan. In the hierarchy of Beings, after the Supreme Being, and the deities, come the ancestors.[68]

Any wonder Parrinder says,

Not only are the ancestors revered as past heroes, but they are felt to be still present, watching over the household, directly concerned, in all the affairs of the family and property, giving abundant harvest and fertility.[69]

What Parrinder says here of West African Religion is also very applicable to the Igbo households. In Igbo society, it is believed that when a person dies, his spirit wanders about till it joins the company of the already departed forefathers. But not all the departed joins this company. For some reasons, some of the departed may not be qualified to join the Revered Company of the ancestors. According to Metuh,

Most African societies accept that death by itself does not turn one into an ancestor. The deceased must have the requisite qualifications, and some process must be fulfilled before he attains the status of ancestor. These qualifications and process vary from society to society. But most African groups make a clear distinction between the departed who are ancestors and those who are not, and have terms and different cults for the two groups. The Igbo, for example, call the ancestors 'Ndichie' and call the departed who have not attained ancestor – hood, 'Ogeli' (wanderer). The former are venerated as good

68 F. Oborji, Trends in African Theology since Vatican II: A missiological Orientation, Rome, 1998, p.146

69 G. Parrinder West African Religion, Op. Cit., p.115

spirits while the later are generally regarded as malignant spirits and are driven away by rites of exorcism.[70]

Similarly, Nyamiti notes,

that a dead parent who was totally bad is no ancestor and has no title to any regular sacred relationship with his offspring. This title is based on the fact that parent was morally good and is – thanks to his death – in a supernatural state. An ancestor whose conduct on earth was totally reproachful cannot be a proto–type of behaviour for his or her descendants and has no basis to the title of mystical communion with them.[71]

These unqualified ancestors are said to wander homelessly and dispossessed, expressing their grief by causing harm among the living. This group, Metuh qualifies as Ghosts. "The term 'Ghosts' could be reserved for the departed who have turned into wandering malignant spirits."[72] Those who are qualified to join the ancestors, says Isichei,

are those who lived "well–spent lives", died in socially approved ways and were given correct burial rites and now living in the world of the dead, which mirrors the world of the living.[73]

These ancestors are capable of doing many things. They are believed to have survived death and to be living in a spiritual world but still taking a lively interest in the affairs of their families.

They jealously maintain discipline in the families, and may inflict punishment on those members whose behaviour threatens the existence and progress of the family. As members of the family, ancestors are invited to be present and participate in most family activities.[74]

They are believed to be much nearer to God and the spirits. According to Mbiti,

The ancestors are bilingual: They speak the language of man with whom they lived until recently, and they speak the language of the spirits and of God to whom they are drawing nearer ontologically. These are the spirits with which African peoples are most concerned. It is through the living–dead that the spirit world becomes personal to men. They are still part of their human families and people have personal memories of them.

---

70 E. Metuh, Comparative studies of African Traditional Religions, Op. Cit., p.136

71 C. Nyamiti, African Tradition and the Christian God, in "Spearhead Magazine", No. 49, p.48

72 E.I. Metuh, Comparative Studies of A.T.R., Op. Cit., p.137

73 Ibid., p.26

74 F. Oborji, Trends in African Theology since Vatican II, Op. Cit., pp.146&147

They are the guardians of the family affairs, traditions, ethics and activities. Because they are still 'people', the living – dead are therefore the best group of intermediaries between men and God, they know the needs of men and have full access to the channels of communication with God directly or indirectly through their own fore–fathers.[75]

The living honours these ancestors who in turn watch over the people. This honour is not however to be understood as worship, as some people misconstrue it. "These good ancestors whom the Igbo people pay reverence are called "Ndi Ichie" which probably means "those of old" or "Nna Anyi" (Our fathers)... In Onitsha traditional society however, 'Ndicie' does not refer to the ancestors but is a social rank higher than that of the 'Ozo' and nearest to the 'Obi'.[76]

In this context, 'Ndi ichie' are ruling nobles; the administrators of the affairs of the town. The ancestors are also called upon at the Igbo prayers and during meals to partake of the meals. These departed ancestors who are invoked in prayers are expected to relay human requests, fears and needs to God.

They are also specifically believed to intercede for man in the land of the spirits while men intercede for them here on earth, hence the common aspect of Igbo prayer after the invocation of the grand fathers and great grand fathers, 'na achulu anyi be ndi muo, k'anyi n'achulu unu be ndi mmadu' (intercede for us in the land of the spirit while we intercede for you on earth). Igbo belief in the ancestors is really strong. The International Theological Commission recently acknowledged this communion and constant exchange between the living and the living dead in African Traditional Religion thus, "The idea of a family union of souls through death is not foreign to many African Religions and offers the opportunity for inter – religious dialogue with them."[77]

1.2.5.2 Prayer (An Aspect of Igbo Traditional Religion)

We cannot bring to an end our survey of Igbo traditional religion without reference to Igbo prayers. It has been observed that man has from time immemorial struggled to find ways of harnessing the forces in the universe to his own advantage but when this failed, man became notoriously religious and reverted to constant prayers and sacrifices. Hence the many religions of the world. And to this fact the Igbo is not an exception. The Igbo traditional religion is therefore not without prayers. Prayer forms an integral part of any viable religious system.

75 J.S. Mbiti, African Religions and Philosophy, Op. Cit., p.83
76 F.A. Arinze, Sacrifice in Ibo Religion, p.19
77 The Irish Theological Quarterly, Vol. 58

Prayer is one of the main driving forces of a religious being, a basic act of religion and it reveals man as expressing some kind of subordination to and dependence on the Supernatural.

For Heiler,

Prayer expresses the faith, life work and ruling motive of the religious believer. It is a sign of religion wherever it is alive – religion in action, and through it, differing cultural identities are revealed.[78]

The Igbo is noted to be deeply religious. And one of the principal factors that manifest this deeply religious nature is his inclination to prayer.

These prayers more than any aspect of religion contain most intensive expression of African traditional spirituality, a study of which takes us to the core of African spirituality and adds valuable dimensions to our understanding of African religion.[79]

Different religions have different objects, practices and ways of expressions. Bastides distinguishes the oral expression of prayers from what he calls the 'materialized prayer' and 'corporal prayer'.

Materialized prayer occurs when the worshipper expresses his basic disposition through manipulation of a material object of some kind e.g. A cult object like 'ofo' cult staff of the Igbo. A corporal prayer occurs when bodily actions such as spitting, dancing or gesturing are used to express communication with God.[80]

Most of the different prayers said by the Igbos are recited by different people in their different official capacities – the priest, the family priest or family head, heads of social groups and, of course individuals. Invariably one sees that prayers are mostly community based and community orientated. Thus as Mbiti says,

A good number of these prayers are set in responsive form which emphasises the group or community participation in prayer and shows also that the concerns expressed in prayers are common or shared concerns. The leader may intone the prayer while the assembled group responds in songs or recitation generally some of the phrases uttered by the leader or a well known formula.[81]

---

78 F. Heiler, Prayer: A study in the history and Psychology of Religion, London, 1932, p.358

79 J.S. Mbiti, The Prayers of African Religion, London, 1975, p.1

80 R. Bastide, L'expression de la piere chez le people san escriture 'La Maison Dieu, No. 109, 1972, pp.106 – 107, in Metuh, "African Religion in Western Conceptual Schemes", Jos, 1985 p.141

81 J.S. Mbiti, The prayers of African Religion, Op. Cit., p.2

In other words, prayers in Igbo land are said communally than individually. Arinze puts it thus, "Besides the traditional morning prayers, public prayer is almost invariably bound up with sacrifice. Individual prayer is not a normal thing except in the form of ejaculations to God, the spirits and the ancestors."[82] This shows that there is a good difference between ejaculation and other prayers. There are special people who say the traditional Morning Prayer and special people in their special capacities also say the other public prayers. Ejaculations, just as the Christian ejaculatory prayers are uttered by people of all ages and by both sexes at any time and at any place and as often as occasion demands them. For instance when a child sneezes, the mother or any person around spontaneously says 'Ndu gi' (Your health). This phrase is a complete prayer asking for protection of life. There are no special prayers said by children, rather they join in the community or family prayers.

The family head, 'pater familia' often says the traditional Morning Prayer of the Igbo. The first and meritable duty of the family head is to thank God for the care and protection of his family through the ancestors and the spirits. The deities, spirits and the ancestors are next in authority to the Supreme Being acting as intermediaries between God and the people offering the prayer. This is a typical reflection of the social pattern of the Igbo people. For one to approach the king, he has to go through the 'Ndi ichie'.[83] So prayers are offered to God through a succession of ancestors and spirits ending sometimes with words of acclamation and support like 'ise' or 'ofor';[84] taken to mean 'Amen' (So be it). This method of the traditional approach to God is more akin to the method more commonly used by the Christians of today especially those of the Catholic denomination. The Catholics believe in the one Supreme God and pray to him but more often through the intercession of the saints.

In Igbo land, the breaking of oji,[85] and the use of 'nzu'[86] normally accompany the traditional Morning Prayer.

---

82 F.A. Arinze, Sacrifice in Ibo religion, p.23

83 "Ndi ichie" – ruling nobles. They are administrators of affairs generally town councillors.

84 'Ise' or 'Ofor' is taken literally to mean Amen (So be it). The use differs according to places. In Anambra Local Government Area, like in Uga, 'Ofor' is more often used.

85 'Oji' is a kind of nut shared between friends as a token of goodwill. It is a kind of hard nut and often bitter. It signifies peace and friendliness; hence oji is not presented to any visitor who is not welcome. 'Oji per se' is sacred. Thus a woman does not pick the pod when it falls off from the tree, what more climbing the tree itself.

86 'Nzu' is a type of white–chalk–like substance. It symbolises goodwill, purity and sacredness. It is very important during worship. Normally the worshipper draws parallel lines on the ground towards the direction of the 'alusi', (shrine). The number of lines to be drawn is determined by one's rank. In Idemili area of Igbo Land, the Chiefs (E-

Oji (kola nut) and 'Nzu' (white chalkish substance) are usually presented first before approaching God and the deities to signify the worshipper's goodwill and friendliness between him and the unseen power. Nzu usually comes before the oji, though each complements the other. Writing on prayer, Arinze says that, "prayer is generally accompanied by the eating of kola nut as an expression of goodwill and as a sensible manifestation of a desire for communion"[87]

When an Igbo is praying, especially in the mornings, certain preparations are to be made or presumed. After he might have sat down, he washes his hands and the next thing he does is to draw some parallel lines on the ground with the nzu and passes it to others around. When this is done, then follows the prayer with the breaking of the kola nut. Whenever prayer is to be offered, ofo,[88] staff is necessity. The family head offering the prayer holds the ofo staff in his hand which serves as a mediator between the spirits of this world and the under world. This practice has a peculiar nature in Ibagwa (North–Eastern Igbo land). There it goes like this,

Each morning at dawn the heads of families and other elder men take hold of the Ofo and ring small brass bell to call Chukwu's attention to their prayer. Having prayed for protection during the day for themselves and their families, they chew some kola and spit upon their ofo saying, "Ofo of the Lord, Chi, creator of every thing, carry all that I am praying now to God.[89]

Ofo may also serve as a symbol of truth and man's innocence of wrong doing against others. It may be regarded as 'god of justice', hence the popular Igbo saying, 'ejim ogu na ejim ofo' declaring one's uprightness about a matter. Then after

---

ze) draw eight lines, the titled men (Nze), draw five, while the non titled men (Okolo) draw four.

87 F.A. Arinze, Sacrifice in Ibo religion, p.23

88 The 'Ofo' sticks are sticks of varying sizes from about two inches long and half an inch indiameter, to something near five inches long and one and half inches in diameter, becoming thinner towards the tail end. They are made out of the Detarium Senegalese tree, one of the special features of this tree is that the branches fall off from the parent trunk when they are fully grown. No cutting of the ofo branch is done. It is believed that Chukwu (the great God) purposely created this tree to be sacred and by the manner its branches fall off, unbroken, He (Chukwu) symbolises the way families grow up and establish new extended families and lineages. Therefore the ofo made out of the branches is the abode of the spirit of the dead ancestors, hence the authority and the sacredness of the ofo, as well as the special place given to it as the emblem of unity, truth, and indestructibility for the individual or the possessing the ofo, (Cf. Edmund Ilogu, Christianity and Igbo culture, 1974, p.18)

89 R. Norton, God, man and the Land in a Northern Ibo village – group, Africa, XXVI, 1, 1956, p.21

the saying of the prayers, he places his ofo staff on the ground and breaks the kola nut.

Generally after the breaking of the kola nut, bits of it are thrown outside, (believing to be offered to the spirits) while the people around consume the other pieces. The better part of the kola nut the 'Obi oji' (the heart of the kola) is believed to be given to the spirits and certain words are uttered such as this, 'Ani welu ihe di nma ka itaa obi oji' (Let 'ani' take what is good and eat). The minor deities like 'Udo' and 'Ogwugwu' are also invoked in prayers. It is believed that the Igbos invoke these deities because none claims to know what they have in mind. However they are generally believed to be wicked but it is not certain whether they destroy or not, hence they are greatly respected.

Igbo prayers are normally made up of the introductory part, the petition and the conclusion. The introduction is a kind of invocation in which the objects of worship are called upon to listen to the petitions. The leader of the prayer calls on God, the spirits and the ancestors. In invocation, says Amponsah,

> *the object of worship is mentioned by its personal name. The name must be honorific. Praise names, Attributes, and proverbs are mentioned as part of the invocation to honour the deity/deities.*[90]

After the introductory part of the prayer comes the petition which is the heart of the whole prayer. The petition comprises more of blessings for his families and curses and damnation for his enemies. On this Amponsah observes that,

> *petition is materialistic; requests are made for material blessings, health, longevity, peace, grace, potency, and rainfall, protection from enemies and death, increase of children, food, flocks or crops.*[91]

And finally comes the conclusion, which is sometimes, and more often ended with a beautiful Igbo proverb.

At this point, it is necessary to observe that some forms of sacrifice accompany all formal and organised prayers. In most parts of Igbo land, prayers are accompanied by the pouring of a liquid usually 'nkwu' wine or gin or some other alcoholic drink depending on the occasion. This is to say that Libation is an integral part of any organised prayer in Igboland. In fact it is a common practice or a characteristic of Igbo prayers to conclude any formal prayer with libation.

---

90 K. Amponsah, Topics on West African Traditional Religion, Vol. II, Cape Coast, 1975, p.38

91 Ibid. p.38

In the capacity of this observation, we shall take a sketchy look on libation as a characteristic of Igbo prayers, for a deep and better understanding of some practices associated with the healing ministry in the local Church in Igboland.

1.2.5.3 Libation (a characteristic of Igbo prayer)

Libation is simply and generally understood as an act of "pouring out of an offering of wine to a god or one's object of worship"[92] The word libation comes from the Latin, "libare" which means to take a portion or to taste. We have observed that it is a common characteristic of the Igbo prayers to invoke 'Chukwu' the Supreme God, the spirits and the ancestors to take part in the kola nut that normally accompanies the traditional Morning Prayer. Arthur Glyn says that,

libation is usual either before eating or drinking, to place on the ground or as the Ibani do, to throw in the air a small portion of food or water and as this is being done, a petition in the following or similar words is addressed to the names on behalf of their descendants, eat, drink and live.[93]

This practice of throwing a portion of food or drink in the air and asking the gods and the spirits to eat and drink portrays so much the etymological meaning of libation as 'to take a portion' or 'to taste'. Therefore, the practice of throwing out some part of the food or kola nut and pouring out of some quantity of wine during prayer is a profound manifestation of the sincerity of the invitation to the spirits and ancestors to partake in the meal or drink. Hence K. Amponsah says that "the pouring of libation is a necessary act because it is a process which tends to keep us closer to our ancestors and to the gods."[94] The gods are really wanted to partake in the eating and drinking. And this could be one of the major reasons why the names of the departed ancestors are mentioned in prayers to remind them of their togetherness with their children here on earth, to protect them from all malign influences. No wonder in Elechi Amadi's book, 'The Concubine', when Anyika the medicine man was called to administer to the sick Emenike, he first demanded for kola nuts and gin. When they were brought, he broke the kola nuts, cut them to pieces, and threw them outside. He then poured out some gin on the ground as libation and muttered as each drop reached the ground:
Gods of night take this
Gods of the earth take this
Ojukwu the fair take this

92 Advanced Learners Dictionary of current English, London, 1962, p.562
93 L.A. Glyn, The Lower Niger and its tribes, London, 1968, p.349.
94 K. Amponsah, Topics on West A.T.R., Op. Cit., p.49

Amadioha king of the sky, this is yours;
And you ancestors, small and great
guardians of this compound, take this.[95]

It was only after this libation that Anyika started to administer his medicine to the sick man. This however shows the importance of the gods and the place of the ancestors in the preservation of health and lives of the individuals.

The Igbo offers libations at any convenient place. There is no special place for this practice. On this Glyn observes:

"This practice as I have seen it in hundreds of other towns of Ibo land is performed religiously and without shrinking even in the presence of white strangers particularly with regard to the presentation of kola nut and palm wine as a mark of welcome and friendship on all special occasions, in addition to the regular routine, as a tribute of reverence and gratitude to the town protector... What is more, no meal is ever eaten and no liquid is ever drunk until this act of grace has been fulfilled.[96]"

This practice of libation goes to manifest the Igbo's knowledge of the omnipresence of God and his recognition of this presence since he carves out no special place or occasion for this act.

The prayer that accompanies libation is generally as important as the libation itself. The content however depends on the purpose for the libation and the occasion in which it is made. It is also important to note that not all libations are accompanied by utterances. "Certain libations are without prayers most especially when two or three people meet to partake of a small drink."[97] In Igbo traditional society, it is common to see little groups gather at a friend's house especially in the evenings after the day's work to recreate and partake of some drinks. In such refreshment gatherings, the act of libation is not forgotten though it is not often accompanied by utterances.

In such cases one simply pours out some quantity of drinks and goes on enjoying himself. None will ever pretend to overlook the presence of the gods and the ancestors.

Through the act of libation, we have seen that the Igbo traditional believers express their belief in the Supreme Being, the veneration of the deities and the ancestors, showing man's dependence upon these supernatural beings. This gives the people confidence and security to go about their daily activities without fear. Through the act they take cognisance of the presence and importance of their dead relatives who are believed to have much interest in their daily affairs.

---

95 E. Amadi, The Concubine, London, 1978, p.6
96 L.A. Glyn, The Lower Niger, Op. Cit., p.350
97 K. Amponsah, Topics on West African Traditional Religion, Op. Cit., p.51

1.2.5.4 Medicines and Charms (Ogwu)

This is one of the areas in Igbo traditional life in which the question of terminology is extremely difficult and confusing. Names for charms and medicines are identical in Igbo traditional society. Their uses are also very common, "There is hardly any distinction made between medicine as pharmaceutical preparation and medicine as charm or purveyor of mystical powers."[98] Writing on mystical powers and magic, Mbiti says, "there is no African society which does not hold belief in mystical power of one type or another. It shows itself or it is experienced in many ways."[99] These mystical powers are believed to be present in words especially that of elder to a younger person. There are also mystical powers, which make charms or medicines to be effective. It is also believed that there are mystical powers, which make people disappear from one position to another, to lie in thorns, to send curses or harm or death on people even from a distance (actio in distans). These objects however play a vital role in the life of the Igbo. According to Le Roy,

> *a charm is an object which by some mysterious immanent and unconscious power is believed to preserve from evil, diseases, bullets or motor accidents or to make one succeed in trade, in a love affair, in fishing, in catching thieves, in passing examinations etc*[100]

V. Ifeanyi defines charms as simply "an object believed to have occult powers."[101] Charms are generally called 'ogwu' in Igbo language, which is also a name for medicines.

'Ogwu' in general, which can mean charms or medicines, can be prepared from roots, herbs, or plants having some real or imaginary powers to give solution to a variety of human problems and sickness. Ogwu as a pharmaceutical preparation can be used to cure different types of sickness beginning from 'isi owuwa' head ache, to 'afo osisa' diarrhoea, and 'Iba ocha n'anya' Yellow fever and 'Okiri ngbawa isi' mental sickness. There are also Igbo pharmaceutical preparations used by traditional Orthopaedic doctors or 'bone setters'. On the other hand 'Ogwu' considered as charms can be used for various purposes as have been identified above.

Charms or Medicines can also be dangerous or destructive depending on their preparation and use. Their powers are believed to be inherent in nature so that

---

98 E. I. Metuh, Comparative Studies of A.T.R., Op. Cit., p.55

99 J.S. Mbiti, African Religions and Philosophy, Op. Cit., p.197

100 A. Le Roy, La Religion des Primitifs, p.272, quoted in F.A. Arinze, "Sacrifice in Ibo religion", p.20

101 V. Ifeanyi, The Catholic Church and the Challenges of traditional system of Health care, Rome 1989, p.61

anyone who knows their make–up can tap them. These charms and medicines are not only prepared from herbs and plants. They can be mixed up or prepared from other objects such as animal parts to give solutions to a variety of human problems and sickness. The Igbo believes too that these medicines and charms work in conjunction with certain invocations. In fact, E. 1. Metuh says that, "it is the ritual invocations which gives dynamism to the mixture and triggers it into action."[102] In traditional Igbo concept, Medicine can be defined as

a recipe of herbal mixtures and some ritual formulae designed to generate some powers which are built into nature by God and other spiritual beings to meet various human needs.[103]

Parrinder who believes that the Igbo heals himself with medicine defines medicine as,

a term that covers both natural healing agencies, leaves, roots and the like and also the invocation of magical or spiritual influences that are thought to be associated with them.[104]

Both conceptions of Igbo traditional medicine bear some common elements. Both acknowledge the power of human words on the objects of nature to release energy or force that can influence human life and nature.

We can therefore conceive medicine in Igbo context as a combination of various natural objects prepared to give solution to various human problems by re–activating the immanent power of God in these objects through the invocation of the same power of God.

Medicines and Charms are both prepared by Medicine men in Igbo society. There are good and bad medicines as well as protective and aggressive or destructive charms. Good or protective medicines are socially approved ones usually used to cure diseases and ward off misfortunes while bad medicines and charms are applied to socially disapproved goals, usually used to bring some injuries or misfortunes to people. People use medicines prepared for protection of their individual persons as well as for the protection of their families and kindreds. Protective medicines can also be used to protect the infection of diseases of one kind or the other. This type of medicine is either eaten or inserted into the body in form of inoculation. Some others are smeared all over the body in form of a lotion. A good deal of the protective medicines is either placed at the entrance of the house or in a corner of the compound. It can also be hung in the

102 E. I. Metuh, Comparative Studies of A.T.R. Op. Cit., p.213

103 Ibid. p.213

104 G. Parrinder, West African Traditional Religion, Op. Cit., p.156

ceiling of the room. There are others that can be buried in the floor of the house or in a comfortable part of the compound.

1.2.5.5 Respect for Elders

'Onye na–amaghi onye toro ya akabeghi' – He who does not know his elder is not yet mature. "If you respect today's King, others will respect you when it is your turn" These are Igbo proverbs relating to respect to seniors, elders and those in authority at the family, town and other levels of social organisation. The respect accorded the elders in Igbo land; derive from their social status and the invaluable services they render to the society. It is said that gray hairs signify wisdom. This wisdom is acquired through years of experience which the elders pass on to the younger generation. They are consultants on issues that require very careful and mature treatment. Thus, when an elder dies, a library is said to have been burnt.

In a family, "the grandfather is the head and the arbiter, the person to whom all matters are referred for a decision. He is therefore regarded with much respect. Chiefs and other elders perform this role in society and such people are also accorded great reverence".[105] When a child is born to the family, the elder is consulted to give a name to the child, which often reflects the history of the family in question. Where the naming of a child is performed publicly, it is the exclusive right of an elder to officiate in the ceremony.

In the customary marriage rites, the elders feature prominently, both in the determination of the "bride wealth"and in the exchange of other marriage gifts. As part of testing the bride's character, "she is expected to be ... respectful towards her elders, obedient and even–tempered".[106]

In the religious sphere, the elders lead in family prayers, make offerings and pour libations to the ancestors. As visible representatives of the ancestors, they are the custodians of morality, of laws and customs. They are embodiments of truthfulness and dispensers of justice. They settle disputes in the community impartially and so maintain peace. They have the power to bless or curse. Because he or she is a symbol of justice, the Igbos says: "*Okenye adi ano n'uno, ewu amuo n'ogbili*"literally – an elder cannot be at home, while a goat delivers in tethers. Metellus Cimber capitalised upon this social status of an elder while speaking about the inclusion of Cicero, an old man, in the plot against Caesar. He said:

105 Kofi A. Opuku, West African Traditional Religion. Lagos: FEB Int. Ltd., 1978 p.50
106 Ibid., p.129

O, let us have him; for his silver hairs
will purchase us a good opinion,
and buy men's voices to commend our deeds:
It shall be said his judgement ruled our hands;
Our youths and wildness shall no whit appear,
But all be buried in his gravity.[107]

There are some other concrete ways of showing respect to the elders. A young person greets him or her on the road by his or her title name, listens attentively when he or she is talking, and offers them seat, where there is none available for them. Also in the community sharing of meat, the elders choose first in order of seniority. special portions of the slaughtered animal are exclusive preserves of elders, such as the eyes, the heart, liver gizzard etc. Again, during the annual festival "*Alom muo*"in honour of all the ancestors, fowls are slaughtered. The following morning, "as an act of homage, the head of the family sends a wing, a leg and the liver of a fowl to the oldest man in the village who is regarded as the visible representative of the ancestors".[108]

The elderly woman is regarded as "Nne ora" – (mother of all) in the vicinity, and is respected by the young brides for whom they serve as advisers. They occupy high positions among the "umuokpu"(daughters of the land who are married). Not to respect an elder might merit the offender a beating, a fine or a curse.[109]

Hence the Ibos hold that he who listens to an elder is like one who consults an Oracle. The Oracles are believed to give the infallible truths, thus the elders are also believed to say the truth and their words and instructions are heeded to for the promotion of good behaviour among the young.[110]

The elders are also taken as the repository of communal wisdom, culture and tradition and are thus conceded leadership in the affairs of the people. The main reason for this is that it is believed that the elders are nearer to the ancestors; in this regard Davidson, B., avers:

legitimate power lay in the office sanctioned by ancestral
norms, not in the person, and the person lost his right to
exact obedience once he abused that office.[111]

---

107 Wifit, D., ed., "Julius Caesar" in The Complete Works of William Shakespeare. London: Hamlyn Pub. Group Ltd., 1982. P.726

108 Opuku, K. A., Op. Cit. p.50

109 Cf. Ikenga–Metuh, Comparative Studies of African Traditional Religions. P.146

110 Onwubiko, O., African Thought and Culture, Owerri: Totan Publishers Ltd., 1988, p.31

111 Davidson, B., The African Genius; Boston, 1969, p.200

The elders, ipso facto, respected their authority and hardly abused their office. The respect for elders helped in the maintenance of law, order, justice custom and tradition.

It is also held by the Ibos that respect for the elders is reciprocal hence he who respects his elders in addition to winning favours from the elders, they in turn would be respected when they become elders. The elders must also live up to expectation by properly executing the responsibility demanded by their office.

Finally, there is also complimentareity in the execution of authority. The Ibos are generally egalitarian in nature and shun dictatorship. Consequently, overwhelming power manifestation on the part of the elders is often met with resistance hence the Igbo proverb: Oke mmadu bu egbe, okorobia bu igu. Ma igu adighi na egbe o naghi ekwu okwu, ma egbe adighi, igu enweghi ebe o ga ano – The elder is the gun, the young is 'igu'. If there is no 'igu' in the gun, it cannot fire and sound. If there is no gun, 'igu' would have no where to rest it thus becomes useless.

This wonderful symbiosis and balance of power shows the typical sense of importance attached to each sector of the societal strata. It is therefore not enough to have only one group. This confines the community solidarity aspect.

1.2.5.6 Respect for Life

The Igbo man has very great respect for life. For him life is the greatest and most precious gift from God, the source and fullness of life. It is the highest good a man can have. For him life is not just to exist. It is the full dynamic existence in which all the good things of life will come. He therefore cherishes life and jealously guards and preserves it. This is manifested in many areas of his life particularly in his prayers and often in the names he gives his children.

The object of Igbo prayers is life. In his traditional Morning Prayer, the family head prays for life, for good health, for recovery from sickness and against death. He also asks for other materialistic blessings for his family. Below are extracts of prayers said by an Ibo.

Petition (Part of Morning Prayer)

Olisah onye oholoho anya	Olisah, the big eyed one
Obu gi ji ji, jide nma	You are with yam and knife
Onye iwanyelu olie	Who ever you give eats
Nye anyi aru ike	Give us health
Nye anyi ogonogo ndu	Give us long life

Nye anyi ihe olili na onunu	Give us food and drink
Gozie umuaka anyi	Bless our children

Prayer at Igbo Traditional Marriage

Omumu bu ihe mbu n'uwa	Childbearing is he first thing in this World
Anasi na madu k'eji aka	It is said that one boasts with life
Chineke chekwaba di ya	May God guide her husband
Fa muta nwoke, oga adi	If they get a son he will live
Fa muta nwanyi oga adi	If they get a daughter, she will stay
K'ime n'esinalu oliaku ike	May the wife be fruitful
Wepulu ya oya	Remove sickness from her
Wepulu di ya oya	Remove sickness from husband
Chineke dobe mu onwem	May God keep me myself
Ana mayo gi odinma nke anyi	I am asking you for the good of all of us[112]

These samples of prayer show us the importance that the Igbo attaches on life. His prayers of petition are full of petitions for long life and prosperity. It is also noticed in Igbo society that at the birth of a child, the parents spend so much as a result of the ceremonies following the birth of the child. There are many of such occasions. Neighbours, friends and relations of the family where a child is born gather to see and welcome the new child and celebrate the birth of a new life. The occasion after delivery is one of the times that prayers are offered at a shrine. In Alor in Anambra State of Igbo land, the ceremony is called 'Izu ahia nwa' (a type of presentation ceremony). The child is taken to the main market of the town where there is the major shrine of the town and certain ceremonies are performed. There are other ceremonies after delivery and childbirth that are highly regarded and take a lot of time and money such as the naming ceremony. However all these go to manifest the great regard for life.

Igbo names also depict this great value and respect the Igbo has for life. We now examine some of such names.

The Igbo names his son: 'Ndu bu isi', which means (Life is supreme),'Nduka' meaning (Life is greater). Both names simply signify that life is worth more than any thing one can think of. He also gives his children names such as, 'Ndu' simply meaning (Life), 'Ndubia' meaning (May life come). There are also names to show that children are loved and appreciated namely, 'Nwamaka' (What a beauty to have a child), 'Ginikanwa' (What is greater than a child), 'Ngozika' (A child is a blessing), 'lfeyinwa' (There is nothing like a child). The last four names are

112 M.C. Obiagwu, Our Praying Fathers, Rome, 1983, pp.39,40,46&47

given mainly to female issues. In Igbo society, male children are more often preferred to females. So parents very often give such names as above to show that they equally, if not more appreciate female gifts from God.

Life is also sacred and belongs to God, hence names like 'Chinwendu' (Life belongs to God) and 'Chikwendu' (If God agrees to life) abound. The Igbo man therefore goes at any length to preserve not only his life but also that of other individuals.

Anything that deliberately goes towards the extinction or obstruction of human life is regarded as wicked and evil. To take away life in any form is a serious crime. People who happen to commit suicide for any reason are not mourned and there is no funeral for them. It is believed that they will not reach the abode of the ancestors. They wander about and are classified as 'akalogeli' (a group of evil spirit). In the traditional Igbo culture they are not even buried. They are thrown away into the 'ajo ohia' (evil forest), as a sign of rejection by men and by the gods. The Igbo culture also forbids abortion, murder, euthanasia, and all other crimes that tamper with life and the dignity of the human person. It is strongly believed that it is a sin against the earth's spirit to take away life and is punishable by either ostracisation or by tit for tat.

1.2.5.7 Marriage and Transmission of Life

Marriage in Igbo society, just as in other human societies plays a significant role in the life of the people. It is a very important event in the life of the Igbo, an objective to be attained by young growing people, male and female alike. For the Ibos, marriage is not just a serious affair but it is also complex with social, economic and religious aspects, which often overlap with one another.

It is not just the affair of the young man and his fiancée, but a long process between both families, entailing the marriage payments by the fiancé, religious ceremonies and sacrifice, and the celebration of the marriage itself.[113]

For the Ibos, marriage is the focus of existence and the members of the communities participate actively and play vital roles in the negotiations, in the payments of the bride price and in the marriage consent itself. In fact no one or any family can ordinarily, single–handedly, give out a daughter in marriage. Any wonder Mbiti says of African marriage,

> *It is the point where all members of a given community meet: the departed, the living and those yet to be born. All the dimensions of time meet here and the whole drama of history is repeated, renewed and revitalised. Marriage is a drama in which every one becomes an actor or actress and not just a spectator. Therefore marriage is a duty, a re-*

113 F.A. Arinze, Sacrifice in Ibo religion, Op. Cit., p.3

quirement from the corporate society, and a rhythm of life in which every one participates. Otherwise, he who does not participate in it is a cause to the community, he is a rebel and a law breaker, he is not only abnormal but 'under human'. Failure to get married under normal circumstances means that the person concerned has rejected society and the society rejects him in turn.[114]

Marriage in Igbo society is looked upon as a sacred duty that every one must perform. Marriage is seen as a God–given gift and Igbos believe that it is God himself who commanded people to get married and transmit life to continue his work of creation. So to live is to transmit and care for life which is the highest good a man can have. This is portrayed in his daily prayers and in Igbo names. Any body therefore who under normal circumstance refuses to marry is considered a useless person. One is not even free to delay marriage after a certain ripe age of his life. Let us see part of the letter of the sister of Peter Obiesie to him when he delayed his marriage to Nneka, narrated by Onuorah Nzekwu in his novel, Wand of Noble Wood. She wrote inter alia:

It is a pity that you have to wait all these years before having the opportunity to marry. Now that Isdor and Chukwuemeka have taken their first steps towards the attainment of the vital goal – marriage. You ought to begin now to search for a girl to marry... I am worried by the remarks you made to me several times before, to the effect that you might one day become a priest. We are no Irish people whose ambition in life seems to be able to trace as many Bishops, Priests, Monks, Reverend Mothers and Sisters as is possible in their genealogical tables. ... Chew upon these words which come to you from your sister Uz'aka.[115]

In choosing a marriage partner in Igbo traditional set–up, the parents often make the choice, sometimes even before the children were born. The normal thing is for parents to choose partners from other households for their children especially from their friends and compeers. Sometimes parents go to a house where there is an expectant mother to put in 'application' in view of a female child to be born. But most of the children engaged in this way do not get married when they grow up. In other cases where the children are grown up for marriage and make the choice themselves, it is still the parents of the male that meet those of the female and they begin marriage negotiations.

Marriage in Igbo society is generally monogamous, though some practise polygamy mainly as a symbol of status or wealth. According to Jordan, "Probably, less than twenty percent of the men were polygamists, so that the normal thing for girls was to be the sole wife."[116] Here it is necessary to mention that the main

114 J.S. Mbiti, African Philosophy and Religions, Op. Cit., p.133
115 O. Nzekwu, Wand of Noble wood, London, 1961, pp.80–81
116 J. Jordan, Bishop Shanahan of Southern Nigeria, London, 1949, p.222

purpose of marriage in Igbo society is to raise children. Life and transmission of life are cherished values in Igbo traditional culture and to live means to be able to transmit life. Marriage and procreation are therefore inseparable. Without procreation, marriage is incomplete holds the Igbo. The Igbo believes he can "immortalise" himself in this world by leaving children behind. This desire obviously makes him have as many children as possible to immortalise his name and memory and live on in his lineage and community. To express his desire for this personal immortality, the Igbo names his children, 'Afam efuna' (May my name never be lost), 'Amaechina' (May my lineage never close down), 'Obiefuna' (May my big household never extinguish).

The greatest hope therefore and the expectation of the individual for himself and of the community for the individual is to get married and beget children.

> *Only on the birth of a child does a woman become truly a kinsman in her husband's group. Only on the birth of a child is a man assured of the "immortality" of a position in the genealogy of his lineage, or even of security of esteem among the important people of his community. Only on the birth of a grand – child is a man in a position to be truly sure that his name and spirit will live in the history and genealogy of his people.*[117]

There is no wonder then, why Obuna tersely puts it that, "to die without a child is to descend into oblivion – forgotten by both the living and the dead"[118] and Ndiokwere says, "a childless marriage as far as Africans are concerned, is indisputably a disaster."[119] And we quickly add that to die without having a male child in Igbo society, is as good as dying without a child. This is also another major reason why some men get into polygamous marriage even today when Christianity has permeated every fibre of the Igbo society. The Catholic Church is over hundred years today in Igbo land.

1.2.5.8 Family Unit and Extended Family System

In Igbo society, the traditional family institution has a much wider circle of members than is observed in most societies of the Western world and in the modern societies of today. The family is the smallest unit in the social structure of every society. As a unit, the family is a firm foundation for the Igbo society. It is generally accepted to be the basis of every human community and is regarded as the nucleus of the society from which larger kinship groups are built. The members are very devoted to the groups to which they are closely bound socially, eco-

---

117 P. Bohannan, African Outline, Penguin Books, Harmondsworth, 1964, p.163
118 E. Obuna, African priests and Celibacy, Rome, 1986, p.30
119 N. Ndiokwere, The African Church today and tomorrow, Vol. 1, Onitsha, 1994, p.39

nomically, and religiously. They are attached to each other and cooperate with one another.

In Igbo society, the family may have a double perception. In one aspect, the family may include all peoples with a common descent the children, parents, grandparents, uncles and aunts, brother and sisters who may have their own children and other immediate relative. The relationship between his wide range of brothers and sisters and their other relations give birth to what Anthropologists called extended families. Green beautifully defines it as

a group of closely related people known by a common name and consisting usually of a man and his wives and children, his brothers and half brothers and their wives and children and probably other relations.[120]

In Nigeria, the law admits, "the extended family is usually a corporate body which may own property such as land in which its members have rights."[121] This extended nature of Igbo family makes the Igbo refer to a distant cousin as a brother 'nwannem'. There is no straight Igbo word for cousin. The Igbo word for cousin is explanatory 'nwa nwanne nne m' (the son of my mother's sister or brother) or 'nwa nna m ochie' (the child of my uncle). Mozia writing on solidarity among the Igbos says,

The extended family is a wider expression of solidarity. It exists for the common good of each individual member of the nuclear family ... There is therefore a broader and deeper consciousness of each individual in the different nuclear families to participate in the social, political , economic and religious life of this larger community – the extended family.[122]

Igbo family on the other perception refers to a smaller group consisting of a household – inmates of a house comprising of the man, wife, or wives, children and probably relatives and other dependants living with him. Writing on the family, Mbiti observes that "it is the practice in some societies to send children to live for some months or years with relatives. And these children are counted as members of the families where they happen to live."[123] With this we can conclude that the Igbo traditional family, in whichever perspective we look at it is made up of a good number of individual relatives. It is not simply made up of a man and his wife with one or two children as is common in Europe and North

120 M.M. Green, Land tenure in Igbo village, London, 1941, pp.2 – 3
121 E.I. Nwogugu, Family law in Nigeria, Ibadan Hienemann, 1974, pp.106–107
122 M.Mozia, Solidarity in the Church and solidarity among the Igbos, Rome, 1982, p.203
123 J.S. Mbiti, African Religions and Philosophy, Op. Cit., pp.106–107

America or some modern Nigerian families. The number of family members may be as high as twelve or sometimes over twelve.

The Igbo family also includes the dead ancestors and the children to be born. Of very great importance to the life in Igbo family are the human spirits or souls in the person of the ancestors referred by some authors as the living–dead. The ancestors are very close to their living relatives.

They expect frequent and regular offerings from the living that in turn expect them to reciprocate by giving them protection and prosperity. Hence the popular Igbo proverb of a man trying to free himself from a difficult moment, 'Ana achu aja ikpe an'ama ndi muo' (We offer sacrifice so that the blame may be on the spirits), is a proverb of a struggling man. The ancestors may also inflict some punishment on their relatives if they are neglected or for misconduct. There is a proverb to show that these ancestors may be sometimes offended: 'Achuba aja ma afuro udene ife mere be ndi muo' (If the vulture does not appear on the scene of sacrifice, we know that all is not well in the spirit land.)

Igbo family has also a special place for the yet to be born children. They are the buds of hope and expectation and each family makes sure that its own existence is not extinguished. That is why you have names like 'Onochie' meaning (the re–incarnated), perhaps meant to replace the dead father or grand father, 'Nwa nonye' signifying 'the companion', (May the child stay with us). The families are happy for new births and prepare for their coming into the world. A family without an issue is therefore regarded as having its lineage terminated.

Igbo family has great respect for seniority. Authority in Igbo family is centred on the father who is the head of the family.

The younger ones of the families "seem to live perpetually as minors, governed even in their personal affairs by the head of the family, even though with paternal benevolence."[124] However, this condition of authority over the younger ones is no more obtainable in the society, since the youth; no longer minors in their outlook have the added incentive to act on their own.

1.2.5.9 Sense of Community

The cultural sense of community is one of the major characteristics of the Igbos that can throw more light on their worldview. The Igbo believes that the attainment of full human life can only be possible through active participation in the communal life of the people. One must therefore be loyal and generous with the living family and community members, and be in loving and harmonious solidarity with one's community in order to be inwardly at peace and flourish outwardly.

---

124 A.E. Onyeocha, Family apostolate in Igbo land, Op. Cit., p.20

A community for an Igbo denotes first and foremost an ontological, moral, religious and effective quality of human relation. It is ontological in so far as all the members of the community are believed to descend from a common ancestor. Every man is linked to his parents, on the natural level he receives life from them, depends on them to grow up. His parents in turn are bound to their grand parents etc. This link which binds all members of the same family by propagation is broadened to include all members of the community or clan, who are believed to be descendants of the same ancestor. Every one thus considers himself a member of a definite community and as part of the whole.[125]

It is therefore clear that one becomes a member of a community from the moment of his birth since one is bound to another by the reason of common ancestorship. No one is free not to be a member of his community but the community in extreme cases has the right to relinquish one of his memberships by expulsion or execution. "To be without or to be cut off from a community is to be alienated. To be is to be with others. Outside the community there is no life, nothing."[126]

Discussing African anthropology, Maimela aptly puts it thus,

> *African anthropology is human centred and is socially oriented. Accordingly, individuals were continually reminded that a fulfilling life cannot be lived in isolation from their human fellows. Rather life is possible only in communal relationships in which individuals try to strike balance between the private life and the social life, thus maintaining the network of relationships with their fellows so that every person is provided with a space to breathe and live a meaningful life. A human being is only human because of others, with others and for others. Hence it was important to teach people to avoid dehumanising and bad relationships, by refraining from activities that are injurious to our human fellows or to threaten to undermine the social fibre and the stability.*[127]

The above quotation is very true of the Igbo community consciousness. Every Igbo needs one another to become a full man. Social life is not anything foreign or imported to his cultural life. Being in community is an essential element of his human worldview. And thus, "I am because we are, and since we are, therefore I am"[128]

Igbo names have a lot too to say about the value or importance of the community life of the Igbo man, 'Ubakanma' (Great number is better), this name is a name mainly given by members of a large family. The new child adds to the

125 L.E. Esomonu, Respect for human life in Igbo Religion and Morality, Op. Cit., p.42

126 E.M.Zuese, African Traditional Religion in Abingdon Dictionary of Living Religions, p.7

127 S.S. Maimela, Religion and Culture: Blessings or Curse?, in "the Journal of Black Theology in South Africa, Vol.5, No.1, May, 1991 , pp.1–12

128 J.S. Mbiti, African Religions and Philosophy, Op. Cit., p.114

strength and esteem of their community. 'Igwebuike' (Community is strength). This is a very common name in Igbo society. It is also used as a popular saying, meaning 'United we stand'. The strength of the individual is in his community. The Igbo society is really a highly structured network of communal solidarity and mutual co–operation such that solitary life of any individual is a dreadful plight and regarded as a vice or sign of wickedness.

1.2.5.10 Sense of Hospitality of the Igbos

Hospitality is part of Igbo culture. It is a very common Igbo trait, generally cherished. It is natural to the Igbo and is a major social obligation. Inability to meet up to hospitality is a humiliating experience for him. His hospitality shows his concern for the human person. Igbo hospitality is a spontaneous affair. One could even go to any degree of personal inconvenience for the comfort and pleasure of another especially a visitor. Hospitality may be expressed in very symbolic ways – supply of necessary information and assistance, exchange of gifts, presentation of kolanuts and palm wine to visitors and strangers and sharing of meals. It is only the unwelcome visitor that is not served with kolanuts.

> *In traditional African culture, where ever there is food to be taken, every one present is invited to participate even if the food was prepared for a less number of people without anticipating the arrival of visitors. It would be a height of incredible bad manners for one to eat anything however small without sharing it with anyone else present, or at least expressing the intention to do so.*[129]

In Igbo culture, a man's worth is very often assessed by his ability to take care of unexpected visitors. Hence the common saying, 'Mberede k'eji ama dike' (the great man is known by his ability to meet up with surprise visits).

For Marius Nkwo,

> *Entertaining a visitor is a pleasant task to Igbos... A visitor's prejudices are respected. The family must make all adjustment necessary for the visitors comfort. It is a must of such situations ... it is extended to people who are entirely strangers.*[130]

Writing on hospitality, Mbiti says,

> *There are morals concerned with hospitality to relative, friends and strangers. Therefore when people travel, they may stop anywhere for the night and receive hospitality in*

129 Okafor, F., Africa at Crossroads, New York, 1974, p.21
130 Nkwo, M., Igbo Cultural Heritage, Vol. 1, University Publication Co., Onitsha, p.24

the homestead. They should not be molested, unless of course they abuse the hospitality that they have received.[131]

The Igbos not only offers and expects hospitality but they demand that hospitality be reciprocated directly or indirectly. The famous Igbo saying, 'Ola nmanya madu, kedu mbosi aga ala nke gi' (Drinker of other people's wine, when shall we drink your own) is a direct demand of reciprocity of hospitality from the less generous ones.

1.2.5.11 Love for Proverbs

When Europe discovered Africa, Africa had no written literature to confront Europe with. Hence Europeans concluded that Africa was no part of history. But there was oral Tradition.

The African people developed legends and folklore. They had proverbs and metaphors. They had their myths and their narratives. They had imagery and elegy. These however were transmitted orally in a language the Europeans regarded as incomprehensible and showed no inclination to learn.[132]

To learn a people's culture, to gain an adequate insight into their thought patterns, their beliefs, Tradition and institutions, to understand their moral values, their philosophy of life and their vision, it is indispensable to know their language, and their proverbs which are part of the former. Language is the carrier of culture and the mother tongue constitutes the warp and woof of the mental life of a given people.[133]

Many definitions of proverbs have been attempted but none has met universal acceptance. Etymologically, the term proverb is derived from the Latin word 'Proverbium' which can be split into "pro" meaning 'forth' and "verbum" meaning 'word'. The Greek equivalent is "paranoima" which means 'way side saying', a form of folk literature.

According to Metuh,

Proverbs are short sayings, full of sense, which have come into common and recognised use... Proverbs spring spontaneously from the people. They are 'vox populi' (the voice of the people) in the profound sense and consequently, should be accepted as a true

131 Mbiti, J.S., Introduction to African Religion, London, 1981, p.177

132 L.N. Mbefo, The reshaping of African tradition, Enugu, 1988, p.78

133 L.E. Esomonu, Respect for Human Life in Igbo Religion and Morality, Op. Cit., p.131

index of what a people regard as true, and are interpretative of their principles of life and conduct.[134]

"Proverbs are therefore trust worthy witnesses of the social, political, ethical, and religious ideals of the people among whom they originated and circulate".[135] They have no specialised occasions for their uses, but proverbs are often involved in speeches and actions on every sort of occasion even in General conversation to embellish, conceal or hint. They are used in different ways and context.

For the Igbos, proverbs are kernels, which contain the wisdom of the traditional people highly appraised in Igbo society. Wisdom is weaved in proverbs and wise sayings, which constitute common vehicles for expressing and conveying religious ideas and feelings. Proverbs embody wisdom and wisdom causes joy. Proverbs are the mark of wise men, for says an Igbo proverb: 'Atualu omanu omalu, atualu ofeke ofenye isi n'ofia' (If you speak to a wise man in proverbs, he understands, but if to a fool, he flings them into a forest). In Igbo society certain truths are so sublime and sacred that they cannot be directly expressed, so they need to be expressed in proverbs.

The use of proverbs is cultivated as an art and cherished as an index of good oratory and acquaintance with traditional knowledge and wisdom. Elders considered as fountains of local wisdom are revered mainly because of their proficiency in using proverbial diction. It is also a mark of a good orator to embellish his speech with sensible proverbs because a speech garnished with proverbs and wise sayings is pleasant to listen to. Hence the Igbo saying, 'Inu bu nmanu eji eli okwu' (Proverbs are the palm oil for saying words). Another Igbo proverb reinforcing the importance of proverbs says. 'Na nwa mara atu inu kwuru ego emere na isi nne ya' (a child who knows how to use proverbs, has justified the bride price paid on his mother).

The special merit of the use of proverbs is that they go back to the pre–colonial days and consequently one can use them to prove that certain ideas, concepts, practices, values, respect for human life, existed among the Igbos before the advent of Christianity and Western civilisation and thus are original Igbo concepts and are not borrowed from foreign culture.[136]

At this juncture we shall analyse a few of Igbo proverbs and express the truths in them:

---

134 E.I. Metuh, Comparative Studies of African Traditional Religions, Op. Cit., p.20

135 J.A. Kelson, Proverbs in Encyclopaedia of Religion and Ethics, Vol. 1, p.415, (ed.) Clark T & J., 1918, quoted in Metuh, "Comparative Studies", p.20

136 L.E. Esomonu, Respect for Human Life in Igbo Religion and Morality, Op. Cit., p.132

'Tupulu ndi muo nni, agbanalu fa ogu fa na nkita' (Throw out food to the spirits and do not worry yourself to settle their fight with the dogs over the food). The truth in this proverb is that one is not expected to prevent the dogs from eating the food offered in sacrifice to the ancestors. The important thing is to offer the sacrifice, which is done in a shrine outside the house and not indoors. What interest the ancestral spirits are the spiritual essence of the sacrifice and the internal Disposition of the offered, and not the material food that may be eaten by animals or insects around. The spirits do not eat physically but in a spiritual and invisible manner. 'Ofu mkpisi aka ruta nmanu, ozue ibe ya onu' (One finger touches the oil that spreads to the other fingers). This proverb simply shows the meaning of community consciousness, that what happens to one person, affects the others in the same community. If one member suffers, all suffer together. If one is honoured, all the others are honoured too and all rejoice together. This also applies in human health. If the finger is hurt, the whole body is sick, but when cured, the whole body is once more at peace or healthy.

1.2.5.12 Death and Dying

Death is a passage to new existence, the transition to new and true life. It is thus an event of the same kind as birth, puberty and marriage. It is not only the most important of all these stages of life but receives the fullest and the most detailed ceremonial expression, all other stages reach their culmination and final conclusion in this. The deceased person is removed from the secular time and laws of this world and placed back in the mythical antiquity. This is shown by the ritual ceremonies performed at death.[137]

The above primitive expression of death by Elliade very much fits into the Igbo traditional conception of death. For the Igbo the belief that death is not the final end of man is very common. "The belief about 'Ndu' (life) is that it is endless even after it has been terminated by death." Death is not regarded as a final farewell; it is all part of a wider plan.

> *Men and women come, they stay for a while, they go, and they fulfil some purpose in their day and Generation, and then they pass on to the beyond, and later reappear again in this world and so complete the cycle.*[138]

Though death is not seen as the final end of man, it is still a threat to life, since it robs man of his greatest gift of God, which is life. It is regarded as one of

137 M.Elliade, From Primitive to Zen: A thematic source book of the history of religion, London, 1967, pp.168&169.

138 G.T. Basden, Niger Ibos, Op. Cit., p.282

the crises of life and people dread to discuss freely about it. Hence the Igbo names his child, 'Onwudinjo' (death is bad), or 'Onwu bu Uya' (death brings lamentation). He normally asks clemency of death. So you have names like 'Onwughalu' (May death allow to exist), or 'Onwuzulike' (May death rest). Death is universal, unpredictable and inescapable and ultimately beyond human control. It takes hold of anyone irrespective of position, sex, or race. He therefore names his child 'Onwuamadike' (Death does not respect a hero, 'Onwuameze' (death does not respect the king). Man has also made fruitless efforts to placate or terminate death, after which death is accepted as both natural and inevitable. Hence names and sayings like, 'Onwudifu' (death exists), 'Agbapuluonwu' (no one can escape death) abound. There are terms used to describe the actual act of dying which show the concept people have about death and dying. The Igbo sees death as a new beginning, which marks a change of status for man. It is only a passage a going home.

The Igbos say that man is on a market trip on earth, and must eventually go home. That is why in Igbo society, when somebody dies, people normally say 'onago ebe osiri bia' (he has gone back to the place from where he came). "The common orthodox belief among the Igbos is that death is a creation of God made for the specific purpose of recalling any person whose time on earth is fulfilled."[139]

For the Igbos, all deaths are not the same. The way people feel and react at deaths of different people differs. The death of a growing and promising young man is not the same as a death after a ripe old age. The death of a man well advanced in years who has reached some recognisable status in life and has got some children and relations to look after him and stay beside his sick bed is counted as blessing to be sought after. Every Igbo prays for such death. It is called 'Onwu Chi', meaning God's death or natural death. In this type of death, people generally do not weep. The death is seen as 'Onwu anuli' or 'Onwu olili' (happy death). It is believed that such good and blessed people go directly to join their ancestors in the spirit world; only to come back later to this life, 'ilo uwa' (re–incarnation). Only good people re–incarnate.

The death of a young man, who has still a lot to fulfil in life, is detested and abhorred. At such death, people lament the havoc done by death and exclaim in disappointment and confusion, 'Onwu di njo' (death is bad). This type of death is classed as unnatural or sudden. Similar to this, is any type of accidental death, such as a death caused by drowning in a stream or one who falls from a tree or dies of a contagious disease like leprosy or small pox. These last groups of death are classified as 'Onwu ekwensu' (deaths caused by the evil spirit, 'Ekwensu').

139 L.E. Esomonu, Respect for human life in Igbo Religion, Op. Cit., p.174

Those who die in any of these ways are believed not to make it to the home of the ancestors.

They are said to be restless, disgruntled, and wandering evil spirits who can bring only mischief to their relations and neighbours because they are embittered because of their exclusion from the ancestral home.[140]

1.2.5.13 Grief

The idea of grief has an important place in the life and culture of the Igbo people. The word brings to mind the idea of the pain of separation that accompanies the loss of a dearly beloved person. But grief is not just that. "Grief is a process and therefore it is always changing and becoming"[141] Experiences that can cause grief to men are many and varied, and such occurs frequently in life. It comes as a normal reaction to significant loss or separation; such losses can be loss of people, places, relationships, objects or even ideas. A person is therefore besieged by grief, when something unpredictable happens to him or when he loses a relation by death, such as the death of a father or son, mother, sister, brother or any other close and beloved relation, loss of good health by attack of an incurable or prolonged sickness or the loss of the means of livelihood by accident or any other kind of disaster. At such occasion of loss one feels empty and forsaken. Life seems almost meaningless to him. It pains him and he suffers the agony. The man is in grief.

Since the Igbo regards death as one of the greatest crisis in life, the death of a relation puts him into grief. He mourns the dead. Mourning goes a long way to express the grief. Though this depends on the closeness of the relationship. The immediate relations of the dead clad themselves in black mourning dresses and shave their hairs as a sign of grief at the loss of the dear ones. The wife of the dead stays indoors for a period of time mourning the dead. Distant relations visit the bereaved families from time to time to be with them and give consolation.

One other loss that causes grief to the Igbo is the loss of his farm crops and animals. The Igbos are notable farmers and a good part of Igboland is known for its agriculture. When there is drought or invasion of locusts on the farmland, crops and animals are destroyed and there is consequently poor harvest. There is famine and people are hungry and sick. This causes grief to many families. The farmers whose crops are destroyed are particularly grieved. There is a general belief in Igboland that draughts is normally a punishment from God as a result of sin, so people generally offer sacrifices and pray to God for mercy and help.

---

140 E.I. Metuh, Comparative Studies of African Religions, Op. Cit., p.254

141 R.S. Sullender, Grief and Growth, New Jersey, 1985, p.25

The Igbos has much respect for life and as such attaches great interest to children. Children are seen as blessing from God. At the same time, any parent with a prodigal son is regarded as childless.

Hence an Igbo proverb which says, 'atulu ji ebunu gba aka nwa' (a sheep that has a male issue is childless), is a proverb for ruffians. It pains parents when any of their children is qualified with this proverb. A bad behaved child is always a disgrace to any Igbo man and so brings grief to parents. There are lots of other reasons that can throw an Igbo man into grief. Today a good number of people in grief retire to prayer / healing centres where they go to pour out their hearts to God in prayers and sacrifices. Some others in grief troop to such centres just to listen to others pour out their sufferings or grief in their testimonies. L. Mbefo once asked a well–read lady why she makes endless pilgrimages to one of the praying centres. Her response confirmed to his embarrassment his evaluation of her intelligence. "According to her, the testimonies of the sufferers have a therapeutic value: through listening to the sufferings of others, she creates enough strength to endue her own"[142]

142 Cf. L. Mbefo, Priests and the Healing Ministry in the Nigerian Church, Seminar Paper on ealing Ministry, Emene, Enugu, 1992, p.2

2. Chapter Two – The Igbos and her Understandig of Life

2.1 Igbo Understanding of Life; Human Suffering and Death

2.1.1 Igbo Concept of Ndu (life)

A brief study on Igbo concept of life, Ndu, will help us to appreciate the next section. The Igbo word Ndu, which appears prominently in their proverbs and personal names, has the highest value. It is the *summum bonum.*

Ndubisi:	Life is the prime necessity
Ndukaku:	Life is superior to wealth
Ndulue:	If life stretches out
Ndukwe:	If life agrees

Through such expression they believe that life has an important value and must be conserved, because any break of the harmony between man, nature, and the spirits of the ancestors would lead to a possible destruction of life in the community. Therefore, religious rituals, moral provisions, and social work of kinship relations are channelled towards the preservation of *Ndu.* Christopher Ejizu has shown the important role which the *Ofo* plays in the whole network of Igbo ritual and worship.[143] *Ofo* is the extension of the ancestral power and judgement for good conduct and conformity to the traditional moral standard, which has as its primary concern the preservation of life and property. *Ilo Uwa,* as we shall, see presupposes that life is a continuous interplay between the two spheres of the one world inhabited by human and spiritual persons. Both spheres of existence make demands of life as a guarantee of non annihilation of the human species and the preservation of generations. The Igbo say: *Ujo bu ndu,* meaning "fear is life." The Igbo man apparently lives in fear of threats to life. These threats are sometimes imaginary, *sine fundamento in re.*

On the other hand *Ndu,* according to Edmond Ilogu, "is not just to exist and be counted at the census. It is the full dynamic existence in which other things; all the good things will come."[144] Therefore whatever has negative effect on this dy-

143 Ofo is a symbol of life and authority. "Eji m ogu eji m ofo." Cf. Ejizu, C., Ofo: Igbo Ritual Symbol (Enugu, Fourth Dimension, 1986), pp.1 – 12.

144 Ilogu, E., Christianity and Igbo Culture (New York, NOK, 1976), p.130

namic existence (life) results in suffering: poverty, depression, disappointment, hatred, abandonment, and death of beloved ones or a parent, childlessness, sickness, lack of shelter or warmth and so forth.

Life, the Igbo believe, is not only for individual persons. Communities, like the lineage, the clan, and even the nuclear family are in their own existence connected with individual life. When the Igbo say *Onye di ndu n'edokwe ihe* (he who is alive will definitely stumble on good fortune or riches one day), they seem to express the philosophy on which all their ethical values are based. They also hold their belief (about *Ndu)* that life is endless, even after it has been terminated by death.[145] Continuation is sought in the male line of children to succeed the father, so as to keep the "family tree" growing strong, branching forth into many lineage subdivisions. Hence the importance of children, especially males, this will be discussed in detail in subsequent sections.

Generally, true human existence is regarded as *Ndu* which we can simply Interpret as life. *Ndu* has a number of connotations and modes. It implies an existence in which a being still functions in his natural mode. That is to say, the principle or whatever is the animating force of this object is effective, is still alive *(odi ndu).* On this, T. U. Nwala in his book *Igbo Philosophy* explained among other things that to say to a man *inwula* (you are dead) means that he has become inactive or incapacitated in respect of a certain function expected of him as a human being. For example, physical or mental weakness, an inability to climb a palm tree, infertility, inability to act reasonably in certain things, inability to engage in intelligent exchange, and so forth–all these may earn the expression *inwula.* To say to a man *idi ndu* (you are alive) means that the person has physical and mental ability to execute the above–mentioned roles.[146] Therefore, to possess Ndu, means to be effective. If a person is physically and mentally alive and actively fulfilling his role (that is, those roles expected of him by virtue of the communal values and ideals), then he/she is alive *(odi ndu).* But if he/she physically exists but ineffective, then he becomes *odi ndu onye nwuru anwu ka mma, living* that is worse than death. *Ndu* is the principle sustaining all existence and also regulating all actions. It operates in all modes of existence (existential), but traditional Igbos is more familiar with the human *Ndu* and all its various aspects than any other thing around them. Basic in the Igbo worldview, therefore, is the belief that life is a continuous process, a never–ending process, although there is a belief that the wicked people may die a complete death in the spirit world, which means a final end to their life. The living are believed to be capable of

145 Nwala, T.U., Igbo Philosophy (Ikeja, Lagos, Literamed Publications Nig., Ltd., 1985), p.26

146 Ibid. p.27

bringing about this fate on the dead by prayer and invocation of the gods and ancestors. Igbos have firm belief that this life (*ndu*) is from *Chukwu* (God). Hence they say, Ndu di n'aka Chi) life is at the mercy of God or life is in the hands of God)

2.1.2 Chi the Author of Life

Igbo theology affirms that Life comes from God and belongs to God. Igbo names illustrate this Ndu si na chi (Osi nachi, for short) meaning "Life is from God." Therefore, it is *Chi* who sends a child into this world, guides and protects the person all through his earthly life and withdraws him at death. From the Igbo theory of pre–existence (of the soul), it is evident that parents do not attribute the life of their children to the mere biological fact of conception.[147] Every life had existed in an antecedent world of a divine master: *Chi.* Hence, parents see their children as a "gift" from *Chi.* This belief is testified in Igbo personal names. There are names expressing gratitude to *Chi,* or praising his goodness for them, the gift to parents:

Chi–nyere ndu: God has given life
Nke Chinyere. – The one given by God
Chi–n'enye ndu. – God gives life
Chi–di–ogo. – God is generous.
Chi–nwe. – God is the owner.
Chi–ekwe. – God has agreed, etc.

A few names categorically state that the *Chi* is the owner of life:

Chi–ji–ndu. – God holds life
Chi–nwe–ndu. – God owns life

But the traditional Igboman, like most Africans, does not believe that this quest for a "fullness of life" is to be sought and achieved in isolation. Rather it is to be sought in the social reality, which consists of man's fellowship with his parents who gave his birth, the village and village–group by which he is identified, the ancestors, the spirits and Chukwu, who caused him to be born and directs every moment of his earthly life.

---

147 Cf. Ezekwugo, C.U., Chi: The True God in Igbo Religion (Innsbruck, Austria, 1973), p.112. Chi (One God) is a concept rooted in ancient Egypt religious text. Cf. Budge, E.A., Egyptian Religion (Routledge & Kegan Paul, 1899), p.23

All these show the importance attached to life by the Igbo. So the birth of a child is not just a single event but a long process which continues long after the arrival of a new life into the world.

> *Nature brings the child into the world, but society creates the child into a social being, a corporate person. For it is the community which must protect the child, feed it, bring it up, educate it in and many other ways incorporate it into the wider community.*[148]

In Igbo society, life is generally protected and preserved because it is seen as the most precious gift of God. It is the most important possession and value to be preserved. This is why Ilogu affirms that 'Ndu' (life) is for the Igbo, the highest good "Summum Bonum".[149] And Temples in turn says that, "the supreme value for Africans is life or force to live strongly. This he calls vital force."[150] And according to Thorpe, "This vital force is preserved and strengthened by prayers, sacrifices, rituals wisdom and proper conduct."[151] His sacrifices and prayers are geared towards preservation and prolongation of his own life, the life of his family and that of his friends and relatives.

The Igbo's desire to preserve life can be seen in many other aspects of his life. An area that is worth mentioning is when he is sick. When an Ibo is sick, one of the first things he does is to go to the diviner who tries to find out the cause of his sickness through the act of divination, before he takes any other step to control or cure the sickness. This can be further explained by the request to a white friend below.

> *This is the strange request of an Igbo Chief who came to my house one day, and after much embarrassment, finally asked if I would not give or tell him of some medicine that would prevent him from ever dying. He went away greatly disappointed at my confession of utter inability to help him there.*[152]

2.1.2.1 Health and Sickness an Igbo Understanding

Health and Sickness in Igbo society are seen as two opposing concepts of life. The Igbo cherishes his health so much that for any serious sickness to attack him means almost the end of life, a big problem from God or an attack from the evil spirits. He regards health as the greatest gift he can have in life and sickness as

---

148 Mbiti, J.S., African Philosophy and Religion, London, 1977, p.110
149 Ilogu, E., Christianity and Igbo culture, New York, 1974, p.129
150 Tempels, P., Bantu Philosophy, Paris, 1959, p.44, in S.A. Thorpe, African Traditional Religion, South Africa, 1992, p.112
151 Thorpe, S.A., African Traditional Religion, South Africa, 1992, p.112
152 Leonard, A.G., The lower Niger and it's tribes, London, 1906, p.150

the greatest evil, an enemy that has to be avoided or extinguished. These two opposing concepts in the life of an Igbo we discuss below.

2.1.2.2 Concept of Health

It is generally accepted in Igbo society that God in various ways provides for his creatures so that their existence may be maintained and preserved. It is also generally believed that, the world is made to be controlled and manipulated by man to attain his goals in life. The Igbo therefore struggles against social, natural, and spiritual forces in order to maintain his well being or life. His struggles in life are therefore to preserve his life, to protect it and to continue to live and have healthy life. This is manifested in some Igbo proverbs and names such as 'Ndubisi (Life is the supreme good), 'Ndukaku' (Life is more valuable than riches), 'Ifeakandu' (Nothing is worth more than life).

The Igbo understands health in terms of physical strength, mental, social and spiritual well being. Hence these phrases 'ahu ike' (good health), 'ahu izu oke' (completeness of the body) are generally in the lips of the Igbo. Any wonder Orji says,

> *A healthy man is one who gets up in the morning strong, and goes to his place of work. He is able to answer whenever he is called up. Such is the healthy man. He is not physically weak. He is not restless on account of worries.*[153]

We can see that for Orji, health involves more than just physical strength. The psychological and spiritual aspects are not neglected. That is to say that for the Igbos, health is also multi–dimensional. Little wonder M. Aguaowo writing on health in Nigeria society says,

> *It is not seen only as the absence of physical pain or suffering but as a total wholeness of man taking into consideration his physical, psychological, socio–economic and cultural environment.*[154]

The Igbo of Nigeria prays for health and offers sacrifices for good health and healing. The majority of his prayers has to do with preservation of life in one way or the other but many are aimed at healing the sick or maintaining health. This is very much shown in his ejaculatory prayers, which are uttered by all and at any time. For instance, when a child sneezes, the mother or any elderly person around spontaneously says *'Ndu gi'* (your health). This short phrase is a complete prayer for good health. In Igbo traditional morning prayers, the family heads do not for-

153 Orji, F.C. A., Personal Oral Interview, Enugu, August 26, 2002.
154 Aguaowo, M.G.U., Health in Traditional Nigerian Society, Leuven, 1985, p.6

get to pray for good health for the whole families. Also when somebody is travelling, particularly to a distant land, prayers are offered for his good health and strength to accomplish the journey safely. All these are to show the meaning and importance that the Igbo attaches to health. For him health is wealth. Health is all.

2.1.2.3 Igbo Concept of Sickness

It is generally acknowledged that sickness with its accompanying pain and suffering is a very common concept of life, which poses a lot of problem for man. The Igbo is not an exception in this regard. For him, "sickness is a diminution of that life, a threat posed to life;"[155] "a big problem from God or the devil or from 'akalogeli' (a type of evil spirit), one of the major enemies of man, an evil that should be avoided."[156]

In Igbo society when one is sick, the first thing he does is to examine his conscience to know whether he has done anything evil. He also tries to find out whether he has done all he is supposed to do such as offering sacrifice to his 'Chi' (personal god) or to his ancestors. He also meditates on what he has eaten, whether he has taken any poison anywhere. While he does this self–examination of conscience, one of his relations goes to the diviner ('dibia ofuzo' or 'dibia afa') who helps him to find out or divine the cause of his sickness. The diviner helps him to know whether the sickness is caused by human beings or by the evil spirits or whether it is as a result of an evil that one might have committed or whether it just comes from the above. Only when the cause of a sickness is discovered, is a solution begun to be sought. There are however certain sicknesses that are not discovered by divination, as believed by the Igbo people. What brings such says Orji,

> *is 'Ibeme'. Ibeme comes as a result of some wicked act perpetuated by someone particularly to maltreat another of which others are not aware. The diviner or the medicine man does not see the cause of a sickness that is brought about by Ibeme. God does not allow the diviner to see the cause of such sickness so that the perpetrator has to suffer for his wicked acts.*[157]

Here sickness seems to assume a penal dimension.

---

155 Onyemenegam, J.O., Pastoral Care of the Sick in Igbo Community of Nigeria, Rome, 1985, p.28

156 Orji, F.C. A., Personal Oral Interview, Enugu, August 26, 2002.

157 Orji, F.C.A., August 26, 2000

2.1.2.4 Igbo Myths on the Origin of Suffering and Death

Igbo myths of the origin of suffering and death fall predominantly into the myths of the failed message. This class is further divided into two subgroups: the myths of the two messengers and the myths of a single messenger. For the purpose of precision 1 shall consider one of the myths of the two messengers:

"God allows human beings and the lower animals to decide among them whether death should exist or not. Except for the crocodile and a few others, the rest held that there should be no death. The dog was sent by their group to tell God there will be no death. Carried away by the sweetness of bones it saw on the way, the dog forgot the message. The tortoise, taking advantage of this, delivered the message that death should exist. When the dog arrived later, death was already created."[158]

In some versions of this myth, the toad is said to have been the animal that delivered the "false" message. This is the version that is reproduced in Anthony Iloanusi's text.[159] It is a good example of an Igbo myth which lacks a direct allusion to the very origin of death as such but is interested in the effort to overcome it. Thus, instead of causing death, the perverted message only sabotages the venture to overthrow it.

However, from the above mythological narrative some fundamental aspects can be deduced: the distinction between the world of men and the world of God; the existence between these worlds of "space" which alters the message, a sort of "black box" which explains the difference between the message when it enters and leaves the system. Notice also the inversion of the relationship between "speed" and "slowness" on the one hand and between life and death on the other hand in passing form the world of God into the world of men. This analysis is not intended to give this myth any rational function. It has value just as a myth, a story believed by people. The message it contains affirms that suffering and death originated due to some failure in nature and not as a design of God. In other words, God should not be blamed as the origin of human sufferings and death. The evil of death, which is the *terminus ad quem* of most human suffering, is attributed to the agency of some creatures in the created universe. In some cases God is said to be an indirect cause of death and other calamities leading to it as we have already discussed.

Among the Igbo world, the concept of the judgment of God is so strong that "the wrath of God" has been conceptualised in a certain divinity. This is the

158 Ekechukwu, A., Op. Cit., p.83

159 Iloanusi, A., Myth of the Creation of Man and the Origin of Death in West Africa (Frankfurt, Peter Lang, 1984), p.218

lightning and thunder divinity, *Amadioha*. It is their experience too, that *Chukwu* let the minor, malignant deities torture them, rob them of their property, kill their children and make trade unprofitable, and render women and land barren and unproductive.[160]

However, their appeals to minor deities at time of distress and despondency do not always meet with immediate response. There could be such a desperate situation that one would willingly accept death rather than find oneself undergoing a prolonged suffering. Death becomes a necessary option to man to end suffering. This kind of beneficent passivity which the Igbo see in God's approach to life's miseries does not lead him to despair. Perhaps his difficulties may be attributed to the influences of *Chi* destiny as we saw earlier.

2.1.2.5 Supernatural Agencies Responsible for Sickness

In Igbo society, it is believed that 'Chukwu' Supreme Being is the first among the supernatural causes of sickness. Chukwu, who is believed to be fundamentally good, may allow man to be inflicted by some physical evil such as illness. But when God allows man to be sick, it is believed to be for the good of the individual and the community at large or for the welfare of the individual as a sign of purge or punishment. When God punishes, the Igbo does not pretend to know the reason in all cases. But he believes that the attitude is just like that of a father to a son, meant not to destroy but to save.

Other supernatural sources of sickness include the ancestors, the evil spirits and some other deities or spirits. The ancestors are said to cause some sickness to their living relations who fail to fulfil their requirements or those who committed one type of taboo or the other, or those who have offended them in one way or the other. Although people fear and believe that these ancestors may cause them some sickness, there is little or no evidence to this belief. Other Supernatural beings that can cause ill health according to the Igbo's beliefs include evil spirits, the deities and some other special or group–spirits. Worthy of mention among this group are the 'Muo mmili' (Aquatic spirits) and the 'Ogbanje' phenomenon.

2.1.2.6 "Muo Mmili" (Aquatic Spirit)

This is one of the mysterious forces or evil spirits believed to disturb people in Igbo land. In the past, the existence of the water spirit was only common in the riverine areas of Igboland such as Aguleri, Onitsha, Ogbaru and Oguta, but "has

160 Obiego, C., African Image of the Ultimate Reality (Frankfurt, Peter Lang, 1984), p.158

in the recent times, become widespread even in places far removed from the rivers."[161] Today the issue of muo mmili is almost discussed in every family in Igboland. Muo mmili is believed to be a female deity, associated with the rivers and lakes, and often associated with wickedness. This spirit believed to be the guardian spirit of the streams and rivers is said to inhabit the beds of the rivers and streams. She is said to be the queen of the water, hence she is called Mammy Water or Queen of the sea. Stories portray her as a very beautiful woman with very long hairs like that of Indian woman.

Water spirits are believed to exist in groups. Many sicknesses or misfortunes that people suffer are considerably attributed to the attacks of the water spirits, sometimes inflicting on people "a strange unknown sickness"[162] Pretty women particularly young ones are said to be prey to the attacks of these spirits. "Thousands of young and unmarried ladies are said to be possessed by the water–spirit."[163] They are believed to inflict sickness on an individual for refusing to grant consent to their request for friendship or marriage with them. Sometimes they are believed to inflict punishment on one who entered into friendship, marriage or other form of partnership with them but failed to abide by the terms of agreement. Some girls possessed by the Muo mmili spirits are said to be princesses to the queen of the sea and are at the service of the queen who send them to the earth on errand to do havoc to people. Here is the case of a girl said to have had a relation with the queen of the sea.

She said, she was a princess to the queen of the water and used to see and serve the queen. She said the queen whom she served used to snatch newly born babies from their mothers here on earth and she used to keep them for her, that there were some other girls doing that work with her but she was in–charge, hence they called her princess[164]

The attacks of the aquatic spirits can come in different ways. Talking about young girls who frequent prayer and healing centres for the said delivery from these spirits, N. Ndiokwere puts it thus:

It is believed that their misfortune in life – inability to get a suitable husband or get pregnant after marriage has been caused by the water spirit. These spirits, like the witches, are believed to enter the bodies of victims and block the reproductive systems. In most cases of the so called diabolical attacks, the queen of the sea is believed to have a

---

161 C. Ejizu, Cosmological perspective on Exorcism, in Chris U. Manus and co (eds), "Healing and Exorcism, Nigeria Experience", Enugu, 1992, p.15

162 L. Odinkemelu, Mammy Water in the Society, Her influence on Igbo Culture, Ihiala, 1986, p.12.

163 N. Ndiokwere, African Church Today and Tomorrow, Vol. 1, Onitsha, 1994, p.14

164 G. Ikeobi, Healing and exorcism: The Nigerian experience, in Chris U. Manus et al., (eds), "Healing and exorcism" Op.Cit., p.61–62

hand. She sends her agents, damned dead people to lay snares to human beings. She applies all types of tricks to trap its victims and is believed to be powerful – ruling in both land and sea. The activities of the water spirits are closely related to those of the Ogbanje or Abiku, the spirit of incarnation.[165]

2.1.2.7 The "Ogbanje" Spirit

The Ogbanje spirit is regarded in Igbo society as one of the most devilish agents of people's misfortune in life. Some people attribute the causes of most of their sickness to the activities of these spirits called Ogbanje. Sicknesses caused by Ogbanje are among the most commonly reported misfortunes in the prayer and healing centres in Igbo society. Writers have different opinions of what Ogbanje phenomenon is, and the different forms of the spirit. Some have argued as if Ogbanje is a chosen way of life or a sickness or disease. That is to say that one is not yet clear of what Ogbanje syndrome is and how to prove its existence. But one thing is certain and undeniable, that for the Igbo people, the Ogbanje spirits are a reality to be reckoned with, whatever it may be, clear, blurred or confused reality.

Chinwe Achebe's deep study on Ogbanje shows that every normal individual born owes allegiance to his 'Chi', a creative force, who is God's representative on earth and co–operates with each individual to work out his life's possibilities and Attributes. But Chi fulfils this function partially since there are other forces that intrude in man's life, some of which are evil and must be placated. Some of these forces or beings are 'Nne mmili' and 'Onabuluwa' who constitute the major forms of Ogbanje. They lure the individual to break the covenant with Chi by offering them some rewards such as excessive beauty, wealth, political powers and success in business to mention but a few. And those who break this loyalty are normally the Ogbanjes. And having upset the ordered balance and broken the faith with their Chi, they are exposed to different sorts of afflictions and harassment since their relation with their Chi is weakened and they are left at the mercy of the deities.[166]

There are other opinions on the Ogbanje phenomenon or syndrome. Lucas, for example, describes the Ogbanje as "a confraternity of spirits who visit the world in incarnate form for a short period, the length of each being pre–arranged. The spirits are born into babies who will die in infancy or boyhood."[167]

It is believed that these evil spirits are arranged in age groups. Some are infants of five years and below, others are children of between seven and fourteen years. Others are

165 N. Ndiokwere, The African Church Today and Tomorrow, Vol. 1, Op. Cit., p.16

166 Cf Chinwe Achebe, The Ogbanje Phenomenon, in Chris U. Manus and co (eds), "healing and exorcism", Op. Cit., p.29–31

167 J.O. Lucas, Religion in West African and Ancient Egypt, Lagos, 1970, p.168

young people of not more than thirty years. Each group binds it's members not to live longer than their age limit.[168]

For M. Iwu, Ogbanje is better described as "a case of repeated infantile deaths in a family."[169] They are believed "to be capable of reincarnating into various 'life–journeys' which lasts for very short time during each trip,"[170] their aim being however "to torment parents with pangs of constant births and deaths of their children, and to leave them childless and frustrated at the end of their child–bearing age.[171] Ogbanje is not only known to torment parents but also young people are reported to be tormented by the malevolent spirits. Some are given to protracted illness or in the case of young girls who cannot get married are said to be the result of the attacks of the spirits. The general characteristics of those believed to be possessed by the Ogbanje spirits is that they behave abnormally, have excessive dreams and hallucinations and above all, they are likely to die a premature death or often fall sick. For the Igbo society, Ogbanje phenomenon is an awesome issue and is feared no matter its manifestation, though many Igbos today do not believe in the Ogbanje syndrome. For many, belief in the Ogbanje phenomenon is a superstition. Hence there are suggestions that Ogbanje beliefs are mystical explanations of the sickle cell anaemia, which have claimed lives of many infants repeatedly in many families in the past due to ignorance of the people on medical and health care matters. There are others who have no explanation to offer on this phenomenon. They neither believe nor explain away the syndrome. According to Chinwe Achebe "the association with Sickle cell anaemia is the strongest interpretation of the phenomenon offered to date."[172] But the investigation she carried out in schools in Awgu in Igboland, on sickle cells and repeated deaths in some families shows that sickle cells contribute little or nothing to the high mortality rate in the group and in the belief in Ogbanje that accompanies it.[173]

The Ogbanje phenomenon for the Igbo people still remains a reality, confused or clear. Sicknesses attributed to it abound and increase in geometrical Progression. Ogbanje traditional priests and healers exist in great number. People who claim to have been possessed or attacked by the Ogbanje spirits especially young unmarried ladies appear in the scene regularly. And those who claim to have been

168 E.I. Metuh, Comparative studies of A.T.R. Op. Cit. p.156
169 M. Iwu, African Ethnomedicine, Snaap press, Enugu, 1986, p.29
170 E. Ilogu, Christianity and Igbo Culture, New York, 1974, p.42
171 E.I. Metuh, Comparative studies of A.T.R. Op. Cit., p.38.
172 C. Achebe, Ogbanje Phenomenon, in Chris U. Manus et al., (eds), "Healing and Exorcism", Op. Cit., p.38
173 Cf. C. Achebe, Ogbane phenomenon, pp.38 & 39

delivered of these spirits continually testify and give thanks during prayer and healing sessions. But we have not enough available data of clear and genuine cases to meaningfully and convincingly interpret the issue of the Ogbanje syndrome.

2.2 Human Causes of Sickness

The Igbo man believes that apart from the Supernatural causes of sickness, certain illnesses are as a result of some human causes. Such could be through the activities of some bad or evil people in the society. Prominent among such people are the witches, sorcerers and other wicked people. All those who use these wicked means to attack others or cause illness to others are regarded as malevolent and wicked by the society. There are no doubt other sources of illness such as poisoning, insatiable quest for wealth and power, bad eating habits and exposition to bad weather. All these can cause sickness to man. But we shall have a look at one major phenomenon believed to be a cause to some kinds of sickness in Igbo society – 'Amosu' (witches and witchcraft). Though we must remark that many people do not hold the belief in the existence of Amosu, yet like the Ogbanje syndrome, it remains a reality to be reckoned with in Igbo Society of the past and to a great extent of the present.

2.2.1 Witches (Amosu) and Witchcraft (Ita Amosu)

Among the fears that beset the Igbo society is the fear of evil and malicious people called 'Amosu' (witches), who are believed to use means inherent in them to harm people and destroy things and persons. Belief in Amosu just as in the case of the 'muo mmili' is not common to every part of Igboland until in the recent past. Writing on the history of Igbo people, E. Isichei notes, "Witchcraft is said to be a new development in Igboland and is not yet found in all parts but mainly among the riverine communities."[174] Stories about witches were mainly only connected with the mid–western part of Igboland across the River Niger and places like Aguleri, Onitsha, Ogbaru and Oguta. This was however many years ago. Today, the stories of witches and their activities are told all over the Igboland even in areas far remote from the rivers and the seas. It constitutes one of the major problems and causes of sickness reported by people in prayer houses and healing centres.

---

174 E. Isichei, History of the Igbo people, Macmilian, London, 1976, p.6

Witchcraft for the Igbo people is fundamentally evil and unjust and any person accused of witchcraft is regarded as being inherently evil. Witches are regarded as one of the greatest enemies of the society performing anti–social deeds. Witches are said to be human beings, usually operating outside their human bodies.

Anthropologists and Sociologists use the term witchcraft to apply to people mainly women with an inherent power by means of which they can abandon their bodies at night and go to meet with similar people (other witches) or to 'suck' or 'eat away' the life of their victims.[175]

But why are witches often conceived as women? M. Gelfad attributes it to the quality of the sexes saying that

men are more trustful, easily provoked, more powerful and therefore tend to be accusers, whereas women are more receptive, weaker, less easily roused to temper and therefore become the victims.[176]

Amponsah in turn adds that

women tend to be fussy, quarrelsome and most of them are unemployed or under–employed and therefore have much time for idle conversation and gossiping. Married women are suspected more readily than unmarried ones and the older the woman the stronger.[177]

However not only women are said to be witches. There are men who are said to be witches too. So the term witch is reserved for both men and women who are accused of nocturnal preying on human beings.

Witches are believed to fly about in the nights in form of night birds like the bat 'usu' or the owl 'ukwukwuu' or they turn to animals like rats 'oke' or cats 'unanwulu'. They are believed to witch hunt people whom they think have disturbed their peace. They are said to belong to clubs of the witches where they meet and plan their attacks. It is believed that a witch attacks by despatching her spirit to capture and eventually devour the victim's soul or part of his flesh. This she does even while she (the witch) is asleep in her house. Generally she attacks while her victim is also asleep, only to wake up and fall ill suddenly as a result of the witches attack. There are a lot of other misfortune that could be blamed on

175 J.S. Mbiti, African Religions and Philosophy, Op. Cit., p.202., G. Parrinder, African Traditional Religion, London, 1958, p.123.

176 M. Gelfand, The African witch, E&S Livingstone Ltd, 1967, p.71 in K. Amponsah, "Topics on West African Traditional Religion," p.84

177 K. Amponsah, Topics on West African Traditional Religion, Cape coast, 1975, p.84

the witches such as failure of crops, unsuccessful business ventures, barrenness and accidents. It is however believed that if any of the birds or animals, which they incarnated into, is killed while on course, the real body of the witch which may be sleeping in her hut will die at the same time.

2.3 Care of the Sick in Igbo Society

The Igbo is basically sociable. This is clearly shown in his interest in marriage and family life. He believes that no man is an island and likes to exist in groups and do things together. Hence the extended family relations are very much practised and encouraged. The Igbos see one another as brothers and care for one another's interests. This interest and care that he has for his brother is not less illuminating in the area of health care. So he also cares for his sick brother.

The Igbo like other people of the world give in much of his time to preserve health. He tries to preserve not only his own health but also that of his brothers and relatives.

Hence around the bedside of any sick brother in Igboland are his relatives to watch over, and minister to him. Any wonder lfemesia notes,

Compassion was deeply felt for the sick or wounded, the less fortunate and the physically or mentally handicapped. And the family took the responsibility for all such persons as a matter of course.[178]

In Igboland just as in other African villages,

disease and misfortune are religious experiences and it requires a religious approach to deal with them. The medicine men are aware of this and make an attempt to meet the need in a religious (or quasi religious) manner whether or not that turns out to be genuine or false or a mixture of both.[179]

When a man is sick, various attempts are made to cure him. First, a diviner who is an agent of unveiling mysteries of human life is consulted to find out the causes of his sickness. Then he is treated to some medicines in the form of herbs and roots. This is usually done by the medicine men or herbalists who prepare medicines from herbs and roots for treatment of ailments. Sometimes sacrifices are offered on behalf of the sick person. Some special men such as the diviners, the medicine men and the priests do this. These special men in their peculiar ca-

178 C. Ifemesia, Traditional Humane Living among the Igbo, Enugu, 1979. p.64
179 J.S. Mbiti, African Religions and Philosophy, Op.Cit., p.169

pacities apply different types of treatment to treat their patients and to assure them that all will be well.

> *Some of the activities involved in dealing with illness may not have overt value but they are psychologically vital and no doubt play a great role in healing the sick or helping the sufferer. In this the means are less important than the end, and that is how both the medicine man and his patient see and experience the situation which brings them together.*[180]

However minor complaints such as headaches, stomach upset, boils and cuts are usually treated with herbs and medicines generally known by almost every member of the society without even going to the medicine men. Besides medical care, prayers are also offered for the sick person for healing.

The medicine man usually prays for the sick man as he administers his medicines. He prays for his medicine to be effective on the person and help heal him from his sickness. He has the strong belief that cure is only given by God.

2.3.1 People Involved in the Care of the Sick

In Igbo tradition and religion, there are people who because of their special offices, knowledge and skills are given special names. They are called such names as special men, sacred persons, and sacred specialists. Among these people are the medicine men, diviners, priests and seers to mention but a few. Such men "serve as links between their fellow human beings and God, spirits and invisible things."[181] They may however be distinguished by the following terms:

> *Priests, those who are attached to temples and offer sacrifices; Devotees or Mediums, those connected with the temples and who give messages from the gods; Diviners, those concerned with oracles and divinations; Doctors or Medicine men, those concerned with healing the sick and preparing magical medicines.*[182]

These special and sacred persons look very similar in their nature and functions.

> *As special persons, they have a language, symbolism, knowledge, skill, practice and what I may call 'office personality' of their own which are not known or easily accessible to the ordinary person whether he is a villager or a scholar in search of knowledge.*[183]

---

180 J.S. ibid. p.169
181 J. Onyenemegam, Pastoral care of the sick in Igbo community, Rome, 1985, p.26
182 G. Parrinder, West African Religion, London, 1975, p.75
183 J.S. Mbiti, African Religions and Philosophy, p.166.

These people are generally considered to be wise and intelligent, talented and gifted with many outstanding capabilities. They play very vital role in Igbo life and society but we are here concerned with their role in the health care of the sick in the society.

2.3.1.1 The "Dibia" (Traditional Doctor)

In Igbo society, the name 'dibia' serves for both the diviner and the medicine man or herbalist. The diviner is generally called the 'dibia ofuzo' Or "dibia afa" (divination doctor), while the herbalist is called the 'dibia ahihia na mkporogwu' (medicine doctor). Foreign writers who simply have in themselves notions that do not match the facts generally give the traditional doctors in Africa a bad publicity. But these people occupy a very important position in African traditional society. According to Mbiti, "they are the greatest gift and the most useful source of help to African societies."[184] They have wide knowledge of the properties of many roots and are able to discover the cause of a sickness, diagnose the nature of the disease and prescribe medicines, which often lead to a complete cure.

> *The traditional doctors deal with the crisis not only by treating the observed or acknowledged problem at surface level, but by probing more deeply to find the underlying spiritual cause. By thus seeking a reason, an answer to the question, 'Why', he or she enables the patient to deal with the crisis more effectively. In traditional a society then, the sufferer is treated in a holistic manner, as if the body, the Psyche and in fact, the entire societies were suffering by extension.*[185]

The name dibia connotes so many meanings in Igbo society. The mention of the name brings to mind one type of dibia to the other. This is because every type of sickness has its own particular dibia, and every dibia has his area of specialisation. No good dibia claims to cure every disease. Though it is generally known that some fake traditional doctors (ofeke dibia) claim to cure all sicknesses. Hence Igbos have sayings like "ife ajuna dibia osi na ya n'agwo". However, a strong dibia can combine the cure of a few diseases.

Among the different types of dibia in Igbo society, the 'dibia afa' is the one that foretells the future. He diagnoses diseases or discovers the root–cause of diseases by means of divination and prescribes medicines or sacrifices to be offered. The 'dibia ogwu' on the other hand has to cure diseases by the use of herbs and roots of plants and trees. There are however some diviners who have also the knowledge and the use of the herbs. They are found in every village in Igboland

---

184 J.S. Mbiti, African Religions and Philosophy, Op. Cit., p.166
185 S.A. Thorpe, African Traditional Religion, South Africa, 1992, p.123

and they are regarded as friends of the communities except a few of them who are malevolent and mischievous. One special characteristics of the dibia is that he believes that cure is given by God. He calls on God while he does his own part of the healing. When a dibia gives drug to the sick, he normally says, 'Chukwu bia nara ogwu nua' (God come and take the medicine and drink) as if it is God who is taking the medicine. He sincerely believes that healing comes from God. He believes that if God accepts the medicine, and gives to the sick person, the sick, recovers. He also calls on his ancestors to come to his aid in the cure of the sick. He therefore says 'unu mara ka unu si agwo bianu nonyere anyi' (if you know how you cure please come and stay with us). Onaiyekan is therefore right when he says that

> *very little is attributed to the skill of the doctor, less still to any healing powers that may be naturally inherent in the material ingredients out of which the remedy is concocted.*[186]

The dibia therefore does not charge much money for his services to the sick. He only receives a little token from his patients. In Igbo society, it is well known that only the fake medicine man tries to enrich himself from the charges of his services to the sick. It is believed that the gift and knowledge to become a medicine man are given gratuitously by God for the service of the community. Hence medicine men are always seen as the greatest gift to any community. It is also generally acknowledged that this gift and skill will not last long as far as the dibia continues to extract money from his patients for his services.

The dibia prepares his drugs according to his area of specialisation. There are drugs for illnesses such as 'isi owuwa' (headache), 'Nsogbu afo' (stomach upset), 'Mgbapia akpili'. (tonsillitis). There are also specialists for children's sickness 'Oya umuaka', Gynaecological cases 'Oya umunwanyi', brain fag 'Okiri mgbawa isi' and so forth. There are also dibias that make charms for insect and snake-bites. We shall see more of the specialists as we proceed.

2.3.1.2 Vocation and Training of the Dibia

The calling of someone to become a dibia in Igboland has no fixed rules. The call can come at any time of the life of the individual. It can come to one as a young man, still unmarried or in the later days of one's life. Both men and women are called to the profession. In some cases, the call is hereditary, in others it is not. The important fact is that one must be called. A special deity in charge of both medicine and divination makes the call. The deity is called 'Agwu'. "Agwu is a

186 J. Onaiyekan, The priesthood in Owe traditional Religion, in Adegbola A.E., "Traditional Religion in West Africa", Ibadan 1983, p.46

special spirit of the ndi dibia."[187] Writing on the vocation of the medicine men Metuh observes that "the call is experienced in the form of a mild mental disturbance (Ala agwu – madness of Agwu)."[188] Little wonder, Arinze describes the agwu deity as "the spirit of giddiness, rascality, discomposure, confusion and forgetfulness."[189] When some of these attitudes are continuously observed in a person, the call is suspected and divination becomes the best means to confirm what is happening to him or her. Through the divination, it is discovered whether or not it is the sign of the Agwu deity wishing to have the person to serve him and the community in a special capacity. It is believed that the call by this deity is never rejected without some disastrous consequences on the individual.

The new dibia or the novice receives training from the old. The training may be formal or informal. What is important is that the new dibia learns the art and various secret of the group from the old. Very often, the training is done by the candidate's own father or an uncle or any close relative who is a dibia. The training is generally "long and expensive"[190], lasting "up to seven years or more"[191] in the case of the diviner, and up to ten years or even longer"[192] in the case of the medicine men.

> *Part of the training involves some kind of apprenticeship. Candidates acquire knowledge in matters pertaining to the medical value, quality and use of different herbs, leaves, roots, fruits, barks, grasses and various objects like minerals, dead insects, shells, eggs and so on, – the causes, cures and prevention of diseases and other forms of suffering (such as barrenness, failure in undertakings, misfortunes, poor crop yield); magic, witchcraft and sorcery, and how to combat (or even use) them –, the nature and handling of spirits and the living dead, and various secrets, some of which may not be divulged to outsiders.*[193]

2.3.1.3 The Diviner (Dibia Afa) in the Care of the Sick

When the Igbo man is sick, it is observed that one of the first steps he takes to cure himself is to know the cause of his sickness. This he does by sending one of his relations to consult the dibia afa who tries to find out the cause of his sickness. "Diviners are said to accumulate a vast store of secret knowledge and have

187 F.A. Arinze, Sacrifice in Ibo Religion, Op. Cit., p.64
188 E.I. Metuh, African Religions in Western Conceptual schemes, Jos, 1991, p.215
189 F.A. Arinze,Sacrifice in Ibo Religion, p.64
190 M.M. Green, Igbo village affairs, London, 1964, p.53; G. Parrinder, West African Traditional Religion, Op. Cit., p.44
191 G. Parrinder, West African Traditional Religion, Op.Cit. p.44
192 J.S. Mbiti, Introduction to African Religion, Op.Cit, p.152.
193 J.S. Mbiti, African Religions and Philosophy, Op.Cit, p.167–168.

a deep acquaintance with human nature"[194] "their main duty being to link human being with the living dead and the spirits."[195] The diviner is known as the wise man of the village, generally accepted, honoured and respected. He is a friend to all and he is very much involved in the daily life of the community.

The dibia afa is "a specialist who seeks to diagnose diseases or discover the solution to problems by means of inspiration and manipulation of objects through various techniques."[196] For Basden, he is "a worker with charms, whereby the spirit foretells the future and gives directions for procedure in the matter of sacrifice."[197] To him people go for most of their problems of life such as during famine and drought, in time of loss or in the case of theft, before and after birth of a child, before a journey and in time of illness. They go to him at other times in life such as at the appointment of a Chief or a King, in times of betrothals and marriages and at any time for guidance and comfort.

The office of the diviner is generally hereditary. The children or the young relations of the diviner as the case may be, learn the art of divination from their parents as they practise the art. Some other diviners are trained privately by other diviners. However, in any of these cases the neophyte in this profession generally receives a call from the deity of divination known as 'agwu', the patron spirit of the diviners.

The practice of divination in Igboland is called 'igba afa'. If a man wishes to obtain any information which is beyond his powers, he consults the dibia afa who consults the oracle on his behalf. In consultation for instance, the petitioner usually asks so many questions about his life, his family and property. He can ask for life for himself and his family and prosperity for every body. He can add, yesterday Ugoye my wife had running stomach, Ikenna my first son was nearly bitten by snake where he was playing with other children. Is it all well? Are you sure nobody is behind all these? At this juncture, the dibia takes up his instruments for divination. These instruments are normally in his bag (akpa dibia). Normally the bag contains so many things. According to Arinze,

the content of the bag includes, Nkwu agwu (statue of agwu), udene agwu (statue of Agwu's vulture) Udu Arobinagu (a small pot, source of his information), egede agwu (a drum), okiliko mbe (tortoise shell), ofo (a cult stick), mkpulu afa (divination seeds, about ten of them), isi anu (head of an animal) abuba nnunu (fat of a bird), uyolo (a sort of en-

194 G.Parrinder, West African Traditional Religion, Op.Cit, p.137.
195 J.S. Mbiti, African Religions and Philosophy, p.171
196 G. Parrinder, African Religions and Philosophy, p.171
197 G.T. Basden, Niger Ibos, London, 1966, p.55

closed basket with pebbles inside so that it can rattle when shaken), and okpukpo (bones).[198]

The content of the bag is a necessary component for divination. The dibia must have them before he can divine. And when he must have fulfilled his divination exercises and the different incantations, the diviner prays for his client and family. The diviner also prays to his agwu every morning. He normally speaks to the agwu in the language he believes it understands.

After the divination, it is the duty of the dibia afa to tell his client the proper spirit to whom the sacrifices and prayers are to be offered. He can also tell him of the impending dangers and means of averting them.

2.3.1.4 The Medicine Man "Dibia Ogwu" in the Care of the Sick

Another type of the dibia in Igbo society is the medicine man or the herbalist generally called the 'dibia ogwu' or 'dibia ahihia na mkporogwu'. He is the doctor that deals with 'ogwu'(medicine) and administers it to the sick person. He is greatly gifted to the knowledge of roots and herbs in the forest. According to Parrinder, "West African doctors have wide knowledge of the properties of many roots, bark, leaves and herbs."[199] They cure diseases with medication from roots and leaves of trees. They are able to choose the right herbs to perform their cures. Their medicines however have other ingredients. "Some animal content is also often needed; a sacrifice or the blood, skin or fur is also used. Alcohol is an important third ingredient."[200]

Like the diviner, a special deity in charge of medicine by name 'Agwu' also calls the 'dibia ogwu'. Agwu "holds the divine port–folio of medicine."[201] The dibia ogwu also receives training in order to practise well. In his training, he is taught to diagnose the nature of diseases and how to apply the right treatment to prevent further sickness. He also learns from an experienced medicine man how to deal with the sick person and his method of approach is both psychological and physical. According to Mbiti, his treatment "assures the sufferer that all is and will be well. The medicine man is in effect both doctor and pastor to the sick."[202] Thus the medicine man may

apply massages, needles, or thorns, and he may bleed the patient; he may jump over the patient, he may use incantations and ventriloquism, and he may ask the patient to per-

198 F.A. Arinze, Sacrifice in Ibo religion, Op.Cit., p.65
199 G. Parrinder, West African Religion, Op. Cit., p.152
200 Ibid. p.159
201 E.B. Idowu, African Traditional Religion, London, 1973, p.200
202 J.S. Mbiti, African Religions and Philosophy, p.168

form various things like sacrificing a chicken or goat, observing some taboos or avoiding certain foods and persons – all these are in addition to giving the patient physical medicines.[203]

We can therefore say that from the way the dibia deals with his patients, some of his methods are psychological. This practice, Parrinder refers to as "sympathetic magic, which is based on the belief that using part of a thing or a copy of an object may affect the whole."[204] Generally, the medicine man gives much time and attention to the sick person, which helps him to dig deep into the psychological state of the person. This type of psycho–medical care is still lacking in most of our modern hospitals up till date. And this has contributed greatly to the reason why many, including the Christians and the educated still very often resort to the dibia in spite of the sophisticated and advanced equipment of the modern hospitals.

The dibia is believed to cure various physical ailments and sicknesses of various kinds. It has also been noted that every particular sickness has its own dibia. Hence the existence of many types of 'dibia ogwu' in Igbo society. These different dibias are specialists in their different areas. Among them are 'Dibia omenka' (bone specialists or Orthopaedic doctors), 'Dibia afoime' (Gynaecologists), 'Dibia ogwu anya' (Eye specialists or Ophthalmologists), 'Dibia umuaka' (Paediatricians), 'Dibia ogwu eze' (dentist) and other types of specialists. A little insight into some of these specialists may be useful to our work.

2.3.1.5 Orthopaedic Doctor "Dibia Omenka"

He is a specialist in the problems of the bones. He treats patients who broke their bones as a result of a fall or any other type of accident. He sets the broken pieces of bone back to their former positions and looks after the patients till they get fully recovered. He is really artful and this is portrayed in his name 'omenka' (the artist). He is very patient since he can work on a patient for weeks or even months. Very often, he sets and re–sets the broken pieces of bones many times in a day, until the bones are well fixed. He uses 'oforo' (straight slices of bamboo stick) usually cut from raffia palm trees, and strip of cloths to serve as bandage to keep the broken bones in a steady position. This device serves for the work of the plaster of Paris of the modern medicine. The dibia omenka also uses "Ushe" on the fractured part or sprained bone and arteries, which helps in the healing of the affected part. Ushe is a light yellowish substance extracted from a tree and mixed

203 Ibid., p.169
204 G. Parrinder, West African Traditional Religion, p.158

with oil. Ushe serves as the modern medical lotion called 'nerve and bone'. He also operates on people who have minor boils 'etito' or tumour 'akpu'.

2.3.1.6 Gynaecologist "Dibia Afoime"

The dibia afoime is a doctor who is a specialist in treating the problems of women particularly pregnant women or those who find it difficult to conceive. He helps those women who have miscarriage (habitual abortion) when they conceive to retain the pregnancy. This he does by means of his medication and advice. He also helps women during delivery especially those who have difficult delivery such as when the child assumes an abnormal position in the womb. We have more of this type of doctors among the women folk.

The few men among them are called 'Ozo igbo ndu' (Protector of the life of the Igbos) or 'Odinma eme ogwu' (the good one that prepares medicine).

2.3.1.7 Paedatricians "Dibia Oya Umuaka"

He is a specialist who cares for sick children. He has his own charisma, which helps him to diagnose little children when they are sick. He specialises in the sickness common to children such as, 'alubala' (measles), 'jadi jadi'[205] (a type of dysentery common among children). They treat many other ailments that disturb the children.

2.3.1.8 Psychiatrist "Dibia Okiri Ngbawa Isi"

He is a doctor who specialises in the care of the mentally sick. Like the modern Psychiatrist, his work is a dangerous one. He has to learn the art of handling the violence of the mentally sick. He uses herbs and roots that act as sedative to calm down the violent ones. The violent and destructive ones are often tied with cloth and twine in the hands and/or the legs to prevent them from causing harm or from running away. Many informants according to V. Ifeanyi indicated that the mentally sick "is smacked with a broom with the intention of beating away the forces responsible for the madness. Often, hot objects like pepper are applied into the eyes and nostrils to drive away madness."[206]

205 "Jadi jadi"– This is originally a Yoruba word.

206 V. Ifeanyi, The catholic Church and the challenges of Traditional System of Health care in Nigeria, Rome 1989, p.143

2.4 The Ogbanje Doctor

Some spirits in Igbo society are believed to be inherently evil. Some of them are incarnate human beings, while others are nonhuman powers. A good number of such spirits are believed to attack human beings in their prospective capacities. Their activities are very closely related. They are believed to cause people different types of misfortunes and illness. Only the special and strong dibias are said to have answers to the menace of these malignant spirits. The Ogbanje spirits are one among these spirits as we discussed earlier on.

The dibias who can heal the menaces or the illnesses caused by Ogbanje are called the Ogbanje dibias. They are also called 'dibia oje na mmili'. They are those dibias whose work is to uproot the 'Iyi uwa' (worldly oath), believed to be the pact made by the Ogbanje with his or her group in the spirit world before coming to the human world. The Ogbanje sickness only affects those who belong to the Ogbanje set or group. The Ogbanje dibia does not belong to the group. He does not use evil machinations to treat the sickness. He uses the transcendental power of God available in common objects such as plants, leaves, rocks etc. The Ogbanje dibia heals the Ogbanje of his sickness by first trying to separate him from the company. This he does by breaking the pact he made with the group in the spirit world by uprooting and destroying the iyi uwa. The dibia locates the iyi uwa through the instrumentality or the co–operation of the said Ogbanje or by the aid of a diviner. The object they use as a symbol of their oath, according to Ifeanyi "can be empty shells (ufuru aku), a smooth pebble, a living seed, or any object"[207]. On the healing of the Ogbanje and the breaking of their link with the spirit world, Chinwe Achebe made a very useful observation,

> *The artefacts and symbols used by the traditional healers in breaking the link with the spirit deity (wooden stools, white cloth, powder, cream, bracelets, combs, mirror, ankle chains, ngasi, ngaladam, ose oji, padlock, animal parts, akwukwo abosi, akwukwa, eggs, oiliest, yam, ebube agu, hair, nails, etc) appear on first glance to be a collection of rubbish. However this is not so. For each time they are used separately or in combination, the diviner activates each through invocation or incantation "to serve as power centres or channels of power" We just remember that this world view believes that all forms both animate or inanimate is imbued with unique force which can be harnessed to the service of man .*[208]

---

207 V. Ifeanyi, The Catholic Church and the challenges of traditional System of Healthcare in Nigeria, p.139

208 C. Achebe, The Ogbanje phenomenon, in Chris U. Manus et al., (eds), Healing and Exorcism., Op. Cit., p.37

The uprooting and the destruction of the Iyi uwa mark the first step towards the recovery and healing of the Ogbanje. Other steps may be taken such as the use of herbal mixtures drunken by the Ogbanje or carved right into his body through incisions. Sometimes the Ogbanje wears charms or hang them in his house.

2.4.1 Witch Doctor "Dibiaamosu"

Among the different types of dibia in Igbo society is the 'Dibia Amosu' (Witch doctor). Within the scope of his function is to heal and release those who are said to have been be–witched. There are stories of wicked people who are said to have the power to change into monstrous birds and animals of various species and go to attack others bringing misfortunes and sicknesses to them. Some sicknesses attributed to them include barrenness, devouring of victim's soul or part of his body and sometimes death. Not every dibia can handle sickness believed to have been caused by the witches. Only very strong dibias are believed to be able to heal such illness. Such dibias are called the 'Amosu dibia' or witch doctors. There is however a predominant conception that the witch doctors are themselves witches. But the power of the witch doctor is stronger than that of the witches. If the witch doctor that is believed to be a witch attacks witches, how can his kingdom stand? It looks like a kingdom divided against itself, which is laid waste and so cannot stand. A witch doctor is therefore not a witch. He is a dibia who cures those that are said to be bewitched.

People go to these expert dibias to obtain help when they feel they are bewitched. They also obtain charms to prevent the attacks of these witches or be able to destroy the witches in their transformed states. People also use certain objects, which are said to be repulsive and dangerous to the witches. One such object in Igboland, is 'Ede' (a type of cocoyam used for preparing soup) and 'Okazi' (a special type of vegetable). There are other techniques believed to be used, to drive away the witches and resist their nefarious activities such as the use of charms and some special sacrifices.

2.4.2 Aquatic Spirit Doctor "Dibia Muo Mmili"

The activities of the water spirit are so related to that of the Ogbanje, so the healing work of the Dibia Muo mmili resembles that of the Ogbanje dibia. The dibia offers sacrifices to the spirits to placate them and make them leave the said possessed person. The objects used in the sacrifice are often similar to those used in the case of the Ogbanje.

The only difference is that at the end of the healing and deliverance sacrifice, the objects of the sacrifice are deposited in the bed of the sea or river where the spirit is believed to inhabit.

2.4.3 The Priest (Ukochukwu) as a Special Person in Igbo Society

The priest occupies an important position among the Igbo people of Nigeria. He belongs among the groups of healing agents in Igbo society. The word for the priest in Igbo society is "Ukochukwu". He is also called the 'Eze alusi' (king of a shrine) or 'Onye isi muo' (head man of a spirit). Generally, when an Igbo is asked, who is the Ukochukwu? He promptly answers, 'Ukochukwu bu onye na agba uko na ebe chukwu na mmadu no,' (Ukochukwu is the one that mediates between God and man), or he tells you that, 'Onye ukochukwu bu onye nchu aja' (he is the one that offers sacrifice to the God/gods). Hence Arinze says that, Ukochukwu "is the official servant of a determined spirit, who offers sacrifice to the spirit and in General ministers to his or her shrine."[209] He is seen as an "intermediary between the God considered mighty and man considered weak"[210] This is to say that the priest is a religious leader consecrated to act as a mediator between God and man by offering sacrifices and prayers. So mediation between God and man is one of the primary functions of the priest, the office which one is appointed to act on behalf of men, in things pertaining to God, that he may offer gifts and sacrifices for sins. (Hebrews 5:1) Any wonder some writers refer to the priest in African context as "one who performs religious duties whether in temples, shrines, sacred grooves and elsewhere"[211]

The Ukochukwu is therefore seen as a religious leader who ministers in and around the temples and shrines. Every spirit has it's own priest and it's special way of worship. There is therefore a priest to minister to any particular 'alusi' (shrine) that has a shrine. It does not however, mean that a priest of a particular shrine 'alusi' does all the work concentrated in and around the shrine. Some priests cannot practise divination. In such cases they should consult the diviner.

---

209 F.A. Arinze, Sacrifice in Ibo religion, Op.Cit., p.63

210 H.H. Grahan, Priests in the students merit Encyclopaedia, Vol. 15, U.S.A., 1973, p.279

211 J.S. Mbiti, African Religions and Philosophy, Op. Cit., p.187; K. Amponsah, Topics on West African Religion, Vol.11, Cape Coast, 1975, p.22

There is an example of the case of "Akagu", the priest of "Oyi", the Chief of Abba. The Chief of Abba a town in Awka province went to Akagu, the priest to ask if he (the Chief of the town) could accept to enter into relations with the British. Akagu the priest had first to consult the dibia who dictated that Oyi decided against it.[212]

Akagu the priest could not dictate what could be done because he is only a priest 'ukochukwu' and not a diviner 'dibia ofuzo'. But there are however some priests who are both priests and diviners. They can divine and at the same time offer sacrifices themselves.

2.4.4 Vocation and Training of the "Ukochukwu"

In Igbo society, the vocation to the priesthood is very highly honoured. Those set apart for divine service receive some kind of a call and training. There are different methods of calling and different types of training a neophyte priest may receive. It is believed that people are called or wanted by the gods sometimes because of their love for them. Some priests are believed to be set apart from their infancy (i.e. hereditary) or may be called to the service by some spiritual possession through an ecstatic trance.

The case of S.C.Onwuka of Oka, Ugiri Mbano Okigwe is a typical example. He writes,

A diviner was consulted according to custom and he told my parents who I was supposed to be and that I was called to be one of the priests to serve at the altar and shrine of Duruamaka, one of our many village jujus. In the belief of our village, he is the god who gives fertility to the women and is one of the four most important deities in our area, almost all of which are connected with the Mbaa stream, the life giving deity. Thus from birth I was called to be a priest.[213]

In a family where the call to the priesthood is hereditary, the eldest son (Okpala) is normally the one to succeed his father. In some places the succession goes to the next senior male member of the family. In very few cases where the deceased priest is the only member of his immediate family left and there is also doubt on who succeeds him, the help of the diviner is sought. Normally those called to or set aside for the Igbo traditional priesthood receive some kind of initiation and training before they take up the highly honoured office. Though there were no organised seminaries for training, they were seriously prepared for the

212 Holy Ghost Fathers Onitsha, Igbo Kwenu, p.3; green M, Ibo Village affairs, p.4), quoted in F.A. Arinze, "Sacrifice in Ibo Religion", p.6

213 S.C. Onwuka, I was a juju priest, in E.A. Adegbola, "Traditional Religion in West Africa" Ibadan, 1983, p.2

office. The future priest, when possessed or called sometimes spends several days without food. He has also to observe temporal chastity especially during training and learn to bear other little hardships. His training sometimes includes instructions in the laws. Hence there are different levels of training,

From very simple to highly elaborate, but the priesthood as a class is distinct and developed ... Their training may include seclusion from the world, instructions in the law and sometimes possession by the divinity.[214]

A good number of other priests also learn by serving as apprentice or messenger to the other priests especially in the case of those whose offices are hereditary. Referring to this group, Arinze writes:

From his childhood to his final initiation, the future priest must have gathered much of the priestly sayings and practices especially with reference to sacrifices. Since the candidate is already known where the office is hereditary, as it almost always is, he gradually learns from his father as he helps him in his duties. He stays at his father's right hand during sacrificial rites and hands over to him those things which are to be offered. He is therefore called oje ozi (messenger). Before his father dies, he would have known practically everything about his function.[215]

After the training or at the death of a priest, the succeeding priest would call a grand feast during which he invites other priests of the shrine in his town, the titled men and some other men and women to the celebration. It is only after the celebrations that the new priest can officially assume his office.

2.5 Ukochukwu and the Care of the Sick

The priest plays an important role in the life of the Igbo. His functions are mainly religious but they are not limited to religious duties, as the name sometimes seems to portray. As the name "Ukochukwu" portrays, he mediates between man and God/gods. This he does in the shrines and other places. Apart from this function of mediation, which may be considered primary among his duties, he engages in some juridical duties and also cares for the needy members of the society such as the sick and the suffering. Writing on the traditional priesthood, Manoukin, notes that "priestly duties include the performance of daily and weekly rites, the offering of prayers for the barren and other needy persons and

---

214 G. Parrinder, West African Religion, Op. Cit., p.75
215 F.A. Arinze, Sacrifice in Ibo Religion, Op. Cit., p.69

making libations"[216] The priest therefore has other functions to perform in the life of the people especially in Igbo society. They offer the sacrifices, which are to be offered to specified deities and spirits on behalf of the sick according to the prescriptions of the diviners. But there are certain priests in Igboland who are also medicine men. While in training, they are taught to discover the causes of some sicknesses diagnose the nature of diseases and apply the right treatment to them. They are also trained on how to prevent misfortunes. Some priests even act as witch doctors since they can help those that are said to have been bewitched in the society.

> *Most people claim that priests who act as witch doctors are witches them–selves who are able to recognise other witches and perceive their evil activities. But the power of the witch doctor is stronger than the witches and as such can control the witch spirit.*[217]

The priests perform an important role in the traditional life of the Igbo society as medicine men. Igbo traditional healing is popular among the people and many believers in traditional medicine and medicine men insist that there are certain diseases that can only be cured by traditional medical practice.

This chapter has examined and explained the concept of life, death, health, healing and care of the sick in Igbo traditional society; the next chapter will consider the popular understanding of Health and Healing; Healing Ministry in the Church in Igbo Society and finally the Christian understanding of suffering and sickness in the light of European culture vis–à–vis human suffering and death.

---

216 M. Manoukin, Akan and Ga–Adangme, People of the Gold Coast, London, 1925, p.46

217 K. Amponsah, Topics on West African Religion, Op.Cit., p.30

3. Chapter Three – Understanding of Health and Healing

3.1 Popular Understanding of Health and Healing

3.1.1 Concept of Health and Healthcare of the Sick

The memorandum submitted to the Eleventh General Programme of Work 2006–2015 a Global Health Agenda of the World Health Organisation 'WHO', Geneva stated inter alia that:

> *Global health security has become a prominent item in the international agenda. Conflicts, natural disasters, disease outbreaks and zoonoses, are increasing in number. ... the spread of HIV/AIDS, which has become a disaster in many countries, is an example. Any serious effort to improve the health of the world's most vulnerable people and reduce health inequities must tackle the key determinants of health. Some of these, such as income, gender roles, education, and ethnicity, are related to social exlusion; others, such as living conditions, work environment, unsafe sex and the availability of food and water are more related to exposure to risks. ...There cannot be any material security, social security or well–being for individuals or nations without health ... the full responsibility of a free man can only be assumed by healthy individuals.*[218]

Many memoranda have stated so many good and admirable ideas that will be of benefit to the World if only human beings would have health. Hence since ages, man has been trying to explore avenues not only to improve his health but also to have complete health for the individual, a task that has remained a problem. In the last past years the World Health Organisation had set up a programme advocating 'Health for all'.

> *In the world's wealthiest countries the search for health is becoming the most important aspect of life. On the other hand, this search is becoming increasingly a life project, which is seen in dynamic and relational terms and conceived as the achievement of harmony (or, rather, continual harmonization), between the different dimensions in which*

218 Engaging for Health 11th General Programme of Work, 2006–2015, A Global Health Agenda, May 2006, pp.14 &17

the life of each and every man comes to obtain fulfilment, namely: the physical, the psycho–social, and the spiritual.[219]

On February 11, 2000 through the Dolentium Hominium created Pope John Paul II the Pontifical Commission for Apostolate of Healthcare workers. By means of this commission, the Pope invited all the episcopates of the world to create their own Health Commission to be a sign of the profound concern the Church has always had for the world of suffering and the sick. But in spite of all the programmes and commissions being set up by the different bodies and conferences, the task for complete health for man remains a problem and sickness an enigma.

> *The World Health Organization in its bulletins tells uns that every year infectious diseases kill about seventeen million, and this is a special charateristic of developing countries. On the onther hand, in the other countries chronic illnesses constitute the principal threat to health. But given that life expectancy levels are rising in developing countries as well and in such societies Western healthcare models are gaining upper hand and becoming ever more dominant, these countries will be increasingly exposed to illness of a chronic character.*[220]

This is to say that while man tries to fight diseases in order to get complete health, nature continues to take upper hand by exposing man to illnesses of a chronic character. In the light of all these attempts, we go to investigate the concept health.

3.3.1.2 Defining the Concept Health

There has always been a continuous attempt to get a complete and balanced definition of the term health. And for a long time now, there has been no widely accepted definition of health. Many writers on health have seen the term as one of the most difficult term that can be given a meaningful definition.

Thus it was said that the concept of health is a complex one and escapes any exact definition"[221] Hence Luciano Sandrin notes that,

219 L. Sandrin, The Church: a healing Community, in "Dolentium Hominum", Journal of the Pontifical Council or Pastoral Assistance to Healthcare Workers, Vatican City, Yr. 13, No.1, 1998, p.71

220 L. Sandrin, The Church: A Healing Community, in "Dolentium Hominum" Op. Cit., p.71

221 M.Norbert, Environmental conditions to promote and defend health, in "Dolentium Hominium", No. 7, Yr III, No 1, p.49

the search for health and thus the state of being healthy is often understood as being fit. It therefore becomes reduced to the merely physical dimension of an individual's life and this involves a spasmodic tension produced by the desire to identify with socially ascendent models of how to live today.[222]

Many other authors have seen the definition as an impossible task to be achieved. Hence many attempts to define health have been seen, as incomplete, merely dealing with the absence of disease or over–generalised seeing well–being as all important and neglecting the spiritual and other dimensions of health. One would not therefore, be surprised why Callahan remarked, "All efforts towards a good conception of health is something naturally frustrating."[223] He adds, "It seems impossible to desire a concept of health which is rich enough to be nutritious and yet not so rich to be indigestible."[224]

Most writers who have attempted a definition of health have met many criticisms. Even the very inclusive and modern definition of health by the 'WHO' (1946 – 1948) has been criticised. The World Health Organisation defines health as "a state of complete physical, mental and social well–being and not merely the absence of diseases or infirmity."[225] This definition has been criticised as being simply bad and as having given way to many evils. Among the evils are,

the cultural tendency to define all social problems, from war to crime in the streets as 'health' problems; the blurring of lines of responsibility between and among the professions and between the medical professions and the political order–, the implicit denial of human freedom which results when failure to achieve social well–being are defined as forms of 'sickness' somehow to be treated by medical means, and the General debasement of language which ensues from labelling everyone from Adolf Hitler to student radicals to the brat next door as sick."[226]

Haring in his turn says that, "the definition overlooked the spiritual dimension of health."[227]

The 1970 American Medical Association (AMA) definition of health which stated that health is "a state of physical and mental well–being"[228] met its own

222 L. Sandrin, The Church: A Healing Community, in "Dolentium Hominum", Journal of the Pontifical Council or Pastoral Assistance to Healthcare Workers, Vatican City, Yr. 13, No 1, 1998, p.71

223 D. Callahan, The 'WHO' defintion of Health, in S.E. Lammers & A.V. Michigan (eds), "On Moral Medicine", Michigan, 1987, p.165

224 D. Callahan, The WHO Definition of Health, in "On Moral Medicine", Op.Cit., p.165

225 Ibid., p.165

226 Ibid., p.165

227 B.Haring, Medical Ethics, St. Paul's Publication, Slough, England, 1977, p.153

228 D. Callahan, The WHO definition of Health, in On Moral Medicne, Op.Cit., p.645

criticisms. According to J.M. Boyle Jr., "This is narrower than the WHO definition in two respects: It omits reference to complete well being and drops all together the category of social wellbeing."[229] On the same definition, Haring remarks that "health cannot be defined from a mere study of the body; we must consider the whole person in his human vocation and final destiny."[230] At this junction however, we have to note that these and other assumptions and criticisms, which sprang up as a result of the various definitions of health, have some significant implications for the use of the word health. We shall therefore not hesitate to look into other definitions and conceptions of health to help us attempt our own conception of the term for the purpose of our work.

Health according to a dictionary definition is seen as "soundness of body" or "a state of strong constitution".[231] Here health has still to do with the physical goodness of the person without considering other aspects or dimensions. Treating the WHO definition of health, an author stated that for him, a good definition of health is, "a state of physical well–being which need not be 'complete' but must be without significant impairment of function."[232] This definition though dealing with physical wellbeing understands health as something even less than physical goodness. It also completely excludes mental and social wellbeing of individual as part of health. According to G. Ikeobi, a Catholic pastor in Onitsha in Nigeria,

> *Health is often regarded as the absence of sickness in Western Culture. This thinking has succeeded in pushing back biological death and its shadows for them (and for many Nigerians who think like them) that as long as they visit their doctors and take drugs they consider themselves healthy.*[233]

By this expression, Ikeobi refuses to agree with the notion that health can be meaningfully talked of solely in terms of absence of sickness or infirmities. Hence he added about those Nigerians that, "their life of greed and competitiveness and fear of death surely mark them out as a very unhealthy group."[234] By this Ikeobi shows that human vices can constitute unhealthy living. It seems therefore that like Ivan Illich, he sees health "as a virtue".[235] His idea of health

229 J.Boyle, The concept of Health and the right to healthcare, in On Moral Medicine, Op.Cit., p.645

230 B.Haring, Medical Ethics, Op. Cit., p.154

231 J.B. Foreman (ed), Collins English Gem Dictionary, London and Glasgow, 1974, p.242

232 D. Callahan, The WHO definition of Health, in "On Moral Medicine", Op. Cit., p.172

233 G.Ikeobi, Sickness, Prayer and Healing in Mulumba magazine, Vol.3, No.1 Enugu, Dec., 1988 – June 1989, p.40

234 G. Ikeobi, Sickness , Prayer and Healing … p.10

235 Ivan Illich, Health as a virtue, in "On Moral Medicine", p.150

also portrays the fact that health is Multi–dimensional. During an oral interview, an informant, Odinanwa B. Igwedinma says,

A healthy man is one who gets up in the morning strong, and goes to his place of work and is able to sleep when he comes back from work. He is able to answer whenever he is called up. Such is the healthy man. He is not physically weak. He is not restless on account of worries.[236]

This definition also portrays health as multi–dimensional. In the light of the above survey, we can now say that health is quite an embracing concept. It is generally conceived to be more than physical fitness. Health embraces social, moral, spiritual, physical, and mental dimensions. In fact a fair conception of health involves the person as an integral entity, able to use his energies for the fulfilment of his total human vocation. In other words, health is a basic and dynamic force in our daily lives, influenced by our circumstances, beliefs, culture and social, economic and physical environment. We shall now discuss different aspects of health that affect man's world in the next section.

3.3.1.2.1 Different Dimensions of Health.

Health concerns the well–being of the man in its various dimensions. Human health, which is lacking in any of its dimensions, is unhealthy. We shall here classify the different dimensions of health of the human person as follows – physical, psychological, social, moral, and spiritual.

3.3.1.2.2 Physical or Organic Dimension

Physical dimension of health deals with man's physical fitness viewed from the point of view of vitality and absence of pain, the conditions which to a great extent is contingent on proper training, good diet and a wholesome life–style. Under this dimension, healthcare emphasizes only the condition of the body of the man as a being with physical structure.

If only this Dimension is put into consideration, the more traditional aspects of healthcare remain central. It becomes necessary to trust the doctor and the health structure, the dependence on others and the tendency to remain passive before the doctor who alone can procure health because only him knows the scientific datas and techniques nec-

236 Akuejiofor O.B. Igwedinma, Personal oral interview, Nri, June 26, 1990; A.O. Obiagwu, Oral Interview, Alor, Janaury 1998

essary to the recovery of physical efficiency. It is his duty to put right the non–functioning body.[237]

But the image of a physically, well body, is a powerful one and if used carefully, "can be suggestive of the kind of wholesome and adequacy of function one might hope to see in other areas of life."[238]

3.3.1.2.3 Phsychological Dimension

The psychological dimension of man is closely related to the physical, but also clearly distinct.

Bodily or physical health of man is far less significant than the Psychological and the spiritual health; we must be mindful however of the dependence of psychological conditions on the integrity and soundness of bodily organs.[239]

Psychological dimension of health is often treated as 'mental' or 'psychic' dimension and care should be taken to avoid "reducing psychic health to emotional adjustment and maturity"[240]

Psychologically healthy persons are in touch with their feelings. They perceive the world of ordinary activity as most people do, without manifesting absurd illusions or projections.[241]

Psychological health here means the ability of one to be aware of one's self and the realities around. He is able to choose between practical alternatives and do not have unrealistic expectations. He is responsible for all his actions and fully capable of moral good or evil. In the case of psychologically unhealthy person, it is a different thing. Psychological sickness is a special field for Psychopathologists and Psychotherapists.

3.3.1.2.4 Social Dimension

Man by nature is a social being and in order to exist properly, man needs the support of the community in which he lives in many regards. "The conditions of work, feeding, relational capacity of the individual and the family environment

---

237 C. Bresciani, Salute – Approccio Storico–Cultuale, in "Dizionario di Teologia Pastorale Sanitaria," Op. Cit, p.1076

238 D. Callahan, The WHO definition of Health, in "on Moral Medicine", Op.Cit, p.172

239 B.Haring, Medical Ethics, Op. Cit., p.115

240 B.M.Ashley and Rourke, Healthcare Ethics, 3rd ed., St. Louis, 1989, p.34

241 Ibid., p.34

are determinant factors to reassure the individual a living "health".[242] Social health therefore,

attests to the cooperation and interdependence of people in the fields of nourishment, housing, pre–natal and childcare education, and care of society's dependence members and the shaping of the physical – psychological environment. As a social responsibility, it appeals to everyone's ability and generosity to serve the fundamental social groups of family and community.[243]

These needs or interdependence, Maslow A.W. Categorised and called "safety 'needs' and 'belonginess' and 'love needs'"[244]

According to him,

the safety needs of man include the needs for dependency, security and protection (especially by the weak such as children). The belongingness and love needs on the other hand include the needs for friends, 'a sweet heart', a wife, or children, the hunger for affection, relations with people in general, and the need for a place in one's group or family.[245]

One should not also neglect the importance of the political and economical development for the promotion of the individual health, hence the importance for the health of the community or the society. It therefore observes,

the potential conflict between the Psychological conception of health, which tends to strengthen the subjective freedom in the use of the body and ambient and the socio–ambiental conception, which instead speeds up from the political and social moment the protection of the environment and so, of health.[246]

3.3.1.2.5 Moral Dimension

"The moral Dimension of health is often considered as an aspect of the social dimension."[247] .But there is however a distinction between the two dimensions. The moral Dimension concerns the ability of the individual to exercise a free, responsible, moral activity. "Only a free man or woman is a person fully capable of either moral good or evil."[248] Hence Haring says,

---

242 C. Bresciani, Saluto – Approccio storico–Culturale, in "Dizionario di Teikigua Oastirake Sanitaria", Op. Cit., p.1077

243 B. Haring, Medical Ethics, p.153; Having, Free and Faithful in Christ, p.48

244 A.W.Maslow, Motivation and Personality, New York, Harper and Row, 1970, p.39

245 Ibid., p.20

246 C.Bresciani, Saluto – Approccio Storico–Culturale, in "Dizionario di Teologia Pastorale Sanitaria" Op. Cit., p.1077

247 B.M.Ashley, K.D. O'Rourke, Ethics of Healthcare, Op. Cit. pp.8–9

248 Ibid., p.34

To poison one's body and mind by the abuse of alcohol, drugs, and nicotine is a grave moral disorder. However, moralistic judgemental attitudes must be excluded. The major part of responsibility often falls on society itself or on those who have failed to provide an education properly directed towards a truly human community and favourable social conditions.[249]

This area of health is a special concern of Lawyers, Political leaders, and Clergy acting as moral counsellors.

3.3.1.2.6 Spiritual Dimension

This Dimension is often seen as intuitive and creative. Among man's basic needs in life are to know, understand, contemplate and to create. This level of need we may refer to as the spiritual. We add the word creative because many people confine the meaning of spiritual to our relationship to God.

A good conception of this dimension helps the sick patient to give meaning to his illness, gain greater self knowledge, advance in the sense of the transcendent, find the reason for living, dying, struggling and to reach God (through the sacraments above all).[250]

Hence the Spiritual dimension of health "can be outlined as the needs of meaning, of scope, of realisation which connotes human life, hope, and the will to live, conviction and faith."[251]

To this dimension of health belongs all activity with a creative element in art or science or political innovation – in addition to religious activity as it extends to ultimate cosmic meaning."[252]

This is an area dealt by inspiring teachers and spiritual directors though the health team is not excluded at this level.

Having distinguished above, the various dimensions of health, it is good to note that though separately considered, they do not exist independent of each other. All are inter–dependent laying within each other the dimensional line crossing each other at one point.

---

249 B.Haring, Free and Faithful, Slough, London, 1981, p.64

250 M.A. Monge, Ethical Practices in Health and Diseases, Manilla, Philippines, 1994, p.11

251 M.Petrini and F. Caretta, Ai Confini del dolore: salutte e malattia nelle culture religiose, Citta Nuova Editrice, Roma, 1999, p.15

252 B. Ashley and K. O'Rourke, Ethics of Healthcare, Op. Cit., p.18

Man should not therefore be considered as a composite of several levels, Such as body, soul, spirit. He is a multi–dimensional unity; all dimensions, distinguishable in experienced life, cross in him.[253]

3.2 The Concept Sickness

Having made an attempt into the understanding of the concept health, we now try to examine the opposite concept of sickness. Sickness in it's simple form is seen as "the absence of health".[254] .Sickness has been a very common concept of life that poses a lot of problem for man. According to a document of the National Council for the Pastoral of Health of the Italian Episcopal Conference, Sickness is

A traumatic experience which makes an attempt on the physical and psychological integrity of man and involves a sharp arrest of interests; it makes one perceive existentially the fragility of human nature, determines a different image of himself and of the world around him.[255]

It has remained an enigma for man. And man has continued to explore avenues to combat or eliminate this problem. But all efforts by man towards the achievement of that purpose had proved unsuccessful. The contemporary man instead talks more of prevention of sickness as a means of evading it. Any wonder why he visits his doctors regularly and faithfully. Man has failed to understand what sickness is. Peoples' understanding and response to sickness depends on their knowledge of the concept. People have seen the experience from different points of view. For a lot of people, a time of sickness literally seems the end of the world. For some, it is a time of trial and temptation. According to L. Sandrin,

In our kind of society, which takes strong, healthy, young, and beautiful beings as its ideal model, illness is often a tragedy, and the same may be said of pain, disability and old age – realities to which it is not possible to give a meaning and which are as a result no longer bearable.[256]

Some people have attributed sickness to the workings of the evil spirit. While some others have considered sickness as a scourge or punishment from God as a

---

253 P. Tillich, The meaning of Health, in "On Moral Medicine", Op. Cit., p.162

254 A.S.Hornby & co (eds), Advanced Learners Dictionary of Current English, London, 1965. p.928

255 Cf. M.Petrini and F. Caretta, Ai Cofini del Dolore ... Op.Cit., p.34

256 L. Sandrin, The Church: A healing Community, in "Dolentium Hominum", Op.Cit., p.71

result of man's faults or sins. Hence human sickness is characterised by the question, why? Why am I suffering from this sickness? What did I do wrong? And such questions very often bring frustration and conflicts in the relation of man and God.

Such presents a serious temptation to the sick person and sometimes obscure the great and beautiful image of God before man. Here Petrini and Caretta refers to sickness as

A crisis of meaning which naturally gives rise to some questions: the patient asks himself the meaning of the symptoms (What do they mean?), He asks himself the implications of the sickness (What will it involve?), he searches for a cause or justification (Why me?), he needs to integrate the threat of the sickness in life, (What is the sense of my life and what can I hope for?).[257]

Sickness constitutes a crisis for man, and "not only for the sick but also for the entire family system. It puts the equilibrium of the person into crisis in his physical, psychological, social and spiritual dimensions, but it also puts into crisis the family in these same dimensions: the sick is a "family crisis"[258] Man often, denies his God because of sickness. Sometimes, it is the family of the sick that offers insult to God. When Job the just man of the bible was struck by grave misfortunes and sickness, the family and friends were all concerned about the gravity of the sickness. His wife said to him, "Do you now still mean to insist in your blamelessness? Curse God and die". (Job 2: 9) Some three old acquaintances of him came to his house, and trying to convince him that he must have sinned seriously, hence his terrible sickness and suffering. Very often too in our life, there are the suspicions that the various states of distress in our life are due to some sins we might have committed. But sickness is not generally because of sin. Even Job himself challenged the truth that identifies sickness with punishment for sin. This he did by recounting the good he did during his lifetime. Today, it is commonly appreciated that many people become sick because they nourish grudges and bitterness in their hearts.

Preoccupied by resentments of one kind or another, they are unable to establish good healthy relationships and thereby become vulnerable to sickness of a psychosomatic nature such as stress, heart attacks and cancer.[259]

---

257 M.Petrini & F. Caretta, Ai Confini del Dolore ... Op. Cit., pp.31–32

258 L.Sandrin, Psicologia della Salute e della Malattia, in "Dizionario di Teologia Pastorale sanitaria", Op. Cit., p.981

259 P.Wilkinson, A Theology of sickness, in T. Coyle (ed), "Christian Ministry to the sick", London, 1986, p.74

All this, as we have seen shows that sickness does not simply mean an absence of physical goodness or state of unhealthiness of an organ of the body. Sickness involves more than this. It involves diseases, unhealthiness of organs, physical weakness, stress, fear of death, greed and the rest of other psychic and spiritual deficiencies, which sometimes are responsible for the weakness of the body.

3.2.1 Understanding Healthcare of the Sick

Health is generally noted as one of the essential necessities for achieving any human goal. When our health or well–being is impaired, we become depressed and sad, our normal rhythm of life is disrupted and our daily activities are slowed down or even put to a halt. Man does not like to be sick. He expresses shock and loses all hopes and aspirations especially when the sickness is a serious one. Sometimes, he prefers to die than to be kept alive in such sick condition. Hence a passage in 'a living will' framed by the Connecticut delegation of the American Medical Association of the Euthanasia society reads:

> *If there is no reasonable expectation of my recovery from physical or mental and spiritual disability, I request that I be allowed to die and not to be kept alive by artificial means or heroic measures.*[260]

The above quotation from the American Medical Association of the Euthanasia society is unchristian and against the will of God, who is the giver and author life.

As a result of the way man feels about sickness, a lot of time, energy and talent is given in by man in order to avoid sickness and preserve health. He does whatever is within his reach to keep healthy and alive. Health is therefore perceived today "as a value and there is in this sense a strong scientific, economical and personal investment to cure illnesses, to prolong life's span and to improve the quality of life".[261] Man thus cares very much for his good health.

The Advanced Learners Dictionary of Current English defines the word 'care' as "serious attention, thought, watchfulness".[262] It may also mean "to be alert, or be careful; and 'to care of'' means to watch over, be responsible, to care for the

260 P.Ramsey, The indignity of death with dignity, in "On Moral Medicine", Op. Cit., p.189

261 L.Sandrin, Psicologia della salute e della Malttia, in "Dizionario di Teologia Pastorale Sanitaria", Op. Cit., p.967

262 Advanced Learners Dictionary of Current English Language, p.142

invalid".[263] Caring does not mean well wishing nor does it simply mean being interested in something or a person. To care for another person in the most significant sense is to help him grow and actualise himself. A mother caring for a child does whatever is within her power to help the child grow. The child needs her and she tries to make herself available.

> *Caring as helping another grow and actualize himself is a process, a way of relating to someone that involves development in the same way that friendship can only emerge in time through mutual trust and a deepening and qualitative transformation of the relationship.*[264]

So to care for someone is to enter into a useful relationship with somebody in such a way that it helps the person to actualize and develop himself in whichever aspect he needed the care. Healthcare of the sick therefore, involves the health carers and the people around the sick person entering into a relationship with the sick in such a way that helps him meet his various health needs.

3.2.1.1 The Integral Care of the Sick

A lot of progress is today being noticed in the area of science and technology. The modern man tends greatly towards finding solutions to most of his problems by scientific and technological means. This quest of the contemporary man is not less glaring in the field of medicine and healthcare. Progress is being witnessed in the various disciplines of medicine and surgery, in diagnostic and therapeutic methods and other branches of healthcare services. But in spite of all these progresses, there is still much quest for more humane treatment of the sick person. By humane treatment is meant the treatment of the sick person in his totality as a human person. A lot of Medical experts and health personals still treat the sick as mere case numbers.

Hence what Alexia, a fourteen year old girl was saying as she was receiving treatment in the University Clinic of Ewing Sarcoma is meaningful: "I am not a patient – I am a Person … she would emphasize the word "person".[265]

Many of the healthcare specialists treat one dimension of sickness to the neglect of the others. This type of treatment of one dimension of the person without attention to the other parts can be injurious to the complete wellbeing of the individual. A sick person is to be assisted in his totality as a human person made up

---

263 Random House Dictionary of English Language, 2nd ed. New York, 1987, p.314.
264 Milton Mayeroff, On Caring, New York, London, 1972, p.1
265 M.A. Monge, Integral Care of the Sick: The role of spiritual help in "Dolentium Hominium", No. 12, Vatican City, 1989, p.10

of the body and the spirit. Man is a psycho–somatic unity and when he grows sick, it is not only the physical body which receives pain that suffers the sickness but the whole self suffers. Any wonder John Paul II says that, "illness and pain are not experiences affecting exclusively man's corporal condition but the whole man in his integrity and somatic spiritual unity".[266] When man grows, it is not the damaged organ that suffers but the whole man. Consequently, the sick person needs to be offered an integral care. His various health needs must be taken into consideration otherwise the healthcare remains incomplete or what Paul Tillich would call 'unhealthy health'. According to him,

> *It comes about if healing under one dimension is successful but does not take consideration of other dimensions in which health is lacking or even imperilled by the particular healing. Successful surgery may produce a psychological trauma; effective drugs may calm down an uneasy conscience and preserve a moral deficiency; the well trained athletic body may contain a neurotic personality; the healed patient of the analyst may be sick through the lack of an ultimate meaning of his life; the conformist average life may be sick through inhibited self–alternation; the converted Christian may suffer under repression which produce fanaticism and may explode in lawless forms; the sane society may be the place where pressure of the principles of it's sanity may produce biological disruption by the desire for creativity.*[267]

Integral care of the sick is therefore that complete care or attention given to the sick person in all the dimensions of his personality, bearing in mind that it is the whole man that is sick and not just an organ or a part.

3.2.1.2 Popular Conception of Healing

The word healing is generally a very much misunderstood term. Many people are sceptical and even afraid when they hear the word. Some others are anxious only to know what one says or what stand one holds when the word healing is mentioned in discussion. Christians particularly understand various things when healing is mentioned. What one understands is invariably different and against what the other thinks about the term. So to write about healing is to delve into a very complex area that generates a lot of reactions. M. Buckley in the introduction to his work on healing wrote inter alia:

> *Healing is an evocative word. A very close friend of mine advised me, 'Write about prayer, theology, anything you like, but for God's sake, don't write about healing, that's a real mine field.' So the word itself, even before you can explain what you mean, it generates all sorts of highly emotional and irrational reactions among Christians ... It could*

266 John Paul II, Motu Proprio, in "Dolentium Hominum" No 1, Vatican, 1986, p.30
267 P.Tillich, The meaning of health, in "On Moral Medicine", Op. Cit., p.164

and should be a source of Christian unity and evangelical power. Sadly this is not so. What one Christian understands by healing as essential to the gospel, and his growth as a Christian person is a problem to another.[268]

This could account for the reason why most of the authors I have consulted on healing and healing ministry have not defined what they understand by healing. We can also see why Thomas and Alkire say,

Although religious healing is a 2000–year–old treasure in the Catholic Church, it has been pastorally ignored for centuries.

Outside of Charismatic circles, few people know what to say about it. When they do speak, they tend to label it a 'marginal issue' right over there next forecasting the end of the world.[269]

We cannot discuss fully the general meaning and the origin of healing without mentioning people like Hippocrates (ca.460–370 v. Chr.) History maintained that he was a great figure to be reckoned with in the field of traditional and orthodox medicine. Among other thing, he asserts that Sickness can be cured through natural means. This position of Hippocrates is still current in the healing process of the sick. Reports emanating from recent medical literature indicates that, there are cases of instant healing of serious organic sicknesses like lungs tuberculosis, cancer etc.

These reports underscores that Natural Medicine plays a great role in the healing process of man.

From the aforementioned, one can say that the process of healing originated from Nature which is one of the attributes of God. That means God is the ultimate Healer.

When we talk of healing we are not talking of merely physical healing of damaged organs in the body, neither are we talking of mere faith healing which principally has to do with physical and emotional cure through the actions of somebody. The healing we shall be discussing includes all these and more. In the words of M. Wilson, "we need a conception of healing which is wide enough to include sickness, sin, famine in the Congo and apartheid between races."[270]

Collins Germ English dictionary defines healing as "an act of making well, to cure, to become sound"[271] Another source says to heal means, "to become or make something healthy again; to restore somebody to health or to cure some-

---

268 M.Buckley, His Healing Touch: Freedom through good relationships, Harper, Collins, London, 1987, p.VI

269 L.Thomas and J. Alkire, Healing as a parish ministry, Notre Dame, Indiana, 1992, p.11

270 M.Wilson, The Church is healing, SMC London, in J.Turner, "The Healing Church", Belfast Dublin–Ottawa, 1978, p.8

271 J.B. Foreman (ed), Collins Gem English Dictionary, p.242

body of a disease."[272] And for Scalan, "healing means that process by which what is wounded or sick becomes whole and healthy. It is a naturally induced process to health."[273] These references or definitions seem to have seen healing more from the context of the physical wellbeing of man. But healing is something much more than that.

When human wellbeing and good health are impaired, God is actively involved in the work of restoration and human beings have the responsibility of sharing in this work of restoration.

Etymologically, the word healing is most frequently expressed by two Greek words, 'therapeuo' and 'ioamai'. Therapeuo means to 'heal' or to 'cure', originally used in profane Greek to mean 'serve' or to be in the service to a superior or of cultic service or to care for (e.g. as a doctor). But in the New Testament, therapeuo is never used in the profane sense to serve. It was not either commonly used in the sense of healing by ordinary medical means as found in Luke 4:23 and 8:43. Therapeuo is most commonly used to describe the miraculous healings wrought by Jesus and his disciples.[274]

For John Turner, "to heal means to integrate the various elements of personality and to reconcile man in all his relationships"[275] This Definition of Turner goes more than just mere physical healing. It concerns itself also with man's relationship with both God and man. Integrating the various elements of personality will concern the various aspects or dimensions of human character, his ways and manner of relating to his neighbour. Hence for Turner,

healing is completeness. It has everything to do with all of man's relationships – with those whom he loves and with those whom he loathes; it affects his attitude to those whom he fears, those whom he resents and to those whom he is indifferent. Healing has something to do with man's relationship with God who is all good and who is the healer himself. It deals with man's environment in which he lives, the condition under which he works and the community of which he is a part.[276]

And for M. Buckley,

Christian healing rests it's power in the person of Christ who restores us to a full relationship with God the father, with our neighbour and with oneself. He saw in healing threefold restoration of broken relationships given the Theological name of 'reconciliation' and noted that every form of reconciliation is a healing and every healing is a form

272 J.Crowther (ed), Oxford Advanced Learners Dictionary, Oxford Press, New York, 1995, p.561

273 M.Scalan, Inner healing, Dublin, 1977, p.5

274 F.Graber and D. Muller, Heal, in "The International dictionary of New Testament Theology", Vol,2, ed, Collins Brown, Grand Rapids, Michigan, 1986, p.163–164

275 J.Turner, The Healing Church, Op.Cit., p.9

276 J. Turner, The Healing Church, Op. Cit. p.8

of reconciliation. The two are inseparably linked together in the mission of Christ and his Church just as reconciliation radically restores relationship with God, our neighbours and ourselves, so healing gives us the means to live this restored relationship in our daily lives. Healing is essential to the Christian life as is reconciliation, just as our continued heart–beat and breathing are necessary for human life... Remove one or the other and there is no living gospel left.[277]

This is as true as "the healings of Jesus substantiate his teachings, just as the teachings extend the meaning of the healing" Healing is therefore not just physical or emotional cure of illness, nor forgiveness of sins but all these and more. We can now say that our understanding of healing or the concept of healing we shall use in this work involves healing a person's whole world – body, soul and environment – social and economical. Christ wants us to be healed and He wants every aspect of our lives to be healed. Christ wants us to appreciate the true meaning of his double mandate to the Church – to preach the gospel and heal the sick. He wants us to appreciate the true meaning of healing. Christ did not come into the world as a divided personality. He therefore does not think of man as a being divided into body and soul but as a whole person with body, soul, feelings and historical background which includes his environment and the community of his family and extended relations. Christ wants every aspect of our lives to be healed because without this healing, we cannot live the new life in abundance. "Our Church and our world need healing today just as much as, if not more so than, when Christ healed so stupendously in Galilee two thousand years ago"[278]

3.2.1.3 Sickness and Healing in the Bible

Sickness as we have earlier noted in this work is a very common concept of life, which with it's accompanying pain and suffering poses a lot of problem for man through the ages. Man has seen the experience of sickness from various points of view. For some people sickness literally seems the end of the world, for others a time of trial and temptation.

Calwer Biblical Dictionary understands Sickness in as:

"a disturbance in the expiry of physical and psychological processes of life which can lead to pain, internal worries, social restrictions and in the extreme case to the death; because also the most insignificant illness is a part of the death"[279]

277 M.Buckley, His Healing Touch, Op. Cit., p.1
278 M.Buckley, His Healing Touch, Op.Cit., p.5
279 Cf Calwer Bibellexikon, Band 1, Calwer Verlag Stuttgart 2003, p.763
"Ihr zufolge ist K. als Störung im Ablauf körperlicher und seelischer Lebensvorgänge zu verstehen, die zu Schmerz, inneren Belastungen, sozialen Einschränkun-

Some have attributed sickness to the workings of the evil spirit, while some others considered sickness as a scourge or punishment from God as a result of man's faults or sins.

In the civilisation surrounding the Jews especially in the Babylonian culture, sickness was considered a scourge from attacks by external forces such as the gods, evil spirits, demons, sin and guilt. Exorcism has been practised to drive away evil spirits and bring about healing. Prayers and offerings have also been used in attempt to appease the deity and even magic has been applied to get a cure from sickness. Medicine was extensively practised by priests. "Documentation within our possession disclosed that recovery of health remained the dominion of the religious"[280]

At the emergence of Jesus in the history of Israel, the picture of sickness began to assume new dimension. He came to fulfil and make perfect the history of the ancient civilisation. Jesus unique ministry consisted of preaching the Good News of the Kingdom and of bringing healing to the sick in mind and body. This is clear in his answer to the disciples of John the Baptist who came to him to know who he is. "Go back and tell John what you see and hear; the blind see and the lame walk, lepers are cleaned and the deaf hear and the dead are raised to life" (Mt 11: 3–5). Jesus approach to sickness was different and sympathetic.

> *While Jesus did not attempt to explain disease, his attitude towards it's presence in the lives of individuals marked a considerable advance in thought on the consensus of Old Testament opinion regarding sickness and disease. Instead of manifesting an attitude of contempt towards the weak and the sick, Jesus showed in his first recorded sermon that his earthly ministry was closely bound up with the frail and feeble of body and soul.*[281]

Hence Jesus was completely hostile to whatever made people sick or destroyed them and so he employed the healing power of his father's creative spirit to bear upon the mental, physical and moral illness of the people. Since then the restoration of the sick formed part of the subsequent apostolic practise in conformity with the expressed will of Christ. In the days immediately after the Pentecost, many healings took place at the hands of the apostles (Acts 2:43; 5:12; 8:7) and the pathology dealt with was as varied as that which had confronted Jesus.

---

gen und im Extremfall zum Tod führen können; denn auch die unscheinbarste K. ist Teil des Todes."

280 D. Casera, in J. Onyenemegam, Pastoral Care of the sick in Igbo Community, Rome, 1985, p.63

281 G.A.Buttrick (ed), The Interpreters dictionary of the bible, an illustrated encyclopaedia, Vol.2. Abingdon Press, Nashville, 1985, p.546.

3.2.1.4 Sickness in the Old Testament

My son when you are sick, do not be depressed but pray to God and he will heal you; Renounce your faults to God, keep your hands unsoiled and cleanse your heart from all sins. Offer incense and a memorial of fine flour and make as rich an offering as you can afford. (Eccles 38:9–11)

To get a clear view of the understanding of sickness and healing in the bible, we have to take a brief examination of how the ancient world of the Jews conceives sickness. In the ancient civilisation surrounding the Jews, such as Babylonians and Assyrians and other areas where diseases and sickness were rampant, much emphasis was given to health and absence of diseases. "For Babylonians as well as Hebrews, health was wellbeing, wholeness, peace of body, mind and spirit, in harmony with the environment and with God."[282]

On the other hand, the ancient Jewish world sees sickness as a harsh and bitter experience and the man is really conscious of the bitterness of being sick and complains of it to God. (Ps 31:11) He looks forward to God the physician for healing and recovering. Sometimes he consults the prophets for advice and treatment. He very much appreciates the great benefit of good health (Sir 30:14–20) and prefers to be poor and healthy than to be a sick healthy man. Life was considered as a gift of the gods and sickness seen as,

an evil, which must be distinguished from physical trials to which man is exposed from without, such as hunger, exhaustion, cold and from moral trials such as grief and afflictions of the heart.[283]

Consequently, therefore, the Old Testament man considered sickness as a scourge from attacks by external forces. Exorcism had been practised to drive away evil spirits and bring healing. Prayers and offerings have also been used in attempt to appease the deity and even magic has been applied to get a cure.

Sickness which is also first regarded as divine punishment from God must have been incurred by some sin (Ps 38; 107:17–20). According to Wiseman,

sickness was commonly considered to be the result of divine displeasure for some sins, wittingly or unwittingly committed, This disease might be classified as 'striking' or 'seizure' or 'the hand of god', usually a deity both as the inflictor and the healer.[284]

282 D.J.Wison, Medicine in the Old Testament World, in B. Palmer (ed), "Medicine and the Bible", Pater Noster Press, Australia, 1986, p.18

283 Sacramentum Mundi, An encyclopaedia of theology, Vol.3, Burns and Oates, W. Germany, 1969, p.98.

Various prayers of the ancient Jews buttress the fact of sickness as punishment for sin:

All the time, I kept silent, my bones were wasting away, with groans day in and day out; day and night your hand lay heavy on me. My heart grew parched as stubble in summer drought. At last, I admit to you I had sinned. (Ps 32)

Other prayers include:

Heal me Lord, for I have sinned against you. (Ps 41:4)
Some driven frantic by their sins, made miserable by their own guilt and finding all food repugnant were nearly at death's door. (Ps 107:17)
Pity me Yahweh, I have no strength left, heal me, my bones are in torment, my soul is in utter torment, Yahweh, how long will you be. (Ps 6: 2–3)

In view of this fact that the ancient Jewish world considered sickness a result of divine displeasure for sins, some authors believed there was little or no room for the physicians among the people.

Sandford for example maintains that,

the healing stories such as that of Naaman by Elisha in the second book of Kings 5 are exceedingly rare exceptions , and that King Asa who suffered painful disease in his feet was reprimanded for consulting the doctors.(2 Chron. 16:12)[285]

In the Old Testament culture, it was also a subject of scandal for the just man to be afflicted by sickness. The people did not realise early enough that sickness might also be a case of trial sent by God to individual in order to manifest a person's virtue. The case of Job is a typical example. When Job the just man of the bible was struck by grave sickness, three old friends of him came to him to offer him sympathy and consolation (Job 1&2). Looking at him from distance, they could not recognise him, they wept aloud after which three series of discussions, (Job 3–14; 15–21; 22–27) emerged, having opposing conceptions of divine justice and the idea of sickness. The three friends made attempts to convince Job that his sickness was as a result of his sins, but Job was able to challenge the truth of the idea, reaffirming his innocence while acknowledging God's power.

---

284 D.J.Wiseman, Medicine in the Old Testament World, in "Medicine and the Bible", Op.Cit.,p.18

285 J.A.Sanford, Healing body and Soul, Kenturchy, 1992, p.13–14

3.2.1.3 Healing in the Old Testament

It has been observed that since ages, man has applied various means to avoid or eliminate illness and maintain good health. Among the ancient Israel, health was a highly prized possession such that "it will appear that health was a divine gift, and along with material prosperity was confidently expected by the faithful in Israel".[286] Any person who had a health problem was first to seek recourse to God, the physician of his people for healing and recovery. He offers prayers and offerings to get a cure. "Pity me, Lord, for I am weak, Heal me for my body is sick, and I am upset and disturbed ... O come, O Lord, and make me well, in your kindness save me. For if I die, I cannot give you glory by praising you before my friends..." (Ps 6: 2–8) God reveals himself as the healer both in words and actions. This is beautifully seen when Moses led the Israelites across the Red Sea to a dry desolate land and the subsequent sweetening of the undrinkable waters of Morah where the Lord declared, "I am the Lord your healer." (Ex 15:26) According to Stephen Hill:

> *The sweetening of the bitter waters of Morah was closely connected with the Ordinance of healing which God immediately proceeded to give to Israel. It is evident that the healing of the water was intended to represent the physical healing offered through the divine promise ... It was at this time that God revealed himself to Israel as their physician. Through the redemptive and covenant name of Yahweh Roph'eka (which is translated as "The Lord that healeth thee" or "the Lord thy physician), God pledged to meet all of Israel's physical needs as they believed and obeyed him.*[287]

The use of personal names among the Hebrews lends support to this concept of God as the true healer; 'Asaya' meaning Yahweh heals.[288]

In spite of the strong monotheistic view of the Hebrews who viewed their God as true healer that (Rophe) "forgives all sins and heals all diseases" (Ps 103:3) It was observed that individuals and groups of individuals dedicated themselves to the care of the sick. "The mention of rational remedies and the emphasis on preventive medicine and hygiene (as in Leviticus) implies a corpus of indigenous medical knowledge"[289] Social hygiene and sanitary regulations in Leviticus comprise 213 of the 613 biblical commands and prohibitions. The Human physician was highly prized by his skill and learning. By 190 B.C. when Sirach

---

286 G.A.Buttrick (ed), The Interpreters Dictionary of the Bible: an illustrated Encyclopaedia, Vol.2. Op. Cit., p.542

287 S.Hill, God's Convenant of Healing, Indiana, (no date), p.14–15

288 D.J. Wiseman, Medicine in the Old Testament World, in "Medicine and the Bible", Op. Cit., p.19

289 Ibid., p.15

wrote his book, professional physicians were well respected in Israel. Thus he writes:

Honour the doctor with the honour that is due in return for his services; for he too has been created by the Lord. Healing itself comes from the most High, like a gift from a king ... The Lord has brought medicine into existence from the earth, and the sensible man will not despise them... He has also given men learning so that they may glory in his mighty works ... My son when you are ill, do not be depressed, but pray to the Lord and he will heal you. Renounce your faults, keep your hands unsoiled...Then let the doctor take over, the Lord created him too and do not let him leave you... If a man sins in the eyes of his Maker, may he fall under the Care of a doctor. (Eccles 38: 1–15)

Some other references in the Old Testament where human physicians were at work include:

Gen 50:2. A physician embalmed Jacob in Egypt.
Jer 8:22 The physicians of Gilead were considered worthless.
Hos 5:13 Ephraim turned for a cure to an Assyrian physician.
2 Chron 16:12 Asa relied on idolatrous physicians.

The sick also turned to priests and prophets for consultation and treatment. Leon–Dufour notes that "man practised exorcisms intended to get rid of evil spirits and implored God's pardon by supplication and sacrifices. Medicine was a function particular to priests.[290]

That prophets and priests, included the role of 'physician' is implied in several references (2 Sam. 12:14; 1 Kgs 14:1–13; 17:18–1 2 Kgs 1:1–4; 4:22; 8:9–10; Is. 38: 1, 21) and ordinary people had recourse to them when local practitioners failed.[291]

Various physicians through various remedies took care of different types of illnesses.

Specialisation though never exclusive of general practice, is found in the Old Kingdom (c.2700 – 2300 B.C.) with doctors known for their work on the abdomen, anus, eyes, teeth or 'inner liquids' and the like.[292]

This is supported by the fact that in Egypt about 420 B.C., Herodotus claimed that, "every physician treats one disease and not many; some are physicians for the eyes, others for the head, teeth, and abdomen or for unknown diseases."[293]

290 Leon Dufour (ed), Dictionary of Biblical Theology, London, 1970, p.543
291 D.J. Wiseman, Medicine in the Old Testament World, in "Medicine in the Bible", Op.Cit.,p.15
292 D.J.Wiseman, Medicine in the Old Testament World ... , p.16
293 Herodotus 11.84, quoted in D.J. Wiseman, "Medicine in the Bible, p.21

There were remedies for wounds, and surgery was also practised. The Egyptians give one remedy for a wound. The first day you (apply) meat (or grease) of an ox until it suppurates; but if it suppurates too much, then you will bandage it with mouldy barely bread until it is dried up ... if it closes over it's effluence then you will prepare grease and bandage it until it's mouth is opened and it suppurates.[294]

"The application of the meat was probably to prevent haemorrhaging and the mouldy bread may have served as an elementary antibiotic."[295] Fractures especially open fractures were considered fatal but when it happens the bones were set in splints. We remember the case of Pharaoh's broken arm in the book of Ezekiel (30:21). Operative surgery was also practised in Egypt and Mesopotamia. "In the second Millennium B.C. in Babylon, a number of Caesarean sections were performed when the mother died in labour and it was suspected that child was still alive."[296]

Mention ought to be made also of the female physicians and the nurses whom we know worked also as medical personnels in the ancient civilisation. Nurses and bandagers supported the doctors in the medical functions and "they were also associated with the art of embalming."[297] A few of the female doctors were named but their function was not indicated. This is probably because of the Jewish conception of women in those olden days when the Jews equated women with household properties and slaves. We know that a true Jew does not pray in the morning without thanking God for not creating him a woman or a slave. We know too that even in the New Testament, women were not included in the number of people. "They all ate as much as they wanted and they collected the scraps remaining twelve baskets full. Those who ate numbered about five thousand men, to say nothing of women and children." (Mt 14:20–21; 15:38; Mk 6:44; 8:9; Lk 9:17 Jn 6:13)

3.2.1.6 Healing in the New Testament

The scriptures of the New Testament have their setting in the Graeco–Roman world of the first century (Oikoumene), and Jesus, the apostles and the disciples were all from Palestine, the eastern angle of the empire.

294 Ebers, 522, quoted in D.J.Wiseman, Medicine in the Bible, p.21
295 D.J.Wiseman, Medicine in the Old testament world ... Op. Cit., p.21
296 Ibid., p.21
297 Ibid., p.16

Palestine had, before the time of Jesus had a fair share of hellenization and orientalization in which people shared almost a common world view symptomatic of a polytheistic society[298]

From our brief survey of the concept of sickness in the Old Testament or the pre–Christian culture, we noticed that in the civilisation surrounding the Jewish world, there were various diseases and illnesses with consequent remedies and physicians to take care of the afflicted. People had their own ideas and beliefs about sickness and diseases. They made a lot of efforts to combat or at least to diminish the bitter effects of diseases and sicknesses on themselves. In the apocalyptic expectations of the final stages of the Old Testament, men looked up to the great day of the Lord when God would come to destroy the power of evil in a great and final battle. (Apoc. 16:14) He will set up a New Kingdom where there would be no sickness or death or even weeping and crying. They were looking up to a time when all will be smooth sailing and everything will come to human perfection. But the great day of the Lord does not promise extinction of diseases and sicknesses. Sickness persisted in the New World of the Jews. According to the witnesses of the gospels, Jesus came in contact with many that were sick in mind, body, and the spirit. His attitude towards the presence of sickness in the lives of the people made considerable advance into the pre–Christian thought of diseases and sicknesses. It buttressed the fact that one of the major aspects of the unique ministry of Jesus consists of the care of the sick. This was such that Jesus was completely hostile to whatever made man sick or destroyed him. He was close to the sick and the feeble and identified himself with them. He healed numerous diseases of the most diverse types. (Mk 1: 32–34; 3:10; Lk 5:15; 8.2; Mt 4.23–24; 8:16; Jn 4–47–53).

There were no limits to the healing power of Christ. He healed men physically, spiritually, emotionally and mentally. He healed men in all their relationships with one another and with God.[299]

It is common in the gospel to see Jesus surrounded by the sick people of various kinds; the blind, the deaf, the lame, the paralytics, lepers, the deaf and the dumb, the insane and the lunatics. (Mk 7:32; Lk 4:40; Mt 11:4–5.) Such was his love for people especially those who were sick that W. Neil had this to say:

One of the basic facts of the historical ministry of Jesus, as recorded on page after page of the gospel record, and one which is given pride of place in the earliest preaching,

298 R.P. Martins, New testament foundations: A guide for students, Vol. 2, Acts – Revelation, Pater Noster press, Australia, Capetown, 1978, p.29

299 J.Turner, The healing Church, Op. Cit., p.9

is that by His power countless pain–ridden, blind, paralysed, deranged mortals were healed of their diseases ... If the gospel records are not to be dismissed as wholly fraudulent, we have to reckon with someone who had this unique power. The gospels merely give a handful of detailed cases out of what must have been thousands of cures.[300]

It was also noticed that,

When the sick flocked to Jesus during his earthly life, they recognised in him a friend whose deeply compassionate and loving heart responded to their needs ... These cures involved more than just healing sickness. They were also prophetic signs of his own identity and the coming of the kingdom of God, and they very often caused a new spiritual awakening in one who had been healed.[301]

The gospels specify that Jesus travelled through out Galilee teaching and healing all kinds of sicknesses and diseases. The admiration of the people was unbounded and they exclaimed, "He has done all things well, he makes the deaf hear and the dumb speak" (Mk 7:37). Even when he left Galilee, the people continued to follow him to other places. "Large crowds followed him, coming from Galilee, the Decapolis, Jerusalem, Judea and Transjordania" (Mt 4:25).

Jesus looked at sickness as an ailment that attacks both body and soul of the man and hence he approached each that came his ways as an integral entity. He was able to see clearly the influence of the body and the mind upon each other. The health or ill health of one obviously affected the other. He therefore uses all within his reach to bear upon the mental, physical and the moral illness of the people. While he was always concerned to heal the sick in body, he invariably paid close attention to the mind and spirit of the sick man. A typical example is shown in the care of the paralytic. (Mt 9:2–6; Mk 2: 3–12).

When some people brought to Jesus the paralytic lying on a bed, he saw their faith and said to the paralytic, 'courage, my child, your sins are forgiven'. And at this some scribes said to themselves, 'This fellow is blaspheming...' Jesus said to them, 'Why this evil thought in your mind...' And to the paralytic he said, 'Get up and pick your bed and go home'. This is an example of the wholistic care of the sick. Jesus demonstrated that he was able to bring forgiveness to a man's soul and health to the body and showing by that, that health in body and peace with God go hand in hand.

He first addressed the inner life of the sick man, giving him interior peace, 'courage your sins are forgiven'. He also took note of the faith and lack of faith of the people who brought the sick man before he concerned himself with the

300 W.Neil, The rediscovery of the Bible, London, in J.Turner, "The Healing Church", Op.Cit., p.10

301 K.O'Rourke, Medical Ethics; Sources of Catholic teaching, Op. Cit., p.134

healing of the body of the sick, 'pick up your bed and go home'. The sick person got what is called complete cure of the person.

The above cure of the paralytic and some other healings of Jesus seem to indicate that Jesus attributed the incidence of sickness to the operation of the evil (sin). 'Courage your sins are forgiven' (Mt 9:2; Mk 2:5) The disciples of Jesus also, very often, attributed physical defect to sin. They asked Jesus, "Rabbi, who sinned, this man or his parents for him to have been born blind?" (Jn 9:2) Here Jesus stated firmly that neither the man nor his parents sinned. "He was born blind so that the works of God might be displaced in him." (Jn 9:3) Another instance is the Johanine episode of the cure of the sickness at the pool of Bethzada, "Now you are well again, be sure not to sin any more, or something worse may happen to you." (Jn 5:14) These episodes mentioned however recognise that, in the New Testament, there is a connection between sin and sickness. But "Jesus breaks through the mechanical dogma of retribution (oepke), which was wide spread in the Old Testament and later Judaism"[302] He grants the sick healing and forgiveness. He did not give room to the old Testament religious problems of sickness which was associated with that of retribution originally conceived in temporal terms (Deut 28:21) nor did he support the concept of disease as punishment due to sin. (Ps 38,107) Jesus not only modified the ancient idea of sickness as coming from sin, but he preaches that his own kingdom will do away with every illness and infirmity as part of his triumph over Satan and sin. Looking closely at the episode in John, where the sick man at the pool of Bethzatha was cured, Gerard observed that "some sicknesses are directly linked to sin, at least to the human eyes: excess in smoking, alcohol abuse, sexual promiscuity, self indulgence in several areas."[303] These sicknesses, G. Ikeobi call "indiscretions and dissipations", and he enumerated them as follows:

over–eating, insufficient sleep, use of stimulants (snuff, cigarette, chewing gum etc), use of intoxicants, sexual excesses, emotional excesses, (fear, anxiety, sense of guilt etc), self centred life, superficial life, life without proper mission etc.[304]

All these can lead to sickness and death. "But this is not sin or sickness which is removed by Jesus in his healing. The healing is radical; and the sin goes beyond the human level and is linked to Satan himself"[305] "Sickness is no where

---

302 J.B.Bauer, Encyclopaedia of Biblical theology, London, 1970, p,847

303 G.Mackrell, The healing miracles in Mark's gospel, St Paul's publication, Slough, 1987, p.25

304 G.Ikeobi, Healing and Exorcism: The Nigerian Pastoral experience, in C.Manus et al., (eds), "Healing and Exorcism", Op. Cit., p.65

305 G.Mackrell, The healing miracles in Mark's gospel, Op. Cit., p.25

explicitly seen as the result of personal sin, even in the Johanine account of the healing of the paralytic (an isolated case in this matter)."[306]

3.2.2 Healing and Faith

"Faith is one of the most familiar words in the Christian vocabulary and yet it is one of the most misunderstood, and nowhere is this more true than in relation to healing."[307] Faith is an essential part of human personality. Without faith, man could not trust the other; man could not enter into relationship, what more entering into a transaction with one another:

> *This faculty to trust another's word and to have confidence in his ability to do as he says is the same faculty that enables us to trust God's word and His ability to do what he has promised.*[308]

So faith is essential in our relationship to one another and in our relationship to God our father. It is the same faith that one has when he goes to a human doctor to heal him medically of his ailment, that he should have when he goes to God our father, to heal him of that sickness which he believes only God can cure him. "For without faith, it is impossible to please God: He that cometh to God must believe that he is." (Heb. 11:6) According to J. Turner, "Faith is believing, it is perceiving, it is receiving."[309] This is particular in relation to healing. We believe that God will heal our sicknesses, a belief in something you do not see but only hope that it will be fulfilled and eventually by the grace of God the gift is imparted to us. God requires this faith in us, this trust in him to release his healing gifts. We remember the occasions of the healings of Jesus in the gospels. The case of the blind Bartimeus who cried out to Jesus from the roadside is a typical example.

> *Jesus son of David have mercy on me! And many rebuked him, telling him to be silent but he cried out all the more, 'Son of David have mercy on me!" And Jesus called him and asked what he wanted. 'Master let me receive my sight'. And Jesus said, Go your way, your faith has made you well (Mk 10:46–52).*

---

306 Ibid., p.25
307 J.Turner, The Healing Church, Op.Cit., p.41
308 G.Wright, Our quest for healing, Grene Hurst Press, Cheltenham Glos, U.K., 1981, p.73
309 J.Turner, The Healing Church, Op. Cit., pp.41–43

He also cured the two blind men by touching their eyes and saying, "Your faith has healed you... (Mt 9: 28–30). With this, it is clear that "it naturally follows that God expects to find faith in those who come to him for healing."[310] But this does not mean that one has no faith when he prays for healing and does not directly receive the healing. There are many dimensions of healings and there are many ways by which one can get healing. By faith said Haring, "one opens oneself to the saving and healing power that comes from God and touches the inner most being, as if a doctor were dwelling there."[311] It also signifies,

the abiding state of authentic Christians, in which context, the function of miracles or healings is to give new stimulus and vitality to the faith which Christians should be living fully.[312]

The onus of believing in order to be healed cannot be put on the sick alone. "God requires faith in those who minister to them as well. Sometimes he requires faith in friends and relatives."[313]

That God requires faith from the sick, his relatives and friends and the Ministers of healing to effect a healing in an individual defines and widens the opportunity given to all Christians to pray for the sick. With this in sight, we shall have a very brief survey on the importance of the faith of the Ministers and that of friends and relatives of the sick, in the context of healing.

3.2.2.1 Faith of the Ministers of Healing

After the glorious resurrection of Jesus Christ, before he ascended into heaven, he appeared many times to his apostles. He showed them himself and handed over to them the work of his father. "Go out to the whole world, proclaim the good news to all creation" (Mk 16:16).

And some signs, he enumerated will accompany those who believe: "in my name, they will cast out demons; they will speak in new tongues. They will pick up serpents... they will lay hands on the sick and they will recover" (Mk 16:17–18). Jesus gave the apostles, who were his immediate successors, the power to heal their sick brothers. Healing of the sick was one of the signs by which they will be known. The onus of healing was never placed on the sick alone but also on the Ministers. God requires faith in these Ministers as well in order to heal be-

---

310 G.Wright, Our quest for healing, Op. Cit., p.73
311 B.Haring, Heling and Revealing, Slough, London, 1984, p.46
312 R. Latourelle, The miracles of Jesus and the thology of miracles, New York, 1988, p.328.
313 G.Wright, Our quest for healing, Op. Cit., p.73–74

cause, the healings, they must do in the name of Jesus. Hence Paul, while recounting the story of their ministry in Jerusalem declared, "What miracles and wonders God had wrought among the gentiles through them" (Acts 15:12), and not what they have accomplished themselves.

The continuation of the work of Jesus can be accomplished only through those who believe. "He that believeth in me, the works that 1 do, shall he do also, said Jesus. (Jn 14:12) We see cases of healings done by the apostles and we realise that they were not left only to the faith of the sick. At Lystra, Paul perceived the cripple had faith and he said to him, "Stand up on thy feet. And he leaped and walked" (Acts 14:9–10). Another typical example of healing where the faith of the minister in the name of Jesus is clear is in the healing of the man who was lame from birth at the gate called beautiful. Peter and John directed their gaze at the lame man and Peter said, "Look at us ... I have neither silver nor gold ... in the name of Jesus of Nazareth, walk. And leaping up, the man stood and walked. (Acts 3:1–8) In this declaration, "Peter professes his faith in the Lord who is alive and present and who carries out the healing"[314] Stephen is another who stood out as a man full of grace and power, did great wonders and signs among the people (Acts 6:8).

> *We shall however note that in as much as faith is required of the ministers of healing, faith never refuse to conform to the requirements of the bible. Faith requests anointing with oil and the laying of hands. Faith presents her request in the plainest possible terms.*[315]

And one may quickly add that faith refuses to believe in the incompatibility of faith and medicine in the healing of the sick and never refuses to conform to the teaching authority of the Church. That is to say that it is not only faith that is required of the ministers of healing. The ministers are required to recognise the ordinary teaching authority of the Church and the importance and effect of medicine in the care of the sick.

When we encourage others to act in faith, we should encourage them well by readily sharing their responsibility with them. We shall encourage them by being deeply sympathetic and empathic and by sharing in their physical inability. We remember the case of Peter's mother–in–law, the first healing miracle recorded in the gospel of Mark. "Now Simon's mother–in–law lay sick with a fever, and immediately they told him of her. And he came and took her by the hand and lifted

---

314 E.Bressainin, Unzione degli Infermi, quoted in spiritual care of the family among the igbos of nigeria after "familiaris consortio" – D.Nwafor Anih, Romae, 1991, p.119

315 Ibid., p.82

her up, and the fever left her." (Mk 1:30–31) At the beautiful gate of the temple, we noticed what Peter did with the crippled; "He lifted up the crippled" (Acts 3:7). "Love never puts all the onus of acting in faith on the sufferer, but accepts its share of the responsibility"[316] So ministers of healing should always share in the fate of those to whom they are ministering unto.

3.2.2.2 Faith of Friends and Relatives

Several times Jesus spoke of the connection between his healing power and the faith of the people he heals. He also pays attention to the faith of the friends and relatives of those he heals of their sicknesses and misfortunes. There are obviously many, who are not able to help themselves when they are sick in whatever capacity. Some completely lose faith in the good God; some others find it difficult to pray at the time of sickness. One of the surest proofs of the evil nature of sickness is that it frequently makes prayer difficult, if not altogether impossible. Many of those who are unable to help themselves need all the help that can be given through the intercession of the others. In such cases, the prayer of faith must be offered by relatives and friends rather than by the sick person.

During the ministry of Jesus, he healed many people who were brought to him by friends and relatives. He also went to visit so many that were sick on the invitation of their friends and relatives. The cries of many touched the sympathetic heart of Jesus and he healed many that were sick and even raised some from the dead.

The healing of the epileptic boy is a beautiful example of Jesus healing through the faith of relatives.

> *And when they came to the crowd, a man came up to him and kneeling before him said, 'Lord have mercy on my son, for he is an epileptic and he suffers terribly; for often he falls into the fire, and often into the water... And Jesus answered, bring him here to me; and Jesus rebuked him and the demon came out of him, and the boy was cured instantly" (Mt 17:14–18; Mk 9: 14–21; Lk 9: 37–43).*

Looking critically at this healing work, one notices that the boy had no faith to believe, but Jesus expected the father to believe. Thus when Jesus said to the father of the boy, "If you can! All things are possible to him who believes", the man cried out and said, "I believe, help my unbelief" (Mk 9:23–24). In the case of the Paralytic, Jesus took note of the faith and lack of faith of the people who

---

316 E.Bressainin, Unzione degli Infermi, quoted in spiritual care of the family among the igbos of nigeria after "familiaris consortio" – D.Nwafor Anih, Romae, 1991, p.82

brought the sick man before he concerned himself with the healing of the sick person.

And behold, men were bringing on a bed, a man who was paralysed and they sought to bring him in and lay him before Jesus, but finding no way to bring him in, they went up to the roof of the house, and let him down through the tiles, into the midst before Jesus. And Jesus said, man your sins are forgiven. And the scribes and the Pharisees began to question... And to tell you that the son of man has authority to forgive sins, Jesus said, Rise up take up your bed and go home. (5:18–25: Mt 9:1–8).

There is also the case of Jesus healing the servant of the centurion on account of the faith of the centurion, instead of that of the servant. Such was the faith of the master that Jesus cried out saying "I have not seen a faith like this even in Israel" (Mt 8:5–13; Mk 7:1–10). There are many other instances in the gospel news where Jesus healed because of the faith of the friends and relatives of the sick.

3.2.2.3 Healing and Medical Help

There can be no doubt that the work of the doctors is abundantly blessed by God; or that suffering humanity owes a very great debt to the skill and devotion of the members of the medical profession; but, on the other hand, there are many who feel that they are lacking in faith if they make use of medicinal remedies.[317]

Any sane believer in divine healing of God who is also aware of the terrible scourge that sickness constitute for humanity will have nothing but admiration and lots of admiration for the progress which medical science is making against the evils of sickness. We have noted earlier in this work, that man tried to harness the forces in the universe to his own advantage and when he failed, he became notoriously religious. Similarly, man has since ages, made several attempts to eliminate sickness in the world but when he failed, he surrendered to the divine healing of sicknesses, thereby giving room to various types of healing ministry all over the corner of the earth. But should resignation to 'divine healing' dismiss every effort of the medical specialists to make use of herbs and medicines for the cure of human sickness?

The significance of this enquiry for a better understanding of the healing ministry of the Church cannot be over emphasised. The fact that some ministers of healing believe in the incompatibility of faith healing and medicine cannot be questioned or doubted. There are also many people who cannot understand why they should seek medical help while they are in prayer; they hold it that their faith will make them whole. It is clear that in spite of the monotheistic view of the He-

317 E.Howard Cobb, Christ Healing, London, Washington, Capetown, 1933, p.79

brews who viewed their God as the true healer that "forgives all sins and heals all diseases" (Ps 103:3), the human Physicians were very highly prized by their skills and learning. Hence Sirach wrote about Professional Physicians,

Honour the doctor with the honour that is due in return for his services; for he too has been created by the Lord. Healing itself comes from the most High, like a gift from a king ... The Lord has brought medicine into existence from the earth, and the sensible man will not despise them... He has also given men learning so that they may glory in his mighty works... My son when you are ill, do not be but pray to the Lord and He will heal you. Renounce your faults, keep your hands unsoiled ... Then let the doctor take over – the Lord created him too – and do not let him leave you... (Eccles 38:1–15)

If the powers of herbs and medicines and the practices of medical doctors were so much held in esteem and honoured among the Jewish society, that almost claimed the ownership of the Messiah, why should Christians of today deny the compatibility of faith and medicine? And yet both are geared towards achieving the same purpose, healing. God has regards for the Physicians, and that is why He too extols the physicians and the power of herbs. "Give the physician the honour due him" (Ecclus 38:1). The book of Ecclesiasticus noted too that the Lord brought medicine into existence and no sensible man will despise them. (Ecclus 38:4) There are other instances in both Testaments of the bible where human physicians were at work with herbs and medicines. They include:

Gen 50:2 – A Physician embalmed Jacob in Egypt.
Hos 5:13 – Ephraim turned for a cure to an Assyrian physician.
Ezk 30:21 – Pharaoh's broken arm was treated by the doctor.
Lk 8:43–48; Mt 9:20–22–1 Mk 5:25–34 – The woman with issue of blood had been bearing the sickness, for twelve years before she came to Jesus for a cure.

In the case of the woman with issue of blood, it is presupposed that she had been taking many medicines for that period of twelve years. For Mark said that "she had suffered much under many physicians and had spent up all that she had and was no better but grew worse" (Mk 5:26). The same experience, we should believe was applicable to many of the people healed by Jesus and even by the apostles during their ministries. Their ailments did not just start at the appearances of Jesus and the apostles.

The enquiry of medical help and faith is a matter that requires careful thought and concern. Many have made mistakes in their judgement of the use of one or both means of healing. Many are still making mistakes and some others will still make similar mistakes tomorrow. The case mentioned by E.H.Cobb in his book 'Christ Healing' is a classical example. He writes

Rev J.T. Butlin mentions such case where the patient was receiving ministration from him, and at the same time holding fast to his medicines. Nothing wrong in that, if he had been using the medicine in the belief that it was the way appointed for his healing. Mr Butlin perceived that, in this case, he was really trying both methods, for fear one should fail; and merely hoping that one or the other would prove successful. He told him therefore that he must choose between them. The patient gave up his medicine, put his whole trust in God, and at once began to recover his health.[318]

Now let us examine this case briefly.

The attitude of the sick man in this example may portray a lack of faith in the ministry of Rev. Butlin especially when it was discovered that the patient was trying both the ministry and the medicines for fear one may fail. Or it may be that the sick man had the faith that the prayers should complement the medicine he was taking, in which case Rev Butlin was wrong to have asked him to choose between his ministration and the medicine even though he began to recover his health when he gave up the medicine. The action of Rev Butlin in effect seems to give credence to the incompatibility of faith and medical help. He is not alone in this type of wrong practice of the healing ministry. Many ministers of today are still prone to the same understanding of the relationship between divine healing and use of medical help. Any wonder Archbishop A.K.Obiefuna clearly puts it thus, in the Onitsha Archdiocesan directives on healing ministry:

Religious healing ministry accompanied by prayer is in the realm of Worship. Therefore those authorised to use the gift if they have it should not persuade their clients to dispense with medical help. The healing ministry is not meant to substitute for the medical care of the sick. The task of the minister of religious healing differs from that of the medical people. Today many healing Ministers not only discourage their clients from seeing their doctors but even directly intrude into the sphere of the medical. This is an abuse and is in direct opposition to the advice of the bible which in the book of Sirach speaks thus: Treat the doctor with the honour that is his due, in consideration of his services for he too has been created by the Lord... The Lord brought forth medicinal herbs from the ground and no one sensible will dispense them (Sirach 38:1–15)[319]

It is known, that some healing ministers or groups hold the view that, some people resort to the use of medicines to heal themselves as a means, to avoid the penalty due to their sins, which is the sickness. This assertion once again brings to mind the wrong notion that sickness comes as a result of sin. It is also saying that man should not fight the scourges of sickness: that man should resign and accept sickness, without looking for a solution, and friends and relatives should not bother about seeing him recover. But how can a Christian stay beside the bed

318 E.H. Cobb, Christ Healing, Op.Cit., pp.82–83.

319 A.K. Obiefuna, Directives of Prayer Ministry and Healing Ministry in the Archdiocese of Onitsha, October 6, Onitsha, October 6, Onitsha, 1996, p.2

of a sick brother and offer no remedial help on the ground that the justice of God must prevail? How can a sensible human being, stand beside his brother wounded in a car accident, dying in pains on the ground that faith and not medicine should heal him? Why then was the Samaritan who bandaged and sent to a doctor, the man who was wounded by the robbers on his way from Jerusalem to Jericho named 'The Good Samaritan'? Why then had Isaiah no hesitation in ordering a poultice of figs for Hezekiah's complaint, though God had promised to heal him (2Kgs 20:1–7)? Why does the traditional Alor man bring home a little boy that fell down on the pathway and wounded himself, washes his wound with local soap and water, and smears the wound with liquid extraction from "Onugbo" leaves (bitter leaf)? Again why does the Nnobi woman run to her food store, brings uncooked cassava paste to smear it on the part of the body of a young girl who got burnt by boiling water while she was preparing the evening meals? All these are remedies applied to alleviate pains and heal wounds.

We must find the balance between this God–given instinct to seek alleviation in times of pain and sickness and prayer for healing. God gave us this instinct. God built the natural healing powers into our body. God gives us the prayer of faith ... Our very humanity demands that we do all in our power to alleviate pain and distress wherever we find it. Not to staunch the flow of blood from a cut artery, not to put a splint on a broken limb, not to bind up a wound after treating it with antiseptic – all of which must not be done if the use of means is contrary to the will of God – is to be false to our God–given nature. Even a dog or cat will sort out the grasses to correct its disorders.[320]

Our trust in God to supply our material needs does not in any way preclude help from man. A beggar who prays in the morning to God to provide his daily needs before he goes out to beg will not refuse helps from people because God has not brought the money directly to him. In the same way one should be mistaken to imagine that if he exposes himself to spiritual therapy, he should avoid all natural therapy or else he should be regarded as showing lack of faith. Such practice "is a dangerous fallacy and often leads to dire results and fanatical practices. The medical doctor is just as worthy of patient faith as is the minister who prays. Both seek the same end by different means, and the recovery comes from the selfsame source"[321]

If our common humanity demands that we do all in our power to alleviate suffering, how much more does our Christian faith? The Christian is the last person to be expected to criticise those who have dedicated their lives to the alleviation of suffering. One who refuses to ease another's suffering other than by prayer should be held in contempt, just as James holds in contempt the person who merely wishes well the brother who is a desti-

320 G.Wright, Our quest for healing, Op.Cit.,p.101
321 Ibid., p.98–99

tute. There is nothing contrary to the Christian way of life in doing everything possible to assist the healing powers of the body; it is what one should expect of the Christian.[322]

3.2.2.3.1 Healing and Suffering

The question of healing and Christian Suffering seems to be indispensable and complementary issues. The knowledge or understanding of either of the concepts enlightens and appreciates our perception of the other. An exaggeration or over–estimation of one or the other destroys the teaching of the Gospels of the two mysteries. Healing is as essential to the Christian Gospel as much as is suffering. And for healing to be of value, suffering must have a purpose. Hence it is said that, "in the life and person of Jesus Christ, the paradox of healing and suffering finds it's clearest expression"[323] Jesus is a healer par excellence. "They brought to him all who were sick and those possessed by the devil" (Mk 1:32) "and he cured them all." (Mtt16:16)

We read frequently from the gospels that Jesus healed all the sick that came to him in faith or were brought to him in faith by their friends and relations. "The healings of Jesus Christ was not just the curing of an ailment; it was releasing a person from bondage"[324] Jesus was an enemy to all those sickness which kept anyone back from loving God his father or from living the full human life. And this power to destroy sickness, he entrusted to his Church through his disciples. This gift and power is still available for the healing of the suffering humanity today. So the will of God for his people is health of body and soul and God himself is the healer.

The fact that God desires us to be healed of physical and emotional Sickness does not mean that we endorse an attitude that neglects suffering or omits the Cross. The gospel preached by Christ and his followers looks on Physical and Psychological sickness as an evil to be eradicated when it damages the quality of life. Suffering endured for the reign of God, suffering that entails transforming and liberating oppressive structures, is to be endured courageously for the sake of the gospel, not for its own sake.[325]

This in essence means that the gospel does not ascribe to any attitude that is exclusive of the other, such as over–emphasising the importance of as a response of a loving God to the neglect of suffering as an absolute evil that must be eradicated from a true Christian. The Gospel does not as well look upon suffering as a

322 G.Wright, Our quest for Healing, Op.Cit., p.101–102
323 M.Buckley, His Healing Touch, Op.Cit., p.140
324 B.M.. Meehan, The Healing Power of Prayer, Ligouri Publications, U.S.A., 1988, p.32
325 B.M.Meehan, The Healing Power of Prayer, Op.Cit., p.31

blessing that one has to look up to. It does not in any way exaggerate the spiritual importance of suffering as in the case of

many saints of centuries past who prayed for more pain and more grace, but never for healing. Healing they thought, would deprive them of the more perfect imitation of Christ and divert them from the path to heroic sanctity.[326]

This type of Suffering, Buckley refers to as "Blind Suffering."[327] God does not want us to suffer endlessly and pointlessly. There are lots of people who suffer needlessly and aimlessly because the gospel of healing was not preached to them or it has not brought it's light to bear on human suffering. Too many people are broken today in a way that neither give glory to God nor to man. They blame God for their suffering and hate him for it, thus adding to their inner turmoil because they have thought that suffering is a good thing sent by a loving God.

Suffering is always with man from the moment of birth to the time of death and it has shown itself a mystery to the Christian and a stumbling block to the unbeliever. It is not only that man does not want to be sick but, man does not want to endue suffering of any type at any time of his earthly life. And in the face of suffering, man has continued to ask, Why me?" But Jesus has given man an example to emulate.

When healing the sick and proclaiming the good news, Jesus in a deep Mystical sense is constantly on the road to Jerusalem, on the way to the cross, knowing that the scandalous history of the murder of the prophets in Jerusalem will be re–enacted in him (cf Mt 23: 33–39). His passion, death and resurrection became the inexhaustible fountain of redemption and healing love for all generations.[328]

Jesus has taught an example of suffering by his own passion and death, and his followers had to follow suit. Suffering accepted in union with Christ fosters both personal growth in holiness and a union with Christ's suffering that has value for the salvation of the world. When we unite our sufferings with those of Christ, we participate in the eternal sacrifice for the salvation of all men and women. We partake in the very type of suffering which Jesus himself bore and not just that physical or emotional suffering that is bone of sickness. Francis McNutt succinctly distinguished between two types of suffering:

The suffering that Jesus bore was the anguish of persecution, the type of suffering that comes from outside a person because of the misunderstanding of others. For example, Jesus warns his followers that they will be persecuted, and thrown in jail, that their

326 M.Buckley, His Healing Touch, Op.Cit., p.149

327 Ibid., p.149

328 B. Haring, Healing and Revealing, Op.Cit., p.29

enemies will be their own brothers and sisters, and that they are to be happy when these evil things occur.(Mt 10:16–33)

Likewise, Jesus suffered inner pain but the source of his suffering was outside himself. Jesus struggled with fear in the garden of Gethsemane; he was mocked, scourged, nailed to a cross, and died. However, Jesus did not suffer from physical or emotional sickness that is destructive to the wellbeing of the human person. Rather this was the type of suffering that He removed from those who came to him in faith.[329]

Through his healings, Jesus showed his mission of doing his father's will. Jesus by his healings showed God's plan for man not only in his own lifetime, but in our own time as well. When we pray for healing with other people, we share with them the good news of God's healing power. As the people of God, the ministers of God's healing love; we become channels of divine compassion, and open to whatever Jesus may do. Sometimes we may experience complete healing; sometimes we may discover a deep peace and a new acceptance of a difficult situation or relationship; sometimes we may reject or block God's healing. To minister then to people who suffer, we must have hope for physical and inner healing through the power of the cross, and resurrection of Jesus Christ. By so doing, suffering becomes joy and God is praised for the gift of healing, a visible manifestation of the resurrection.

3.2.2.3.2 Healing and Salvation

Whenever Jesus heals sick people, not only those who directly experience his healing love and power but also all who witness this event of God's nearness and power or who hear of it are called to a decision of faith: to Salvation. Just as in Christ, salvation and healing form an indivisible twofold offer, so the faith – response should not be to either health alone or to transcendental salvation alone. Christ calls for an integrated response in openness to salvation and health, loving adoration of God, healthy personal relationships and entrance into the kingdom of God–which is also a kingdom of saving justice and healing love.[330]

The call to salvation is essentially a call to faith. And we have earlier observed that one cannot talk of healing without faith. The person that needs healing has to believe that he should be healed before going for healing. Healing and salvation are so interwoven and they cannot be separated just as we cannot truly talk of healing without paying due respect to faith. To think of healing is therefore to think of salvation. Even the holistic expression "salus" of the Latin lan-

329 F.McNutt, Healing, Ave Maria press, 1974, in B. Meehan, "The healing power of prayer", p.31

330 B.Haring, Healing and Revealation, Op.Cit., p.16

guage is the origin of the Italian "salvezza" meaning salvation and "salute" meaning health.

In Christ Jesus, salvation and healing form an indivisible entity. "Thanks to Jesus, the healing of the Spirit and of the body becomes an evident sign that the kingdom of God is about to come."[331]

Any division of healing and salvation falls short of wholeness and deprives all around the scene of healing of the profession of faith and gratitude to God. Precisely why Jesus always heals both body and spirit. In the healing of the Paralytic who was brought to him by his relations, Christ healed the spirit "Your sins are forgiven you" (Lk 5:20; Mt 9:2) before he healed the body "Take up your bed and go home" (Lk 5:24; Mt 9:6). Similarly, M. Petrini observes that,

> *when Jesus cures a leper or proclaims the parable of the Good Samaritan, he shows compassion for those who suffer, but there is something more. His gesture announces a new life of the kingdom, the total and permanent cure of the human person in all his dimensions and his relations.*[332]

In the ministry of Jesus Christ, it is obvious that preaching, teaching and healing went together and each was an integral part of his offer of salvation. Hence his injunction to his disciples: As you go, proclaim that the kingdom of heaven is close at hand. Cure the sick and raise the dead, cleanse the lepers, cast out devils. (Mt 10:7–8)

The Church participates in Christ's struggle against evils and furthers his desires to bring salvation, healing and freedom as well as victory over suffering and death. So the life which the Church is called upon to preach is

> *the fullness of the gift of grace which fills the total life experience of man, taking on his vocation to health in order to transfigure it into a vocation to salvation and taking on his vocation to salvation in order to turn it into a service of love for man, the whole man and all men.*[333]

Hence the woman who pushed her way through the crowd to be healed by Jesus heard the words "Woman your faith has made you whole." (Mt 9:12; Mk 5:28) And whenever the Church teaches the good news of Jesus and bring healing to man, they

---

331 M.Petrini, Medicina e Pastorale in "Dizionario di Teologia Pastorale Sanitaria", Op. Cit., p.710

332 Ibid., p.710

333 L.Sandrin, The Church: A healing Community, in Dolentium Hominum, Op.Cit., p.73

radiate both joy of the gospel and healing love and diakonia and people are effectively called to faith, to salvation in all its dimensions, including a higher level of wholeness, healthier personal and social relationships, a healthier life style and a more wholesome form of public life.[334]

This is very evident in his healing works. Christ heals the sick and also forgives him of his sins – a total healing expressed very well in the etymology of the word salvation. The etymology itself indicates that health and salvation are inter–related and can be understood only in a holistic vision, though that does call for careful distinctions. Christ came into the world so that men may have life and have it in abundance. (Jn. 10:l0) This is the wholeness desired by God for men but man alienated himself from God by his sins and lost the wholeness which is only healed by God by the forgiveness of sins.

Alienation or separation from God (sin) leaves the individual and his or her relationships to others and the environment unprotected. This makes the person vulnerable to disease (or disintegration) and death (Gen 3:19).[335]

There is therefore the need for one to, first receive Jesus Christ as the bearer of Salvation, which indeed brings healing. "Christ does this by his double work on the cross: forgiving, redeeming and reconciling on one hand; healing (re–integration) on the other hand."[336] The case of the healing of the paralytic is a beautiful example. (Mk 2:5–12) The Psalmist also expressed that well "Praise the Lord, my soul and do not forget how kind he is. He forgives all my sins and heals all my diseases." (Ps 103:2–3)

3.2.2.3.3 Healing and Exorcism

The mission of Jesus Christ entrusted to his Church entails also the driving out of the evil spirits or casting out of demons generally known as exorcism. "He summoned his twelve disciples and gave them authority over unclean spirits with power to cast them out and to cure all kinds of diseases and sickness (Mt 10:1; Mk 6:7). Writing on healing, G. Mackrell says "it would be difficult to find a more dramatic and more apt beginning to the healing ministry of Jesus than the exorcism described in the first chapter of Mark's gospel."[337] In their Synagogue just then, there was a man possessed by an unclean spirit, and it shouted, "What

---

334 B.Haring, Healing and Revealing, Op.Cit., p.17

335 E.A.Allen, Wholeness, Salvation and the Christian Health Professional, in Eric Ram (ed), "Transforming Health", Marc publications, U.S.A. 1995, p.20

336 E.A.Allen, Wholeness, Salvation ..., Op. Cit., p.21

337 G.Mackrell, The Healing Miracles, Slough, England, 1987, p.32

do you want with us, Jesus of Nazareth? Have you come to destroy us? I know who you are, the Holy One of God." But Jesus said sharply, "Be quiet! Come out of him!" And the unclean spirit threw the man into convulsions and with a loud cry went out of him. The people were so astonished that they started asking each other what it all meant.

"Here is a teaching that is new", they said, "and with authority behind it" he gives orders even to unclean spirits, and they obey him." (Mk 1:23–27) So among the first healing works of Jesus was the case of exorcism. Exorcism is categorised as one of the three major types of the healing miracles of Jesus. We therefore cannot do our work on healing in isolation of exorcisms. Many authors and source books have treated the two terms in close connection with one another.

While discussing healing, one author sees exorcism as "referring to the use of prayer or charms to expel evil spirits and so bring about restoration – a healed state."[338] Exorcism is also defined as "the ceremonial or ritualistic expulsion of an evil Spirit"[339] and to exorcise means "to drive out or rid somebody of an evil spirit by prayer or magic".[340] That is to say that exorcism is an act of driving out demons or evil spirits from persons, things and places in order to bring sanity to the desired person or object. "The exercise consists in prayer to God to effect the expulsion of the evil one. Such prayer may be public – that is in the name of the Church or private"[341] Prayer is essential in the life of the minister of exorcism. The exorcist as a healing minister must heal himself before engaging in the practice of exorcism. The case of the epileptic boy in the gospel says much on this. The boy was both epileptic and demoniac. The father first went to the disciples of Jesus for cure but they could not be of any help. On the arrival of Jesus, the man pushed his way through the crowd to Jesus asking that his son be healed, adding that the disciples had tried in vain to heal the epileptic. Jesus then asked for the boy. But the crowd reported that he was dead as the boy was lying like a corpse after the convulsions. (Mk 9:26) "But that was only a stage of the epileptic attack."[342] The boy's father indicated this by saying that the demon was always

---

338 R.Eya, Healing and Exorcism: The Psychological aspcts, in Manus C. et al., (eds) "Healing and Exorcism: The Nigeria experience" Op. Cit., p.44

339 Encyclopaedia of Witchcraft and Magic, p.81, in Ikeobi ,Healing and Exorcism: Pastoral Experience, in "Healing and Exorcism: Nigeria Experience", Op. Cit., p.57

340 Oxford Advanced Learners Dictionary, p.403

341 M.Eneja, Goodwill Message, in "Healing and Exorcism: The Nigeria experience", Op.Cit., p.164

342 John Richards, But Deliver us from evils, pp.98–99, in G. Ikeobi, Healing and Exorcism, The Nigeria pastoral experience, in "Healing and Exorcism: The Nigeria experience", Op. Cit., p.68

slow to leave him. It was at this stage that the master took up the boy by hand and helped him up and he was able to stand. (Mk 9:27) Later the disciples asked why they were unable to achieve this, and the reply of Jesus was, "This kind cannot be driven out by anything but prayer and fasting". (Mk 9:29)

Some human problems, complex as they are in their nature, give way to, and suggest the use of the act of driving out of evil spirits. They cut across all levels of society and span all facets of life. According to Haring,

> *In many tribes and traditionalist cultures, there is still a widespread fear of witches and all kinds of witchcraft. Whenever serious afflictions come in form of sickness, sterility, miscarriage, the death of a beloved one or other calamities, they tremble in fear of evil spirits and look for 'evil men' or women who might be agents of evil spirits (witches) acting out of jealousy, enmity or vindictiveness... This is surely an atmosphere in which the prince of darkness can use their weaponry of deception and hatred.*[343]

"As a reaction to all this, in many regions anti–magic processes have been devised, systems of divination to discover the witches, the rite and sacrifices meant to dictate vicious omens or placate the spirits".[344] C. Ejizu has similar notion on the activities of these spirits and how they can be attacked and driven away. He says,

> *All forms of misfortunes, including sickness, barrenness, mental illness, failure of crops, drought, premature death, unhappy family life etc are explained by the activities of ubiquitous evil spirits, angry gods, revengeful ancestors and evil forces operating through man and nature. They are all together negative. And man must resist them with all the resources available to him, including placating gods and spirits.*[345]

The fact that Jesus practised exorcisms during his ministry is not disputed. The fact that He gave the authority to his disciples to cast out evil spirits is not under debate. What some people contended in the time of Jesus was the authority with which He drove away the malign spirits. Some of the official Jewish religious groups accused Jesus of casting out devils through the power of Beelzebub, the prince of Devil (Mt 12:24). If Jesus casts out demons through the power of Beelzebub, his kingdom cannot stand because a kingdom divided against itself cannot withstand the attacks or onslaught of the enemies.

But Jesus noted that his miracles including the exorcisms were evidence of the presence of the kingdom. "But if it is by the finger of God that I cast out demons, then the kingdom of God has come upon you" (Lk 11:20; Mt 12,28).

---

343 B.Haring, Healing and Revealing, Op.Cit., pp.65–66

344 Ibid., p.66

345 C.Ejizu, Cosmological Perspectives on Exorcism and Prayer–healing, in "Healing and Exorcism:The Nigeria Experience", Op.Cit., p.18

The activity of Jesus as an exorcist is quite consistent with the Messianic kairos, for the destruction of the reign of the demons was to manifest an essential aspect of God's final victory over evil. The expulsion of demons was to 'signal' the arrival of the kingdom.[346]

In the world today, what is under debate is not whether evil spirits exist or whether they can be cast out, The issue in question is whether what people claim to be the attacks of evil spirits are actually true possession of the evil ones, and the acclaimed expulsions, actually exorcism. The authenticity of some methods of exorcism today is also under great debate. Christ casts out demons with firm and authority such that people were astonished at how he gave orders to the evil spirits who promptly obeyed him. "Jesus can display a gentle bedside manner in his healings. This seldom applies to the exorcisms. Here he goes into the attack immediately"[347]

Having briefly explained the concept of Healing and Exorcism, we shall now endeavour to x–ray the history of Exorcism vis–à–vis Miraculous Healing.

According to Lexikon für Theologie und Kirche, "exorcism is derived from the Greek word exorkizein which means the ritual expulsion or exile of evil powers or spirit from persons, living beings or objects. Its method can be used or proved in all cultures and serve totally as cleansen or healing process. The exorcist assume a special and antagonising image to drive away the evil forces. Who does this must be gifted such persons are for example: Priests, Schamanan and the medicine men. And this process of healing or exorcism is performed in the name of God through prayers powerful words, laying on of hand ..."[348]

Hence, "Catholic exorcisms begin, Adjure te, spiritus nequissime, per Deum omnipotentem ... which means "I adjure thee, most evil spirit, by almighty God

346 R.Latourelle, Theologie de la Revelation, 471–472, in R.Latourelle, "The Miracles of Jesus and The Theology of Miracles", Op. Cit., p.42

347 G.Mackrell, The Healing Miracles, Op.Cit., p.32

348 Exorzismus ist die rituelle Vertreibung od. Verbannung böser Mächte od. Geister aus Personen, Lebewesen od. Gegenständen. Praktiken des E. sind in allen Kulturen nachweisbar u. dienen der ganheitl. Renigung bzw. Heilung. Der E. setzt die Vorstellung antagisierender Kräfte bzw Gewalten voraus. Wer ihn ausübt, verfügt über eine besondere Begabung, etwa Priester, Schamanan, Medizinmänner; sie sind im Kontext der jeweil. Religion "göttl. Menschen". Im Namen od. Im Auftrag der überlegnen Macht wird durch bestimmte Worte (Formeln, Zaubersprüche, Gebete), Gesten (Handauflegung, Anblasen, Tanz), Materiallen (Wedel, Arznein) dem Einfluss der unliebsamen Kräfte präventiv od. kurativ Einhal geboten. – L.Thk Bd 3, 1995, pp.1125 &1126)

... (in Lewis,J.)"[349] The Catholic Church considers possession as an integral part of their spiritual practices.

Hence Martin Ebner writes in his (Jesus – ein umstrittener Exorzist) "An exorcism is a force between two powerful entities. Humanly speaking is an obvious confrontation between the exorcist and the person possessed"[350]

The word which is not itself biblical is derived from *exorkizo*, which is used in the Septuagint (Genesis 24:3 = cause to swear; III(I) Kings 22:16 = adjure), and in Matthew 26:63, by the high priest to Christ, "I adjure thee by the living God ..." The non–intensive *horkizo* and the noun *exorkistes* (exorcist) occur in Acts 19:13, where the latter (in the plural) is applied to certain strolling Jews who professed to be able to cast out demon. Expulsion by adjuration is, therefore, the primary meaning of exorcism, and when, as in Christian usage, this adjuration is in the name of God or of Christ, exorcism is a strictly religious act or rite. But in ethnic religions, and even among the Jews from the time when there is evidence of its being vogue, exorcism as an act of religion is largely replaced by the use of mere magical and superstitious means, to which non–Catholic writers at the present day sometimes quite unfairly assimilate Christian exorcism. Superstition ought not to be confounded with religion, however much their history may be interwoven, nor magic, however white it may be, with a legitimate religious rite.

The Word demon originated from the ancient Greek word *daimon* which referred to beings with special powers which placed them between people and the gods. The beings could bestow benefit or carry out the punishment of the gods. (in Microsoft Encarta, 1994) The questions arise, "Do demons exist?", "can they possess a person's body and cast away the person's soul?". In affirmation Martin Ebener asserts:

> "Demons are understood like squatters in a House. They depend on a foreign body to exist: on the body of an animal or a person"[351]

Every major religious and cultural tradition worldwide has espoused the idea of spirit possession and the need for some form of exorcism. The rites of exorcism have included the use of prayers, commands, fumigations (burning of dung), holy water, hellebore, rue, salt, and roses. The Old Testament shares, "David took a harp, and played with his hand: so Saul was refreshed, and was well, and

---

349 Lewis, J.R., Encyclopedia of Afterlife Beliefs and Phenomenon, Detroit, MI: Visible Ink Press, 1995, p.138

350 Ebner, M. Jesus – ein umstrittener Exorzist in Bibel und Kirche, 61. Jahrgang 2. Quartal 2/2006, p.73

351 Ibid., p.73

the evil spirit departed from him" writes in Wickland.[352] In some cultures the exorcist functioned in much the same way doctors do now; people would visit the exorcist seeking a cure for illness, misfortune, or bad luck.

Our historical journey of spirit possession takes us back to the beginning of civilization. All forms of sickness, both physical and psychological, were attributed to possessing spirits in ancient Mesopotamia. The number of possessing spirits and demons waiting to attach to a person were so great it lead to a fear described by Sargant as "one of the most important factors in the daily life of a Babylonian"[353] Ancient Babylonian priests served as exorcists who performed the ritual by destroying a clay or wax image of a demon meant to destroy the attached spirit (in Microsoft Encarta, 1994). Assyrian tablets offer the first written accounts for the treatment of illnesses. Treatment included incantations and prayers to the gods, as well as direct challenges to the demons which were believed to inflict diseases of every type.

Jesus was the premier exorcist of his time. As much as ¼ of Jesus' healings were exorcisms. The ability to cast out evil spirits was a sign of true discipleship among the apostles. At least 26 references to exorcisms by Jesus may be found in the bible, including, "Jesus preached and cast out devils," Mark 1:39. "Jesus gave his twelve disciples the power against unclean spirits, to cast them out," Matthew 10:1. "The evil spirits went out of them," Acts 19:12. "Jesus rebuked the foul spirit, saying unto him, Thou deaf and dumb spirit, I charge thee, come out of him, and enter no more into him. And the spirit cried, and rent him sore, and came out of him: and he was as one dead, insomuch that many said, He is dead. But Jesus took him by the hand, and lifted him up; and he arose," Mark 9:25–27 In the exorcism of a madman Jesus had cast out the foul spirits; the spirits then entered into a herd of pigs that in turn ran over a cliff and drowned in the waters below.

In many parts of the world spirit possession is strongly related to cultural and social conditions. Considered to have originated in Ethiopia varying forms of *zar* (sometimes called *sar)* possession are known to occur. *Zar* spirits typically possess women whose husbands are considering marrying an additional wife, or where other domestic conflict is present. Exorcism of the *zar* spirit entails an elaborate, and costly, dance ceremony for the victim. After the expensive ceremony wives have been known to threaten a relapse if their demands are not met; consequently extorting further economic sacrifices from their husbands. Posses-

352 Wickland, C.A., 30 Years Among the Dead, USA: Newcastle Publishing Co. Inc. 1974, p.18

353 Sargant, W., The Mind Possessed: A Physiology of Possession, Mysticism and Faith Healing. New York: Penguin Books, Inc. 1973, p.59

sion due to unmet needs and exorcisms which function to meet those needs is not uncommon. The "*zar* possession strategy" to get needs met has been adopted by women (and some men) throughout the world: Muslim Somali, Muslim Sudan, Egypt, parts of North Africa, Arabia, East Africa, Arabia, South America, China, Japan, SE Asia, Ceylon, Tanzania, and Cairo[354].

Accounts from the 4th century AD depict gruesome portrayals of exorcism. Zeno of Verona describes, "His face is suddenly deprived of colour, his body rises up of itself, the eyes in madness roll in their sockets and squint horribly, the teeth, covered with a horrible foam, grind between blue–white lips; and limbs twisted in all directions are given over to trembling; he sighs, he weeps; he fears the appointed day of Judgment and complains that he is driven out; he confesses his sex, the time and place he entered into man…."[355]

The middle Ages (500–1500AD) saw a revival of ancient superstition and demonology. The treatment of mental illnesses was primarily left to the clergy who believed evil spirits were the cause. The devils were exorcised through a variety of techniques which caused physical pain, including scourging. The Roman Catholic Church continued developing the formal rite of exorcism during the medieval era. By 1614 the *Rituale Romanum* was complete; it is still in use today. Between 1970 and 1980 the Catholic Church conducted over 600 exorcisms.

Epidemics of spirit possession have been known to occur. One famous epidemic of demonic possession took place during the 17th century at Loudun. Numerous nuns came down with the affliction. Sister Jeanne des Anges wrote in her memoirs (1640's), "My mind was filled with blasphemies and sometimes I uttered them without being able to stop myself. My thoughts were often bent on devising ways to displease him (God) and to make others trespass against him…As I went up for Communion the devil took possession of my hand, and when I received the Sacred Host and had half moistened it, the devil flung it into the priest's face. I know full well that I did not do this action freely, but I am fully assured to my deep confusion that I gave the devil occasion to do it."[356] One of the exorcists of the Loudun possessions, Father Surin, wrote to a friend, "I have engaged in combat with four of the most potent and malicious devils in hell."[357] A lucid outbreak of demonic possession also occurred at a convent in Madrid during the same century. Upon reviewing the Loudun case Aldous Huxley concluded that what began as hysteria turned into an epidemic of demonic

354 Lewis, I.M., Ecstatic Religion: An Anthropological Study of Spirit Possession and Shamanism, Baltimore, MD: Penguin Books Ltd., Baltimore, 1971.

355 Sargant, W., Op. Cit., p.47

356 Sargant, W. The Mind Possessed: A Physiology of Possession, Mysticims and Faith Healin. Op. Cit. p.51

357 Ibid., p.51

possession due to the actions of the exorcists who played on the nuns heightened suggestibility; the same explanation was put forth by an author of that time who wished to remain anonymous.

Today, science has become the only solution for every kind of problem. No room for anything not based on "proofed" facts. But there should be room for faith. Faith can help people go through crisis where pills become useless. That is why Bettina Eltrop maintained in 'Wunder – Geschichten von Gottes Kraft' that "Miracle is an event that cannot be explained by natural law or a violation of the order of nature".[358] In other words, it is when the impossible happens. It is when doctors have given up on a sick child and for no scientific reason that child gets well. Faith is part of human nature and therefore shouldn't be negated.

Having discussed healing and exorcism, we shall now focus our attention on the catholic charismatic renewal in the Igbo society.

3.2.2.4 Catholic Charismatic Renewal in the Church in Igbo Society

Preamble:

> Charismatics read and pray the Scriptures so avidly because they find that the Scriptures interpret for them what God is doing in their hearts. By the grace of "baptism in the Spirit" in fervent faith and love they have "come alive" to Christ and the Holy Spirit and God is present to them working in their hearts.[359]

The Tradition of divine healing within the Church as we have seen has been long and well documented. Christians in all the ages believed in the miraculous intervention of God to heal. We cannot adequately discuss any Charismatic movement or renewal without tracing it's origin from the divine healing or healing gifts of the Church just as we cannot fairly discuss the healing ministry today without talking of the Charismatic movement or the Charismatic renewal. The history of Catholic Charismatic Renewal anywhere in the World cannot be adequately treated without tracing the history of the Pentecostal and Charismatic movements in America. The Catholic Charismatic Renewal of Nigeria just like the American Charismatic Movement and any other Charismatic Renewal in the world is a direct descendant of the Pentecostal Movement which was initiated in America by Charles Parham, the father of the twentieth–century Pentecostal Movement. The Pentecostal Movement was the offshoot of the later Nineteenth

358 Eltrop,B., Wunder – Geschichten von Gottes Kraft in Bibel und Kirche, Verlag Katholisches Bibelwerk, 61. Jahrgang 2/2006 Stutttgart, p.63

359 Paul Hinnebusch, The Bible in the Charismatic Movement, in W.R.Farmer and co. (eds), "The International Bible Commentary", Liturgical Press, Collegeville, Minnesota, 1998, p.156

Century Divine Healing Movement in America, a movement that was formed as a result of the scattered demonstrations of healing within various religious communities in the 17th and 18th centuries. "The significance of the movement lies in its uniqueness to popularise in America a concept of Salvation that includes health and healing as an integral part."[360] The healing Movement or Faith Healing, Faith Cure or Divine Healing as it is often called,[361] refers to that group of people who maintain the belief that physical disease or illness is cured by the Supernatural intervention of God in response to the prayer of faith... Since the inception in America of the Pentecostal movement and the later Charismatic movement, divine healing has been an integral and universal part of their Gestalt of doctrines.[362]

3.2.2.4.1 Pentecostal Movement

Charles Parham is the father of the twentieth–century Pentecostal movement. Parham began his healing ministry in 1897, some months after he was healed of a major heart problem in Ottawa, Kansas. In 1898, he moved his ministry to Topekas, Kansas where he established a divine healing home to which people came from all parts of America to receive healing and "mighty miracles", took place there. He also ran a Bible College there named Bethel Bible College. Desiring to learn through other healing ministries, he travelled to Chicago in 1899 to visit Dowie's healing home; to Nyack, New York to visit Simpson's Berachach home; and to A.J. Gordon's work in Boston. By 1901, his Pentecostal message made him notorious at his Bible College, but that did not last so long. In his message, "he insisted that the speaking in other tongues is an inseparable part of the baptism of the Holy Spirit and was the only Bible evidence for this experience."[363] By 1903, the new Pentecostal message was already accepted. He succeeded in combining divine healing and the Pentecostal message of the Baptism in the Holy Spirit.

As his ministry developed and grew, he began to open branches in various parts of America, using the disciples he trained in his Colleges. Very prominent among his disciples was a black Holiness Minister William J. Seymour who attended Parham's College at Houston (opened 1905).

He was sent to Los Angeles to share the Pentecostal message with the Local Church of a black woman there, a meeting that gave birth to a centre popularly

360 P.G.Chappell, Healing Movements, in Burgess S.M.&McGee G.B. (eds), "The dictionary of Pentecostal and Charismatic Movement," Grand Rapids, 1988, p.353

361 Ibid., p.353

362 Ibid., p.353

363 P.G. Chappell, Healing Movements, Op.Cit., 368

known as the Azusa Street Revival, which attracted people nation wide. From the Azusa Street Revival, the Pentecostal message was spread world wide, and from 1906 until 1932 Pentecostal denominations were formed across the country.[364]

The Azusa street revival ministry grew so much that W. Seymour, from 1906 was requesting Parham to assist him in the ministry at Los Angeles. On one of his visits to Los Angeles, Parham had to visit Zion, a city with splintered and disunited people in September 1906. His visit to Zion made Zion the second most significant centre in the world for the spreading of the new Pentecostal movement.

> *Parham travelled to different branches of the Christian Catholic Church throughout America and Canada and was successful in converting most to the Pentecostal doctrine. Some of Parham's Zion followers were responsible for planting the Pentecostal message in different countries such as South Africa, Australia, Holland, Switzerland, Jamaica and India.*[365]

So with Parham, Pentecostal movement began to penetrate the walls of the Catholic Church. Here we must note that the movement was not easy sailing for Parham. "His Pentecostalism suffered a set back when it was condemned by the World's Christian Fundamental Association in 1928 as a threat to the Christian Church."[366]

3.2.2.4.2 The Catholic Charismatic Renewal of Nigeria

The Catholic Charismatic Renewal of Nigeria (C.C.R.N) and not Catholic Charismatic Renewal Movement (C.C.R.M) came into being as a result of prayer groups formed at the University of Ife and the Dominican Community at Ibadan by some Dominican priests and brothers in 1972. The formation of these groups was credited to two Dominican priests, Fr. Richard Farmer and Fr. Chukwubikem Okpechi. Richard Farmer initiated the prayer meeting at the University of Ife in October 1972.

Soon after, in March 1973, Bro. Stephen, also a Dominican, Mr. Paul Anie and some others established the "Upper Room Community Prayer Group" in

---

364 Ibid., p.368

365 P.G.Chappell, Healing Movements, p.368

366 Any new movement in the Church is always looked upon with some caution especially by the authority of the Church. The Pentecostal movement was not a exception. Sometimes some of the new movements are often radical and seen as a threat to the life of the Church. The World Christian fundamental Association was not therefore a coward to sense the Pentecostal Movements a threat to the Christian Churches.

St. Dominic's Parish Yaba. From these first groups, the renewal began to grow and spread gradually to other parts of the nation.

The Catholic Charismatic Renewal received greater national publicity and impetus in 1974 with the visit of Francis MacNutt and his team.

Francis MacNutt (PhD, from Harvard and former priest), whose ministry and books on healing have had a significant impact on the ministry of healing in America, was influenced by the ministries of Agnes Sandford and Rev. Alfred Price (one of the Episcopalian founders of the healing ministry, The Order of St. Luke the Physician).[367]

Fr. Francis visited Nigeria between October and November 1974 and his team criss–crossed Nigeria holding Retreat–Seminar on the Charismatic Renewal. The team travelled to Jos, Uyo, Onitsha, Benin, Ife and Ibadan, at which some 1,500 persons including priests, sisters and two bishops, were prayed for 'baptism in the spirit'.[368]

The Catholic Charismatic Renewal as it were, became popular and spread to every nook and corner of the society.

The Catholic Charismatic Renewal from its inception was seen as a Welcome Church Society[369] that would contend with the 'encroachments' of Pentecostals and other sects on the Catholic Church that had led to the defection of some Catholics to such groups.[370]

Yet it had its initial teething problems, because of the attitude of some of its members who were so to say over–enthusiastic and less informed. According to J. Faniran:

Members became more and bolder in the demonstration of their Charismatic gifts. Ultra–Pentecostal teaching and practices began to circulate, particularly among the students members in the tertiary institutions of learning. These soon graduated and while on National Youth Service, some of them became itinerant teachers and spread newly acquired Pentecostal teachings and practices. Their belief was that after a false trial followed for two thousand years, the true Church, the Church of the Spirit, is now in the process of being born, and they have been anointed to bring about this new Church. The cherished Tradition of the Catholic Church, Ecclesiastical offices, the sacraments and the various devotions, particularly those to Mary, the mother of God came under violent at-

367 G.P.Chappell, Healing Movements, in Dictionary of Pentecostal and Charismatic Movements, Op. Cit., p.373

368 Bradley P. Bolt, Healing in the Charismatic Movement: "The Catholics in Nigeria, Religions, Nsukka", Vol.,2, No.2, Dec., 1977, p42

369 The Catholic Charismatic Renewal in Nigeria do not like to be addressed as a society or movement. Just call it a renewal

370 R.Diala, Phenomenon of Healing Ministry in Eastern Nigeria, Unpublished Ph.D. Thesis, Rome 1997, p.77.

tack. This led to tension, confusion and general malaise in the Church in many parts of the Country.[371]

With some of these developments found among some of the Charismatic Renewal members in Nigeria, the Renewal did not gain any easy acceptance within the Catholic Church in the area. The Church Hierarchy, the priests and most informed lay faithful were afraid of what the group would turn into. This is not common with the Nigerian Church only, as Louis Nwankwo unfortunately observed in one of his write–ups. According to him:

> *CCR was started in the United States of America in 1967. It was welcomed by the American priests, the hierarchy and the people. Here in Nigeria, it came into existence by the middle of 1970. It was brought into the country by some American and European priests. The lay people in Nigeria welcomed it, but ironically the priests and the hierarchy rejected it. In fact, some Nigerian priests treated the renewal as an Out cast that must be killed. The Nigerian Parish Priests as if all had a meeting refused to allow the operation of the Renewal in their Parishes, even though the Parishioners were ready to belong to the Renewal.*[372]

This is an over–statement on the part of L. Nwankwo. The Hierarchy and the priests of Nigeria did not reject the Renewal neither did the lay people embrace it without asking questions. It is only the ignorant and the uninformed that would welcome such a new movement without asking questions. Nwankwo should have understood that the Hierarchy and the priests were only trying to "guard and preserve the religious Tradition"[373] handed down to them as he rightly observed somewhere in his writing. So nobody should blame the other for moving cautiously. No one is to be blamed for fearing the end–result of some of the activities of the Renewal since it was new and in some cases over–enthusiastic and radical in actions, and more so as it was a full descendant of the Pentecostal movement. In fact, the Hierarchy and the priests will be blamed by the same source, if they have quickly and without exercising enough caution embraced the Renewal and allowed it to cause havoc to the Church with its Pentecostal doctrines and teachings. In the United States, the CCR did not even gain any easy acceptance by the

---

371 J.Faniran, Charism and Authority: A case study of the Charismatic Renewal in Nigeria Church; "Nigerian Journal of Theology, Vol.7, No.1" June 1993, p.71

372 L.C.Nwankwo, Nigerian Priest and Catholic Charismatic Renewal of Nigeria (CCRN), in A.N.O. Ekwunife et al., (eds), "Renewal of Priestly life and Ministry", Op. Cit., p.241

373 Cf. L.C.Nwankwo, Nigerian Priest and Catholic Charismatic Renewal of Nigeria, p.240: Writing on who is a priest, Nwankwo noted that the priest is a man chosen from men to serve God and His people. He has the task of guarding and preserving the knowledge of the religious traditon.

priest, Hierarchy or the people of America. The Charismatic movement went ecumenical in the 1950's only to become Catholic in 1966, after Sixteen full years of careful observation and self distinction by the Catholics of America. And that was too; after the Catholics have seen the Pentecostal movement (the grandfather of the Charismatic movement) operate in the area for more than half of a century. In fact we can even say that the Charismatic Renewal in Nigeria did not experience much problem penetrating and permeating the whole corner of the society as was the case in America. The CCR in short gained an easy access into the Catholic Church in Nigeria and was warmly welcomed.

The Catholic Bishop's Conference of Nigeria issued guidelines for the operation of the Charismatic Renewal in 1991. The booklet published, contains the directives under which the Renewal will be allowed to operate freely in the Church, while safeguarding the Catholic doctrines and tradition.

> It states vividly also the aims and objectives of the Catholic Charismatic Renewal, one of which is to deepen the Spiritual life of the individual through the reading of the scriptures and participating deeply in the sacramental and liturgical life of the Church.[374]

Having passed through this trial period, the Catholic Charismatic Renewal of Nigeria has been since recognised and accepted within the Church and is today found in almost all the dioceses of Nigeria in general with ever increasing number of members. It has since organised many national conferences. Prominent among them are the 3rd National conference in Benin in 1980, the Owerri Conference in 1983, Enugu in 1986, Kaduna 1991 and Uyo in 1994. In Igbo land, the Catholic Charismatic Renewal is flourishing in almost all the parishes of the thirteen dioceses of the land. The Renewal is today alive and active as vibrant soldier of the Church. Though there are still a few abuses here and there due to the attitude of some fanatical, over–enthusiastic, power–conscious and a few money minded members of the renewal. The Renewal has come to stay with its National headquarter at Iselle – uku in Igboland.

3.2.2.4.3 The Healing Ministry in Igboland

The emergence of signs of healing ministry in the Catholic Church in Igboland and the rate and manner at which it develops and spreads continues to generate excitement and concern within the Catholic Church in the area. Similar trial period as was with the Charismatic Renewal is today facing the prayer and healing ministry in the Catholic Church in Nigeria. The ministry at its inception seemed

---

374 C.BC.N., Guidelines for the C.C.R.N., in N. Ndiokwere, The African Church Today and Tommorrow, Vol.1, Onitsha, 1994, p.22

to have been a much welcome and loved aspect of Christ's injunction finding the much desired fulfilment in Igbo society. But recently the ministry is rearing much abuses and questionable practices, which kept agitating the mind of many members of the Church, including the Hierarchy. There are found within the ministry, not only some encroachment of some Protestant and Pentecostal teachings, beliefs and practices but also some questionable practices of the Igbo traditional diviners and healers that are contrary to the traditional theology of the Church. Here we intend to trace the earliest signs of the healing ministry and the pioneer ministers and prayer/healing centres of this unique, novel and much–loved ministry.

In Igbo society, man has the tendency to turn to the gods, the ancestors and spirits in the search for help in times of need and insecurity. People seek for answer to problems and protections from witchcraft and evil spirits in the special powers of the diviners and medicine men. Today the current has shifted its wave. People turn to religion for answers to most of their problems of whatever kind and standard, be it sickness, poverty, barrenness, attacks of the spirits and witches. The answer given by religion is more of expressed in the context of spiritual healing or faith healing.

> *Comparatively late in Nigeria is spiritual healing properly understood. This was initiated by the indigenous Churches and embellished by American–baked Pentecostals of assorted persuasions. The Alladura, Cherubim and Seraphim, Alleluia Churches and Sabbath healing missions, which are found in almost every town in Nigeria, are the most articulate of these groups:*[375]

We cannot therefore talk of healing ministry in the Catholic Church in Igboland without making mention of the first centres of healing ministry in the Eastern states of Nigeria (Bakana in 1909) and in Igboland in particular (in Ufuma), which so to say, indirectly motivated the establishment of the first known prayer ministry by the Catholic priests in Igbo society, precisely in Enugu diocese in 1973.

3.2.2.4.4 The First Healing Ministries in Igbo Society

We have tried above to justify our reflection on the Healing Ministry in general Igboland by situating it within its proper context – Healing. Now we shall endeavour to discuss its first impact in this society.

375 G. Ikeobi, Priests, Healing and Prayer Ministry: The Nigeria Situation, in A.N.O. Ekwunife et al., (eds), The renewal of priestly life and ministry: The Nigeria experience, Op. Cit., p.214.

Apart from the riverine areas of Eastern Nigeria, the Calabar and Efik countries where the innumerable water spirits forced defensive mechanisms on the Christians, the upland Igbo people comparatively saw little of the indigenous Churches before the war. The presence of Odozi Obodo, Cherubim and Seraphim, Sabbath Missions and Healing homes was negligible. Where they existed, people laughed at them and called them "Uka Akulu Aka" (Church of Clapping Worshippers) .Some calls them "Uka Alleluia". The irony of it was that in spite of these factors and because of them, some "Orthodox" Christians went to them under the cover of darkness for healing and exorcism. The Catholic priests all over the country continued their Latin Sacramental exorcisms at Baptism quite unknown to the majority of Christians.[376]

Healing ministry as well understood to mean prayer service to restore broken man to equilibrium in all his relationship with God and man, originally started in the Eastern states of Nigeria, not with the Catholic Church nor the main line Protestant Churches but, with "the African independent Churches in Bakana in 1909,"[377] and by 1915, there were healing sessions taking place in Bonny and Opobo.[378]

The first of the religious movements inspired by a prophet and marked by an emphasis upon prayer and healing seems to have been associated with the name Garrick Braid, a charismatic figure who discovered his gifts while a member of the Niger Delta Pastorate in 1909.[379]

Later on, other prophets came up with their own groups. The 'Aladura' (in Yoruba language of Western Nigeria, means 'One who prays') which is today, "the largest independent prophetic – religious movement in Nigeria emerged as a result of schism from the Anglican Church in 1918 following the dissatisfaction of it's African members with the Church's failure to help them".[380]

The other groups followed still, either as a result of problems within the local Churches or for socio–political reasons. Some groups however sprang up purely on religious or health grounds. Hence one of the leaders of the Church of the Lord (Aladura) notes:

We Africans feel insecure in many ways – health, success, money etc. We have charms and witchcraft and evil powers and influences. But the established Churches are institu-

---

376 G.Ikeobi, Healing and exorcisms: The Nigerian pastoral experience, in C.U. Manus et al., (eds), "Healing and Exorcism: The Nigerian experience", Op.Cit., p.58

377 H.W.Turner, History of an independent Church:The Church of the Lord (Aladura), Vol. 1, London, 1967, pp.6–8

378 Ibid., pp.6–8

379 Ibid., pp.6&7

380 Ndiokwere, N.I., Prophecy and Revolution: The role of prophets in the Independent African Churches and in Biblical tradition, SPCK, London, 1981, p.57

tions devoid of spiritual power to repel these evil powers. The independent Churches did not come out of African Culture but were formed to give spiritual power to individuals.[381]

In Igbo society properly, these prayer/healing groups and centres were not popular until after the middle twentieth–century precisely in the 1970's. As have been earlier mentioned, the upland Igbo saw little of these groups before this time. But with time there spread all over the place, houses of different shapes and sizes known as prayer or healing homes.

> *Called by different names in Nigeria – 'Mushroom', 'hand clapping', 'band–beating', or 'vision–seeing' Churches – any attempt at reaching the approximate number of these Churches or their adherents is impossible. There is in–fact, practically no little village in southern Nigeria where one type of these Churches or another does not exist.*[382]

Most of the attendants or adherents of these healing or prayer Churches were Catholics and Protestants Christians who lost their own faith for these Churches. Many of them eventually end up as prophets or Senior Apostles and in many cases they end up founding their own Churches. It is on record that one of these prayer centres (the Ufuma Prayer band), had a remarkable effect on the Catholic Church around the Old Onitsha Archdiocese.

The first attempt at healing/prayer session by a Catholic priest at Onitsha was said to have been made, as a means of helping Catholics that were lured out of the Church in quest of healing.

3.2.2.4.5 The Ufuma Praying Band

This is one of the most prominent of the early prayer or healing houses founded in Igboland of Nigeria. The Ufuma Praying band as it is popularly known was founded by one Madam Nwokolo in the 1960's in a small town in the old Onitsha archdiocese called Ufuma. Ufuma is now in Awka diocese, which was carved out of Onitsha in 1978. The adherents of the praying band are made up of people from different religious faith without denominational discriminations.

The Ufuma band claims that it is not a Church but just a praying centre. The founder saw her ministry "as a praying band that was out to help people from all walks of life to come to terms with their spiritual, physical, social and psychological problems."[383] She never advised the members of her band to abandon

---

381 H.W.Turner, History of an independent Church: The Church of the Lord, (Aladura), Vol. 11, London, 1967, p.367

382 Ndiokwere, N.I., Prophecy and Revolution, Op. Cit., p.56

383 R.Diala, Phenomenon of healing ministry in eastern Nigeria, Op. Cit., p.52

their Churches or neglect their leaders but rather compelled them to get their religious duties right with their different Churches and their respective leaders. Any wonder, R. Diala says, "the band was only for rescue operations and not a 'permanent force' intended to oust the established Churches."[384] But G. Ikeobi notes that

this one single group triggered the pastoral problems many parish priests have today ... The question arising from this particular new approach of Madam Nwokolo are many. For the fact that she refused to claim the title "CHURCH" which others of her type answered made her harmless and her insistence on her members being in "good standing" within their respective Churches, unlike other groups, marked her out not as an open enemy but as a sympathetic religious leader. Attempts made in isolation by some parish priests in dissuading the Christians from going to Ufuma, even by imposing sanctions, met with stiff resistance as these attempts were seen as acts of jealous men than as justified pastoral action.[385]

Having x–rayed the popular understanding of health, healing and the healing ministry in the church of Igbo Land, we shall now occupy ourselves in the last section of this chapter with the Christian understanding of suffering and sickness in the light of European culture.

3.3 The Christian Understanding of Suffering and Sickness in the light of European Culture

3.3.0 Introductory Remarks

Here we shall examine the Christian view vis–à–vis European culture and attitude towards Suffering. Sickness and Death in comparison with African conception which is in the Sections already discussed.

We shall also see how difficult it is for man to accept the salvific meaning of suffering. How man always pose the question why God cannot prevent this Human suffering if he is All Powerful. And why He should not prevent it if He is all Love? It is not always easy to accept the Reality of this phenomenon. But Faith has always shown a way out of the woods.

384 R.Diala, Phenomenon of healing ministry in Eastern Nigeria, pp.52&53

385 G.Ikeobi, Catholic response to the Challenges of Prayer Houses: The Origin of Tuesday Prayers in Onitsha, in V.A. Nwosu (ed), "The Catholic Church in Onitsha", Onitsha, 1985, pp.266–267

3.3.1 The meaning of Human Suffering in the official documents of the Church

3.3.2 Suffering and Sickness in Human Life explained

'Suffering'. The term Suffering is very difficult to give a definite definition. It is so because Suffering does not exist, only the suffering man. Suffering is disgusting only when it visits us. It contradicts and disturbs the nature of man. Accompanying this harsh reality, critical questions regarding the cause and meaning of suffering is as old as humanity: – why must we suffer? Why my specific nation or group? And, why me, in particular? What did we (or I) do to deserve this? And, why is it that some are left debilitated by experiences of suffering, while others are enriched, somehow made more whole, more human? Moreover, can we learn from Suffering? Should we strive for a life that is pain free?

These and other questions have forced their way in the thought of man over donkey years. The chronic physical and emotional eilments and numerous deaths and tragic accidents are part and parcel of human experiences.

Anne Sexton captures some of our sense of the search for meaning in suffering in her poem "The Big Boots of Pain":

There can be certain potions
needled in the clock
for the body's fall from grace,
to untorture and to plead for.
These I have known
and would sell all my furniture
and books and assorted goods
to avoid, and more, more.

But the other pain ...
I would sell my life to avoid
the pain that begins in the crib
with its bars or perhaps
with your first breath
when the planets drill
your future into you
for better or worse
as you marry life
and the love that gets doled out
or doesn't.

I find now, swallowing one teaspoon
of pain, that it drops downward
to the past where it mixes
with last year's cupful

and downward into a decade's quart
and downward into a lifetime's ocean.
I alternate treading water
and deadman's float.

The teaspoon ought to be bearable
if it didn's mix into the reruns
and thus enlarge into what it is not,
a sea pest's sting turning promptly
into the shark's neat biting off
of a leg because the soul
wears a magnifying glass.
Kicking the heart
with pain's big boots running up and down
the intestines like a motorcycle racer.

Yet one does get out of bed
and start over, plunge into the day
and put on a hopeful look
and does not allow fear to build a wall
between you and an old friend
or a new friend and reach out your hand,
shutting down the thought that
an axe may cut it off unexpectedly.
One learns not to blab about all this
except to yourself or the typewriter keys
who tell no one until they get brave
and crawl off onto the printed page.

I'm getting bored with it,
I tell the typewriter,
this constantly walking around
in wet shoes and then, surprise!
Somehow DECEASED keeps getting
stamped in red over the word HOPE.
And I who keep falling thankfully
into each new pillow of belief,
finding my Mercy Street,
kissing it and tenderly gift – wrapping my love,
am beginning to wonder just what
the planets had in mind on November 9th, 1928.
The pillows are ripped away,
the hand guillotined,
dog shit thrown into the middle of a laugh,
a hornet's nest building into the hi–fi speaker
and leaving me in silence,
where, without music,
I become a cacked orphan.

Well,
one gets out of bed
and the planets don't always hiss
or muck up the day, each day.
As for the pain and ist multiplying teaspoon,
perhaps it is a medicine
that will cure the soul
of its greed for love
next Thursday.[386]

In the light of the following poem how then can one speak of human suffering responsibly and compassionately, since the experience of suffering lead to critical questions about God, oneself, oneself in relation to God and to others. Related to this experience is the problem of communicating what is meant by the words itself. Despite the fact that the experience of suffering is common it is not very easy to give a concise, all–dimensional account of this experience. In a detailed and erudite study on global torture, Elaine Scarry, too, highlights the difficulty of conveying an experience of physical pain to another when she contends "whatever pain achieves, it achieves in part through its unsharability, and it ensures this unsharability through its resistance to language."[387] What can be so difficult for sufferers is that while they experience their distress as a prime reality, as the very focus of their lives at times (as in the case of torture or domestic violence), others do not and truly cannot know what it is.[388] This inexpressibility of suffering and the split between one's sense of one's own reality and the reality of other persons is best shown by Scarry's own words, based on a extensive analysis of reports from Amnesty International on torture:

> So, for the person in pain, so incontestably and unnegotiably present is it that "having pain" may come to be thought of as the most vibrant example of what it is to "have certainty," while for the other person it is so elusive that "hearing about pain" may exist as the primary model of what it is "to have doubt." Thus pain comes unsharably into our midst as at once that which cannot be denied and that which cannot be confirmed.[389]

---

386 Anne Sexton, "The Big Boots of Pain," in The Complete Poems (Boston: Houghton Mifflin, 1981) pp.547–

387 Elaine Scarry, The Body in Pain: The Making and Unmaking of the World (New York: Oxford University Press, 1985) p.4

388 Simone Weil, Waiting for God, trans. Emma Grauford (New York: Harper & Row, 1951) p.120

389 Scarry, ibid.

One can know that a person is in pain and is suffering, but not what it is about this specific person that leads to the suffering.[390]

As with the experience of falling in love, suffering in its resistance to language is more akin to a mystery that we encounter rather than a puzzle to be solved. Writing in *The Cuture of Pain,* David B. Morris notes "... a mystery, as distinguished from a puzzle, might be defined as whatever refuses to yield up all its secrets to common sense."[391] Try as one might to find a "correct solution" to a mystery (such as suffering) through the use of common sense and reason, it consistently resists closure and retains an essential open–endedness to definition and explanation.

He elaborates:

> A true mystery, as opposed to a puzzle or riddle, cannot be known apart from the veil that separates us from a full understanding. The veil in a sense is what make the mystery visible; it gives a presence or appearance to the unknown. ... A mystery, then, is not something that exists principally to be solved. In fact, it transcends or eludes every normal technique of solution.[392]

One might expect, then, in pursuing definitions of and responses to the experience of suffering, that no one answer exists and that any "solution" will have its inherent limitations.

Mysteries also disrupt accepted and familiar ways of handling a situation, and often put one in a state of questioning everything, including simple answers to profound questions. Perhaps, this native elusiveness of suffering is also one reason why so many in search of religious meaning for suffering find many traditional theological responses unsatisfying when juxtaposed beside the scale of massive suffering in this century.[393]

---

390 Eric J. Cassell, "Pain and Suffering," in Encyclopedia of Bioethics, vol. 4., ed. Warren Thomas Reich, rev. Ed. (New York: Macmillan Library Reference USA/Simon & Schuster Macmillan, 1995) p.1900

391 Morris, p.152

392 Ibid., 24

393 Lucien Richard, What Are They Saying about the Theology of Suffering? (New York/Mahwah, N.J.: Paulist Press, 1992) p.5 Cf. Paticia L. Wismer, "For Women in Pain", in In the Embrace of God: Feminist Approaches to Theological Anthropology, ed. Ann O'Hara Graff (Maryknoll, N.Y.: Orbis Books, 1995) 138 – 58.

3.3.3 Suffering defined

A simple way to enter into and begin an inquiry into any mystery is by consulting some knowledgeable source at hand. According to Merriam–Webster's Collegiate Dictionary, to suffer is "to endure death, pain, or distress," "to sustain loss or damage," or "to be subject to disability or handicap." The implication here is that one is vulnerable to that which is out of one's control, and this vulnerability can lead to an experience of pain or distress.

Further, to suffer is to take on that which is difficult, to "labour under" or "bear," as well as "to put up with that which is unavoidable or inevitable." Although experiences of suffering come unexpectedly, at times, and involve our vulnerability to the world, choice in how we react or respond to suffering is implied here. We can decide "to take on" or "to endure" versus to deny, evade, or suppress these experiences.[394]

Conversely, these definitions show that in some situations suffering is also associated with *loss of choice*, or agency, due to the necessity of submitting to or enduring something or someone more powerful than oneself –as in to suffer is "to submit to or be forced to endure," to be made to do what one does not choose or want to do because of another."[395] Examples of this can be seen in experiences as varied as the consequences of war to those of disease to those of discrimination of all sorts, as well as forced prostitution, rape, and domestic abuse.

The various connotations of these dictionary definitions range from a nagging or chronic pain caused by disappointment or the consequences of disease to a sense of longing over missed opportunities (e.g., associated with sorrow); from a deep sadness or regret to the unbearable quality of extreme suffering which involves anguish of body and mind (as with affliction, torture, anguish). Not only physical experiences, such as bodily pain, are involved, but also psychological distress, such as dread and anxiety or an inconsolable grief or misery (as depicted the term "woe"). As can be quickly observed, a constellation of synonyms and related concepts is frequently associated with suffering, including pain, affliction, distress, anguish, sorrow, lamentation, woe, agony, torment, torture, grief, and a sense of loss and /or of being victimised.

---

394 Helen M. Luke elaborates on this definition by providing a sense of suffering as similar to the image of the undercarriage of a vehicle – that which bears the weight of one's life. "Suffering is that which carries the weight we carry in full consciousness." See Luke, The Way of Woman: Awakening the Perennial Feminine (New York: Image Books/Doubleday, 1996) pp.56, 57, 59.

395 *Merriam – Webster's Collegiate Dictionary*, 10th ed. (Springfield, Mass.: Merriam–Webster, Inc., 1994) p.1177

Beyond these common dictionary definitions, both religious and non–religious alike have attempted to define and understand suffering. For some, "suffering can be any experience that impinges on an individual or on community's sense of well–being."[396]

It can involve "the disruption of inner harmony" of an individual as the result of physical, mental, emotional, and/or spiritual forces.[397] In this sense, suffering is not just a physical sensation but is also a subjective experience involving the "whole" person. For some, this whole person can be defined as a composite of physical, historical, cultural, psychological, socio–political, and spiritual dimensions.[398] Rarely, for example, does the person in anguish suffer without some relation to her past, present and future and/or to the social matrix of which she is a part. Accordingly, since the "whole" person affected in the experience of suffering, authentic Christian responses to suffering must address not only one aspect or dimension of a person but the total person within her social/cultural context. So, if one addresses the suffering of women, one must consider not only that women might suffer differently than men in a patriarchal context, but that women will also differ amongst themselves in how they suffer because of their different socio–cultural contexts.

In addition, suffering afflicts not only individuals but entire communities. The "whole" community, as well as the "whole" person, can be involved, for example, in the effects of dropping the atomic bomb in Hiroshima on present and future generations. Racism provides another example of how not only an individual is affected by, say, a violent act, but how such an act ripples through an entire community – becoming an historical lightning rod for future acts of aggression and protest against such violent incidents.

Thus, both personal and communal suffering can occur, and are often interwoven. With the help of selected scholars who have looked closely at suffering from a variety of viewpoints we can comfortably conclude that Suffering and Sickness belongs to the Nature of Man. It can also take several shapes and forms. One is downfouded when one find oneself faced with a mystery which one thinks negates the idea of a source of all goodness and therefore of the divine origin and meaning of life. The idea of all goodness and divine origin and meaning of life as an attribute of God for these people admits no suffering. That is why they contend that if God existed, Suffering would not be there, and if Suffering exists,

396 Sparks, p.950

397 Mary Ann Fatula, "Suffering," in *The New Dictionary of Theology*, ed. Joseph A. Komonchak, et al. (Wilmington: Michael Glazier, 1988) p.990

398 Cassell, "Pain and Suffering," 1900

then God is either not there or is weak and therefore not all powerful. For them God and the concept of suffering are incompatible.

A renowned theologian, Karl Rahner sees the *Why* question from another point of view. He said: God, in christian faith is incomprehensible Mystery and the incomprehensibility of suffering is a point to unintelligibility of God.[399] For him God seizes to be God in the moment we understand his Being whole and entire. It belongs to the qualities of God that we do not understand Him. In short we do not have final answer to the question of why God should allow suffering in the World. According to him in this way we should understand and accept God and let him be.

God and Suffering as a Mystery should remain as it is. This is also the opinion of St. Paul in his letter to the Romans. He writes "But you – who do you think you, a human being, are, to answer back to God?"[400]

After all said and done, the very reality of suffering jolts our faith and belief in God. But it is also the way we come to know God better. Just as in Life the degree of Sacrifices one makes for the other is the degree of Love and affection. In actual fact suffering feels terrible, but it can help us appreciate what we have. The death of a loved ones is devastating, but it makes us aware of how precious life is. We truly appreciate material possessions for example, only by knowing what it means to lose them. We value our health only when we know how easily sickness can take its place. Illness humbles us and erodes our sense of invulnerability.

As Aiken rightly points out:

> There are many levels on which we can find meaning in our painful experiences. For example, we can appreciate being spiritually cleansed in this World or developing our faith and character through afflictions of love. We can develop deeper levels of empathy when we know what it's like to be in someone else's shoes. Firsthand experience can sensitize us to others in ways that living an easy life cannot, and it makes us more credible when we give hope and reassurance to others.[401]

The understanding of Human Suffering and meaning of life requires further elaborations. To help realise this end, we dare to ask whether suffering has a meaning or not. How can one arrive at a proper understanding of this meaning in the very context of his ordeals? That is in his human physical and mental agonies.

---

399 DIFÄM – Deutsches Institut für Ärztliche Mission – Gelbe Beilage: Januar – März 1999 p3

400 Röm. 9,20

401 Aiken, L. Why me, God?: A Jewish guide for coping with Suffering. Northvale, New Jersey London, p.36

Further experience of suffering as with most mysteries are those that life thrusts upon us in such a way that we cannot evade dealing with them on some level.

In recalling the events surrounding the death of his father Thomas Merton wrote:

> Indeed, the truth that many people never understand until it is too late, is that the more you try to avoid suffering, the more you suffer, because smaller and more insignificant things begin to torture you, in proportion to your fear of being hurt. The one who does most to avoid suffering is, in the end, the one who suffers most: and his suffering comes to him from things so little and so trivial that one can say that it is no longer objective at all. It is his own existence, his own being, that is at once the subject and source of his pain, and his very existence and consciousness is his greatest torture.[402]

It seems, as indicated by Merton, that the more one tries to avoid suffering, the more one becomes separated from one's self as a human person and falls into the banal and the trivial. If we try to evade suffering, perhaps we are trying to evade a basic human condition and a part of the reality of what it means to be human. Perhaps, then, suffering is constitutive of human persons.[403]

Interestingly, Morris also notes that painlessness may be more of a curse than a blessing, as indicated by the rare medical and psychological case studies of pain–free individuals. In these cases, pain–free children die early and are more prone to inflammation and infection, and often, the individual becomes more of an outsider or side–show wonder.

A life immune from the pains that flesh is heir to can lead one to constant vigilance over minor physical activities, indifference to the pain of others, and social isolation.[404] So, the goal of a pain–free life may not be the ideal that one might assume.

However, as expressed by Lucien Richard, and many other theologians, sociologist, and cultural critics, characteristic of post–modern European and American cultures is this very desire to evade and deny the experience of suffering in our midst – perhaps, due in part to our current awareness of the overwhelming degree of global suffering. Based on the work of Robert Lifton and Eric Olson, Richard notes the vast desensitisation to suffering in our culture. This "psychic numbing," as it is often called, is characterised by an "overwhelming attempt to eliminate negativity ... marked by the repression of pain and the consequent inca-

---

402 Thomas Merton, The Seven Story Mountain (New York: New American Library, 1948) p.86

403 Cf. Lucien Richard's discussion of Stanley Hauerwas's view of ethics and suffering, in *What Are They Saying about the Theology of Suffering?*, p.104ff.

404 Morris, 12–4.

pacity to suffer ... incapacity to confront and appropriate the reality of suffering".[405]

Furthermore, this contemporary condition of denial and avoidance is also characterised by personal and collective narcissism and a lack of empathy, which, when severe enough, becomes apathy on an individual, as well as a national, scale. Sölle also raises this concern regarding contemporary Western culture and defines apathy as the very inability to suffer. She understands it as "a social condition in which people are so dominated by the goal of avoiding suffering that it becomes a goal to avoid human relationships and contacts altogether."[406] When an individual or a whole collective avoids suffering, there is a corresponding lack of vitality, passion, and intensity, as well as a lack of awareness of one's own suffering and that of others. Not only does this lead to political apathy, cynicism, and alienation but also to an uncontrolled consumerism and a value system of self–indulgence, as noted by both Richard and Sölle.[407] One only needs to spend a day in the late–twentieth–century San Francisco Bay Area or to examine the history of post–World war II U.S. foreign policy to discover the validity of these claims.

However, if one agrees with theologian Walter Kasper, perhaps there is a greater mystery that we are led to through this experience of finitude:

> No one has experienced humanity to the full unless he or she has experienced its finiteness and suffering. But then experience becomes a way of leading into an open immensity, into a mystery that is ever greater and never to be completely plumbed.[408]

It is in this understanding that physical suffering cannot be totally meaningless. We shall take a typical biological example of a physical pain in the abdomen. This can be the warning sign of an inflamed appendix or a peptic ulcer and many other conditions. Some of these conditions need surgical intervention if life is to be saved, and others need surgical operation for the elimination of the diseased organs. The experience of this surgical operation can be unbearably painful. But it is a pain that leads to a healthier leaving, therefore in other to live without a deceased organ or an inflamed Appendix it is only natural and necessary that one looks at the pain as inevitable. It leads to higher good. The logical

405 Richard, 10.

406 Dorothee Sölle, *Suffering*, trans. Everett R. Kalin (Philadelphia: Fortress Press, 1975) 36 Cf. Sölle, *Strength of the Weak*, 24–30

407 Richard, 22 Cf. Sölle, *Strength of the Weak*, 11–9; Ernest Becker, The Denial of Death (New York: The Free Press, 1973)

408 Walter Kasper, The God of Jesus Christ (New York: Crossroad, 1984) p.84

conclusion is "in some circumstancaes, therefore, physical pain is an effective warning system essential for the survival of the body."[409]

In other words suffering and life belongs together and that suffering helps us to appreciate values of life and persons. God sometimes expresses His love for us in pleasant ways; at other times, He does it by sending us difficulties and tragedies. Finding meaning in our suffering helps elevate us above it so that we can transcend it. Even in our worst tragedies, God is not absent. We have to know that He is especially close to us at those times when we seek Him the most. The more we want to relate to Him, the more intense our relationship can be.

To enhance our intimacy, He sometimes reminds us how artificial the security of worldly props is. Our health, money, friends, family, homes, and possessions can disappear in a moment. The only thing that is permanent and can truly take care of us is the Almighty. He is the end and beginning of all things – alpha and omega. *Oka 'ka* Igbo people will say.

A beautiful story cited in *Why me God*? Illustsrates this idea: A man died and went to heaven. There, he and God watched a videotape. One side of the frames showed the events of the man's life, while the other half showed God's and the man's footprints side by side in the sand on a beach.

As the film showed every crisis that the man had gone through, the two sets of footprints symbolized that God had stayed steadfastly by his side. But as they viewed the man's most painful tragedies, only one set of footprints remained. The man felt devasted and began to cry. "God," he plaintively asked, "I always had such faith in You. How could You have abandoned me in my time of greatest need?"

God gently replied, "My beloved child, I would never abandon you. When you see only one set of footprints is where I picked you up and carried you."[410]

But it is unfortunate that our society has tendency to regard suffering as foreign to human condition and therefore it must be alleviated if not conquered. This, in fact, is an obstacle to a balanced understanding of human suffering. Those who cut themselves off from suffering also cut themselves from their fellow men and from the World. In essence they erect walls between themselves and others. This escapist mentality is in opposition to the nature of man as a social being. The human environment other or the human civilisation will remain stagnant without man taking the pains to improve its frontiers. So that any meaningful development that is the efforts to bring about a reasonable and meaningful changes that are geared to the overall betterment of the human situation must

409 Dominian, "The Meaning of Suffering," in The Tablet, Vol. 236 no. 7409, 10 July 1982, p.692

410 Aiken,L., op. Cit., p.37

necessary include suffering and be realised through it. In short, suffering is only another name for the World; a World without suffering loses its name.

The Holy Father, John Paul II underscores the above assertion thus:

> nevertheless what we express by the word "suffering" seems to be particularly essential to the nature of man. It is as deep as man himself, precisely because it manifests in its own way that depth which is proper to man, and in its way surpasses it. Suffering seems to belong to man's transcendence: it is one of those points in which man is in a certain sense "destined" to go beyond himself, and he is called to this in a mysterious way.[411]

It has been well established that sufferings are necessary part and parcel of human condition. However, suffering indicates a lack of what should be. It shows that all is not well. The question now is can one make it up or put things right?. Or are there things that must be endured? Our sucessful grappling with meaning of human suffering will depend in part on clarity of vision. The problem we have in defining and coping with suffering is that man never resigns himself to the inevitability of sufferings. Dr Colston urges us to make a distinction between those sufferings to be corrected and those that must be endured. In other words, we must respond exactly "to doing what we can about the situation... There are other things that we cannot do and must accept... The cross of Christ recapitulates the human experience of suffering in the world."[412]

It follows from the above citation, that certain types of suffering can and should be alleviated. "God made man upright, but people made many inventions" Therefore there are man–made suffering which is unnecessary and can be avoided. Most people suffer because of what we do to each other and to ourselves. For example people start wars, oppress each other, kill, rob, rape, cheat, and the like. God doesn't directly create evil. We do, though, when we act as if He is absent. He then witholds obvious punishments so that we don't fell always compelled to do what is right.

God wants us to preserve our health, but He doesn't force us to do it. And in fact, most people do not live healthily. The overwhelming majority of sickness today happens because people do not take proper care of themselves.

The main causes of adult death (heart, lung, and liver diesease, cancer, and strokes) are largely preventable. For example, cigarette smoking is the single largest preventable cause of death, lung cancer, and chronic lung disease. Another source of death and untold hardship on our people which could be pre-

---

411 John Paul 11, Apostolic Letter On the Christian Meaning of Human Suffering, Press Kisubi Uganda, 1984, p.4

412 Colston, L.G., "Meaning of Human Suffering" (International Ecumenical Congress, University of Notre Dame, April 1979) cited by Flavian Dougherty, in Hospital Progress, May 1981 in Onyenemegam, J.O., Op. Cit p.43

vented is the road accidents. It is caused due to reckless driving and ignorance of the road signs and regulations. The experience of Wars and conflict among the nations and the individual and the sufferings that come through these experiences are glaring examples of suffering that can be avoided. The perennial war and conflict in the middle east and the recent Kosovo war along with the conflict between Ethiopia and Eriteria and so many other countries in Africa and other parts of the World can at least be avoided. The volume of human sufferings and agonies that came as a result of this conflict is a challenge to the 20th century claim of civilisation.

In reference to the unpleasant consequences of these conflict and wars the Holy Father asserts: "One thinks, finally, of war. I speak of the last two World Wars, the second of which brought with it a much greater harvest of death and a much heavier burden of human sufferings."[413]

Such undeserved suffering should be prevented. Human concern should guide us here. To achieve this intense and sacrificing love Dominian advises thus:

> At the international level, everyone agrees that we should not let People perish as a result of famine, exposure to cold and heat, poor sanitation, flood ... that we must recognise the important principle that people should not suffer when they are helpless victims of natural disaster. But we have gone further and try to protect the innocent victims of war, of other adverse circumstances, ... our doing so is a good example of suffering being conquered by human concern, which can broadly be called love.[414]

This in brief is Solidarity with the Suffering, which we are called upon to translate into reality in our lives. Our life missions are not only to grow personally but also to help others who need strength and support to find meaning in Suffering as a christian. We are aware that all men and woman who suffer in their lives are not all christians. But the Christian solidarity especially with the poor and the needy, in their situations is exemplary, and responds most adequately to the obvious human need of Love, which knows no boundary of faith. We are all children of the same father. The suffering of one among us affects the rest. We are linked to one another with an inseparable strings of love and oneness. That is why no one lives alone for himself. We are responsible to one another and to God.

---

413 John Paul 11, The Christian Meaning of Human Suffering: Apostolic Letter – Salvifici Doloris Marianum Press Kisubi, Uganda,1984 p.13

414 Dominian, J., "The Meaning of Suffering," in Pastoral Care of the Sick by Onyenemegam , J.O., Rome, 1985 p.43

3.3.4 The Christian meaning of Human Suffering.

According to Dorothee Sölle, German Feminist Theologian, all true theology begins in the experience of suffering. "Theology originates in our need for more, in our sense of failure, in our awareness of life destroyed. Its locus is suffering or the disregard for life that we experience all the time."[415] For her, Christian theology grows out of the paradox or constrast between life experienced as finite and constricted by negative forces and the promise of abundant life given in the Gospels (e.g., John 10:10):

> Theology begins with experience and sets experience over against the promise of a whole life, the promise of the Kingdom of God. It confronts these statements with the genuine life that has been promised to us, which is no more nor less than everything for all of us.[416]

Echoing this reality, that is the power of salvific suffering, the Apostle Paul says:

> "In my flesh I complete what is lacking in Christ's afflictions for the sake of his body, that is, the Church."[417]

The aformentioned statement is the Apostolic letter *Salvifici Doloris* of the Supreme Pontifex John Paul II to the bishops, Priests, Religious families and to the Faithful of the Catholic Church on the christian meaning of Human Suffering. This document shows that Suffering is a part and parcel of human history and has a salvific undertone which is illuminated by the Word of God. These words have as it were the value of a final discovery, which is accompained by joy. For this reason St. Paul writes: "Now I rejoice in my sufferings for your sake"[418] The joy comes from the discovery of the meaning of suffering, and this discovery, even if it is most personally shared in by Paul of Tarsus who wrote these words, is at the same time valid for others as followers of Christ. The Apostle shares his own discovery and rejoices in it because of all those whom it can help just as it helped him to understand what the Holy Father calls the salvicfic meaning of suffering.

In essence, suffering is an element of human life that deepens our awareness of dependence on God. The book of Genesis indicates a brokenness in human life which offspring ultimately will restore (Gen. 3.15). The book of Deuteronomy warns the Jews of disobedience to Jahweh: "He will inflict you with the plague

415 Dorothee Sölle, *The Strength of the Weak: Toward a Christian Feminist Identity, trans.* Robert and Rita Kimber (Philadelphia: Westminister Press, 1984) p.90

416 Ibid., 91.

417 p.3

418 Ibid

until it has consumed you on the Land which you are entering to make your own" (Deut. 28:21). Suffering and illness are described as a test for the people of God. Job's fidelity was tested. "But stretech out your hand and lay a finger on his possessions; I warrant you, he will course you to your face" (Job 1:11) We read in the book of Judith: "We shall be grateful to the Lord our God, for putting us to the test, as he did our forefathers ... Not for vengeance did the Lord put them in the crucible to try their hearts, nor has he done so with us. It is by way of admonition that he chastises those who are close to him" (Judith 8:25 & 27).

From the foregoing, suffering obviously contributes to the growth of human wholeness. Isaiah speaks of the healing influence of suffering on individuals thus: "On that day Yahweh dresses the wounds of his people and heals the bruises his blows have left" (Is. 30:26). Here we see the integrative function of suffering in which the acceptance of human brokenness heals the human condition destroyed by pride. Moreso, the book of Wisdom points to the same truth when speaking of the destiny of good men: "Slight was their affliction, great will their blessings be. God has put them to the test and proved them worthy to be with him" (Wis. 3.5).

Therefore we can see that pain and suffering also enter into the spiritual realm and ask for a readjustment in our relationship with God. By them humans are placed in a new position which in turn demands a new response to the wholeness of our being.

The Pope affirms that Suffering seems to belong to man's transcendence: it is one of those points in which man is in a certain sense "destined" to go beyond himself, and he is called to this in a mysterious way. ...It can be said that man in a special fashion becomes the way for the Church when suffering enters his life. This happens, as we know, at different moments in life, it takes place in different ways, it assumes different dimensions; nevertheless, in whatever form, suffering seems to be, and is almost inseparable from man's earthly existence.[419] We believe in the redemptive life and death of Jesus and thus we accept without hesitation that suffering has the power of atonement. Isaiah writes of the suffering servant of Yahweh: "On him lies a punishment that brings us peace, and through his wounds we are healed" (Is. 53:5). This text teaches us the interpersonal meaning of suffering. Let us look at the Gospels for greater clarity. The story of the rich man and Lazarus shows that suffering is not necessarily a result of sinfulness but that it belongs to a human condition as stated. Suffering offers Lazarus the opportunity for personal acceptance and the rich man the opportunity for practical expression of love. St. Luke tells us that Lazarus lived up to his vocation while the rich man did not (Lk. 16:19–31). The spiritual values in their earthly life thus became the basis for self–realization in their life after death.

---

419 John Paul 11, op. Cit., p.5

The atonement aspect of suffering is particularly strong in narratives of Jesus' suffering and death. Van der Poel comments on it thus: "The totality of Jesus' life is interwoven with many forms of suffering. He knew fatigue, hunger, and thirst. He experienced opposition, rejection and loneliness. In all these we see his oneness with human nature and his effort to teach us how to let God's presence fill our daily life. These human experiences also touch on reconciliation of the human with the divine. Jesus' life in its human setting was totally filled with God's presence and love. In him God's love was accepted in the human reality, and the human was accepted by the divine majesty."[420]

In sum Jesus gave meaning and importance to human suffering. He also united human existence with God and opened the way for all who participate in human nature to participate also in God's life.

Albert Keller in his Book titled *"Schmerz–Leid–Tod"* writes on Suffering. Hence the Dispute between Leo and Johanna:

Leo: Please turn off the Television.

Johanna: Turned the TV off and asked: Why? Are you not interested in this programme?

Leo: What is interesting about this? Can't you see an innocent child dying before us and you are asking me; *Why?*. Let me tell you, this picture makes me sick. When I watch this type of scene without being able to do something about it, I feel guilty like those murderers.

Johanna I think we are making the matter worse by not watching it.

Leo: Who benefits when you only watch? You are worried; but it does no one any good.

Johanna: I think when one ignores the suffering of people one is making his or herself guilty. This is just like those who watch it without doing any thing concrete.

Leo: You may be right but it disturbs me on one hand to see how people are suffering. Unfortunately, people who are capable of helping do nothing.

Johanna: Which people are you referring to? Can you not help?

Leo: Have you forgotten how we helped the refugees from Vietnam financially?

Johanna: Yes, that is only contribution. That does not put an end to the sufferings in the world.

---

420 Cornelius Van der Poel, "Suffering and Healing: The Process of Growth" , in Hospital Progress, February 1981, in Pastoral Care of the Sick in Igbo Community by Onyenemegam, J.O. p.45

Leo: There is no end to suffering in the World. It will never be a Paradise.

Johanna: You are not suppose to say that as a Christian.

Leo: Christianity has never promised a rosy world or paradise in our earthly life.

Johanna: No! When you say that it means that God is responsible for all these sufferings in the World. Who do you believe then? Why can he not help? Can he not. Is he incapable? Or do you mean that the agonies of these people does not perturb him. He loves without limit as or unconditional as you claimed. Look millions of people are dying of hunger and of natural disaster and you do not care to ask your loving God why. Where is your Love?

Leo: Listen! Calm down

Johanna: Why? I can not understand how you believe that God is love. Love? He is Love but he allowed your sister and her son to be burnt up in a car accident. I will never forget how Reinhard is called and told that: Hilde and Stefan were burnt up in a Car.

Leo: I can not understand how you bring this incident into our discussion. Do you think I did not think of Stefan when I saw that Child killed in the TV report.

Johanna: That not withstanding I think you did not think deeply about it – you should have posed the question why should God permit such a thing to happen? She believes in God as you do. What type of God is that? What type of Belief?

Leo: In any case let my faith help me to come out of this ordeal.

Johanna: I think you do not have feelings anymore. God has blocked your sense of feeling and sympathy. I have also the impression that nothing shocks you, you and your Belief.

Leo: Johanna, that one has no feeling is not because one believes. But when one believes, one knows that no matter what happens one is not abandoned by God.

Johanna: Do you know that or do you believe that?

Leo: I know and I believe that.

Johanna: Well then, Leo, now tell me your stand: How can you believe in such a God. A God who is good and almighty and at same time permits suffering, immeasurable evil in the World. Either he can not prevent them; that means he is not almighty or he does not want to prevent them; that means he is not good. Does it remind you of something?[421].

---

421 Keller, A. Schmerz–Leid–Tod: Verlag Butzon &Bercker Kevelaer, 1980. Pp.15–17

The original text of the above dispute reads: Disput zwischen Johanna und Leo. Ein Fernsehbericht über Vietnam–Flüchtlinge

Leo: schalte das doch bitte aus.

Johanna: Warum? Interessiert dich das nicht?

Leo: Was heißt "interessiert"? Da stirbt ein Kind vor unseren Augen, und du fragst, ob's mich interessiert. Du kannst dir doch so etwas nicht anschauen und sagen: "Das ist aber interessant." Mich jedenfalls macht es ganz krank, wenn ich mir so etwas mit ansehen muss und nur stumm dabeisitzen soll und nicht helfen kann. Ich fühle mich dann fast mitschuldig.

Johanna: Ich glaube, wir machen uns wirklich mitschuldig, wenn wir die Augen davor verschließen, wenn wir abschalten oder wegsehen.

Leo: Und wem nützt's, wenn du zuschaust? Dich quälen doch solche Bilder auch bloß – und wirklich geholfen ist keinem.

Johanna: Ich finde, wenn einer das Leid und Unglück um sich herum nicht wahrhaben will oder wenn er es verharmlost, dann macht er sich vielleicht genauso schuldig wie andere, die sehen und nicht helfen.

Leo: Gut, das mag ja sein. Mich bedrückt es auch, wenn da auf der einen Seite eine solche Not herrscht und andererseits so viele Leute gleichgültig bleiben. Und ich frage mich auch: "Warum wird da nicht mehr getan, und warum hilft keiner richtig von denen, die es könnten?"

Johanna: Und wen meinst du damit? Hilfst du denn?

Leo: Das weißt du doch, dass wir für die Vietnam–Flüchtlinge gespendet haben.

Johanna: Ja, spende nur schön. Damit ist deren Elend doch nicht aus der Welt zu schaffen.

Leo: Du wirst das Leid auch nicht ausrotten können und auch nicht die Gleichgültigkeit. So sind die Menschen nun einmal – und aus der Erde wird nie ein Paradies.

Johanna: Das dürftest eigentlich du gerade als Christ nicht sagen.

Leo: Wieso? Hat das Christentum jemals ein Paradies auf Erden versprochen?

Johanna: Nein! Aber wenn du sagst: "Das Elend lässt sich nicht beseitigen, die Welt ist nun einmal so", dann müsste für dich doch Gott für all das verantwortlich sein, an den du glaubst. Warum hilft der denn nicht? Kann er es nicht? Oder meinst du, der ganze Jammer dieser Menschen lässt ihn überhaupt kalt? Er liebt sie doch nach deiner Meinung grenzenlos. Da kommen Tausende um und Millionen verhungern, und du fragst deinen lieben Gott nicht: "Wo bist du denn lieb?"

Leo: Hör mal bleib doch auf dem Teppich, und wird nicht geschmacklos!

Johanna: Wieso ist das geschmacklos? Ich finde es geschmacklos von dir, an einen lieben Gott zu glauben, Lied? – Lieb soll der sein, und er hat deine Schwester und ihr Kind umkommen lassen? Mir geht es nicht aus dem Ohr, wie Reinhard angerufen und gesagt hat: "Hilde und Stefan sind im Auto verbrannt."

Leo: Ich verstehe nicht, wieso du jetzt ausgerechnet diesen Unfall ins Spiel bringst. Glaubst du, ich hätte nicht eben, als ich das sterbende Kind sah, sofort an Stefan gedacht?

Johanna: Und trotzdem hab' ich fast den Eindruck, du hast dir aus deiner Schwester nichts gemacht, sonst müsstest du dich doch mit der Frage herumschlagen, wie Gott so etwas zulassen kann. Sie hat ja ebenso an ihn geglaubt wie du. Was soll denn ein solcher Gott, so ein Glaube?

Leo: Mein Glaube hilft mir jedenfalls, über so einen Schicksalsschlag hinwegzukommen.

Johanna: Mir scheint eher, er stumpft dich ab und macht dich gefühllos. Ich habe fast den Eindruck, dich kann überhaupt nichts mehr erschüttern, du mit deinem Glauben.

Leo: Johanna, man ist doch nicht gefühllos, nur weil man glaubt. Aber wenn einer glaubt, dann weiß er eben – egal was auch passiert –, dass Gott einen nicht im Stich lässt, so oder so.

Johanna: Weißt du das, oder glaubst du das?

Leo: Ich weiß es, und ich glaub' es.

Johanna: Also, Leo, jetzt sag mir doch endlich: Wie kannst du so etwas glauben. Ein Gott, der gut ist und allmächtig und der doch das Leid zulässt, dieses unermessliche Leid, das es überall auf der Welt gibt? Entweder kann er's doch nicht verhindern – dann ist er nicht. Fällt dir darauf was ein?

From the above conversation we can see how difficult it is to discern the divine will in the midst of disaster and evil in the world. Within each form of suffering endured by man, and at the same time at the basis of the whole world of suffering; there arises inevitably the question "why". It is a question about the cause, the reason, and equally, about the purpose of suffering, and, in brief, a question about its meaning.

We are convinced that suffering is bad, that suffering is evil but at the same time we are expected to see it as part and parcel of our Christian life. How is it possible? How can one reconcile it? His Holiness responds to this seemingly contradiction in the following brilliant way, thus:

Both questions are difficult, when an individual puts them to another individual, when people put them to other people, as also when man Puts them to God. ... And it is well known that concerning this question there not only arise many frustrations and conflicts in the relations of man with God, but it also happens that people reach the point of actually denying God. For whereas the existence of the world opens as it were the eyes of the human soul to the existence of God, to his wisdom, power and in a radical way, especially in the greatness, evil and suffering seem to obscure this image, sometimes daily drama of so many cases of underserved suffering and of so many faults without proper punishment. So this circumstance shows perhaps more than any other the importance of the question of the meaning of suffering; it also shows how much care must be taken both in dealing with the question itself and with all possible answers to it.[422]

The above viewpoint emphasises the importance of the search for the *why?* and meaning of suffering in human life. And moreso that suffering is one of the most frequent experiences of daily life and one which constantly prompts questions as to its meaning and purpose. In fact those who wish to attack the idea of God challenge believers with the paradox that a God who is all–loving nevertheless lives with and permits so much suffering in the world.

In the face of difficulties in the life of man by way of mental and physical handicap, sudden transition from normality to ill health, the pain of loss, the ultimate tragedy of death, are our constant reminders that suffering is never far away. Suffering becomes more inexplicable when a young person with special gifts is struck with some disabling diesease or dies; when a gifted child is attacked by a malignant illness before its talents have matured. How can one explain these tragedies of Life?

In the Gospel of St. John, the teaching of Christ ends with the solemn statement: "You will suffer in the world. But take courage! I have overcome the world" (John 16:55; 1 John 5:5). For the true Christian suffering has a new meaning. "All I want is to know Christ and to experience the power of his resurrection; to share his sufferings and become like him in his death, in the hope that I myself will be raised from death to life." (Phil. 3:10–12). St. Paul understood his suffering in the light of Christ's suffering, and could express his feeling as he did.

Christ freely chose a particularly painful sort of death. In this way he made sure that there was no form of human suffering which he had not embraced and therefore transformed. Everything he touched, including suffering, was invaded by his love and thereby made purposseful and creative. To perceive the true answer to the "why" of suffering we must go – to the revelation of divine love for we are conscious of the insufficiency and inadequacy of our explanations. Hence Albert Keller's contribution:

422 John Paul 11 Op. Cit pp.14 –15

We only have to see it (suffering) as a task proposed to us. ... From this aim in our life, we can say in a christian way: There is nothing that is not meaningful as long as it is in accordance with the love of God and the love of Neighbour – and everything is without meaning when it opposed to the love of God and love of Neighbour: that applies to suffering and also not less and not more to other things we experience in our lives.[423]

Meditating on this subject with christians, the Holy Father , Pope John Paul II writes:

We must above all accept the light of Revelation not only insofar as it expresses the transcendent order of justice but also insofar as it illuminates this order with love, as the definitive source of everything that exists. Love is also the fullest source of the answer to the question of the meaning of suffering. This answer has been given by God to man in the Cross of Jesus Christ.[424]

It is important to note here, that suffering and sacrifice is the only means to show our love of God and love of neighbour which is the summary of our christian life. As christians we are bound to love because without love our christian life is meaningless. Without love we are dead spiritually because love is life. St. John rather puts it thus: "For God so loved the world that he gave his only Son, that whoever believes in him should not perish but have eternal life" (Jn.3:16).

What lessons do we learn from what we have so far discussed?

Christ's suffering is a model for our suffering. Concerning the Sick and the Suffering one reads in Vatican Council II Document thus:

Christ's words show them that illness has a meaning and a value for their own salvation and that of the world. They are also aware that during his life Christ loved the sick and that he often healed them. ... Christ still suffers and undergoes torments whenever we his followers suffer.[425]

We see at its centre separation from experience of the of the Father, the Incanation and the ultimate reunion to his Father. However, the ultimate criterion of love is the maintainance of relationship. Christ while maintaining his relationship of love with the Father, met suffering face to face. He met it in the human condition, and his life , death and resurection constitute the event which has trans-

423 "Wir müssen es nur als eine Aufgabe betrachten, die uns gestellt ist. ... Von diesem Ziel unseres Lebens her läßt sich aber christlich sagen: Nichts ist sinnlos, solange es im Einklang mit der Gottes– und Nächstenliebe steht – und alles ist sinnlos, wenn es ihr widerspricht: das gilt für das Leid nicht mehr und nicht weniger als für irgendeine sonstige Gegebenheit, die uns begegnet" Keller, A., Op. Cit p.61

424 John Paul II., Salvifici Doloris ... No. 13

425 Vatican Council II., Introduction to the Rite of Anointing and to the Pastoral Care of the Sick, S.C.D.W., Hominum dolores, 7 December, 1972. p.15

formed suffering. Now suffering has become creative and part of the evolution of man towards God. It cannot be escaped and the world needs it for its progress. Therefore whether suffering is peculiar to us or to the society in which we live, it has to be handled with a loving response on our part because of its benefits in our lives.

Van der Poel shows us how suffering reveals our capabilities and limitations:

> *1. It makes us aware of our dependence on others.*
> *2. It makes us appreciate the concern of others for us.*
> *3. It opens our minds to the needs of others; and*
> *4. It inclines our heart to extend love to those in need.*
>
> *Suffering also teaches us respect for the weaknesses of others and for the efforts they make to rearrange their lives. It makes us sensitive for a power beyond our control, and thus it directs our minds to God ... and it provides us with opportunity to make God's love real to those in need.*[426]

We shall now examine the Human suffering in typical European background.

3.3.5 The meaning of Human Suffering in a typical european background

The Igbo people and indeed all Africans have been recognised by both foreign and indigenous authors as being very religious, family–tie, *umunna,* togetherness, life of sharing, and these aspects of their lives reflect in the way they understand pain, human suffering and death in their lives. The Igbo people in particular share their joys, pains and sorrows with neighbours. When one suffers in a family all members participate in this ordeal.

The same applies in some of the European countries especially in Germany. where families and relations play a greater role in care of their ageing, sick and the dying members of their families. According to a report of the Statistisches Bundesamt 2005 which among other things maintained that:

"The importance of family and other private means of supporting and helping the weak, old and sick people of the society are indisputable. 68 percent of more than two million destitute people who are in need of care and support are being catered for in their homes and families".[427]

---

426 Cornelius Van der Poel, op. Cit., pp.44–45

427 "Die Bedeutung von Familie und weiteren prvaten Netzen für die Unterstützung hilfe– und pflegebedürftiger Menschen ist unbestritten. Von den über zwei Millionen pflegebedürftigen Menschen leben 68 Prozent im eigenen Haushalt und werden von Familienangehörigen und anderen Migliedern des privaten Netzes vollständig oder zum Teil versorgt". – Bundesministerium für Familie, Senioren, Frauen und Jugend,

In Igbo land in Nigeria togetherness plays a vital role in caring for the sick and the suffering people in the society and the same system obtains in Germany.

And moreover, what both Societies shares in common is the fact that all means availabe are explored to reduce and to avoid pains and suffering, especially the unnecessary ones as already discussed above. Ibos would put it this way, 'ejiro afufu anya isi' – one should not parade and show–off suffering.

The Germans will say like the Ibos that Krankheit hat in unsere Leistungsgesellschaft keinen Platz. the afore–discussed situation leads naturally to the next section: european understanding of human suffering and death.

3.3.6 European understanding of Human Suffering and Death

In most of the european countries, especially in German Society, Sickness is viewed as a weakness and a disturbance to the Economic progress of the Society. The Germans are very hard working and anything that disrupts this disorgnises the system and should be avoided by all means. Generally illness is not seen as something positiv. Sickness expresses, that one is not fit and thereby not equal to the environment. This picture is portrayed more in Radio and Television advertisements. What dominates the european Media is youthfulness, fitness and beauty. How one can remain ever young and strong through medication. Sick person disrupts the work process.

However, whether we wish to acknowledge it or not, it is not unusual for humans to attack and /or blame the one who suffers. As Simone Weil remarks:

> *Men have the same carnal nature as animals. If a hen is hurt, the others rush upon it, attacking it with their beaks. ... our senses attach all the scorn, all the revulsion, all the hatred that our reason attaches to crime, to affliction. Except for those whose whole soul is inhabited by Christ, everybody despises the afflicted to some extent, although practically no one is conscious of it.*[428]

Fünfter Bericht zur Lage der älteren Generation in der Bundesrepublik Deutschland, Berlin im August 2005, p.313

428 Weil, 122. "Research in the field of victimology reveals that the initial universal reaction of human beings to victims of violence is to reject them." Joy M.K. Bussert, Battered Women: From a Theology of Suffering to an Ethic of Empowerment (New York: Lutheran Church in America, Division for Mission in North America, 1986) 31. Cf. Marcia Alpert and Susan Schechter, "Sensitising Workers to the Needs of Victims: Common Worker and Victim Responses," Victimology: An International Journal 55 (1979) 385 – 9

In these ways, suffering is, perhaps, the quintessential solitary experience. Consequently, this inherent loneliness heightens the suffering in that isolation can become its outcome.

Hence Cassell writes:

Because the sufferer's loss of connection with the group is one of the most important aspects of suffering both from the standpoint of its origins and its opportunities for relief, the loneliness of the sufferer is not only the feeling of being alone but an absence from the general "we–ness" of the world, from a shared participation in spirit.[429]

Connection and communication with others breaks down and one enters into a state of alienation wherein one's condition is not easily or totally conveyed to nor understood by others. One notices a similar situation in some societies where people live without family or friends or loses the one they have simply because they are sick. Sickness means then total solitude and isolation. No one wants to be infected, they claimed as one of their reasons. In this society Suffering is avoided by all means within human power. The relationship between the Healthy and the Sick is often very deplorable and unfriendly. Some families avoid and isolates any sick member and are ashamed to identified with or talk about them in Public. Many do not seem to understand the religious purpose of suffering.

Another important aspect of this section is the help rendered to the Dying. In english speaking european countries it is called "terminal care" This concept means the assistance given to a person or persons in their last stage of their earthly existence. It embraces all the medical, physical, social, and psychological care offered to the sick–dying patient.

This concept Hospice was first used in the Middle Ages. Norbert Hofmann described this word "Hospice" as a special community of persons who took a solemn vow to serve the needs of pilgrims and travellers in the Middle Ages.[430]

Down to the middle of this century, the concept of "Hospice" focused its attention more on the Christian hotels in the big cities which was organised by the Protestant churches and which is comparable to that of the Catholics in the Kolpinghauses.[431]

---

429 Cassel, 1902

430 Im Mittelalter "wurde das Wort 'Hospiz' dafür benutzt, spezielle Gemeinschaften von Personen zu beschreiben, die ein feierliches Gelöbnis ablegeten, den Bedürfnissen von Pilgern und Reisenden zu dienen".
Hofmann, Norbert, Hospiz zum hl. Franziskus in Recklinghausen–süd, Recklinghausen 1990, p.35

431 Bis zur Neubegrundung der Hospizidee in der Mitte dieses Jahrhunderts stand der Begriff Hospiz dann für christliche Hotels in den Großständten, die von der evangelischen Kirchen getragen wurden, vergleichbar mit den Kolpinghäusern in der Ka-

For a number of reasons, hospice care is somewhat difficult to define. This is in part because the term "hospice" dates back to the Middle Ages and over the years has had different meanings. Furthermore, present day hospice care is characterized by its diversity. Therefore we shall give various definitions of Hospice.

In Webster's New World Dictionary (1972) hospice is defined as an inn for travelers, especially one kept by a religious order, and secondarily as a home for the sick or the poor. Stedman's Medical Dictionary (1982) defines hospice as an institution that provides a centralized program of palliative and supportive services to dying persons and their families, in the form of physical, psychological, social, and spiritual care. Such services are provided by an interdisciplinary team of professionals and volunteers who are available at home and in inpatient settings.[432]

In 1978 the National Hospice Organization (NHO) adopted the following definition: Hospice is a medically directed, nurse coordinated program providing a continuum of home and inpatient care for the terminally ill patient and family. It employs an intedisciplinary team acting under the directionof an autonomous hospice administsration. The program provides palliative and supportive care to meet the special needs arising out of the physical, emotional, spiritual, social and economic stresses which are experienced during the final stages of illness and during dying and bereavement.[433]

Etymologically, the term "Hospice" originates from Hospitium a latin word meaning hospitality and lodging. This word Hospice means more than hospitality and lodging, it entails the whole conern and care given to the dying patients and their relatives.

The hospice movement describes therefore not only the activities involved but also the solidarity with one another. Here one should correct the wrong idea that Hospice movement concerns itself only with the "dying clinical complexes". The movement aims and touches all segments of man.

Although the basic idea and practice of hospice movement dated as far back as the time before Christ, it was officially inaugurated in 1967. There were already in the early Middle Ages about 750 hospices in England, "40 in Paris alone and in Florence 30. It came very late in the Federal Republic of Germany be-

---

tholischen Kirche. Vgl.: Godzik, Peter, Die Hospizbewegung in der Bundesrepublik Deutschland, in: Godzik, Peter, Pfister, Karl Dietrich, Pleitner, Henning (Hg.) "... daß die Gemeinde zum Hospiz werde", A1–A103, (Diakonisches Werk der EKD Stuttgart 1992) A3

432 Zimmerman, Jack M., Hospice: Complete Care for the Terminally Ill, Urban & Schwarzenberg, Baltimore–Munich, 1986 p.17

433 Background materials provided to the author by the staff of the Maryland Hospice Reimbursement Commission,1981 in Zimmerman, Jack M.: ibid: p.17

cause of oppositions from the two big churches. They refused the establishment of "Sterbekliniken" The churches were afraid that the dying will be deported and dishonoured. The cause of this scepticism was a film showned in the Television by the ZDF on June 10th 1971 about Pater Reinhold Iblacker "still 16 days ... klinic for the dying" which reported about life in St. Christopher Hospice in London. The German film producers maintained that the "klinic for the Dying" has led to many irritations and oppositions in many sectors. The aim and aspiration of this Hospice movement was doubtful and suspicious. People were saying among other things that the founders wanted to commercialize and institutionalise the dying.[434] And also to this Film Anton Szekely writes: it is a pity, that such a Film exist. It is unwanted and intrusive. The dying humanity is taken as a job, it is inconceivable. Through this movement we have lost our sense of love, sympathy and responsibility. For a example a son left his dying father and for a football match without quams of conscience.[435]

Secondly, the good social system and the health insurance programme in the Federal Republic of Germany contributed immensely to its late take–off. Unlike other countries where one has to pay for all one's Hospital bills without state assistance. So countries like USA saw this Hospice movement as a financial and a social help/relief.

These were among the reasons for the late take–off of the Hospice Movement in the Federal Republic of Germany. The first attempt of this model station was opened with 5 patients for Palliative therapy in the Surgical department of Uni-

---

434 In der Bundesrepublik Deutschland hat die Hospizbewegung erst sehr spät Fuß gefaßt. Noch Mitte der 70 Jahre lehnten Fachkundige aus beiden großen Kirchen die Gründung von "Sterbekliniken" ab. Es wurde eine Abschiebung und Ghettoisierung der Sterbenden befürchtet. Anlaß dieser Skepsis war bei vielen der vom ZDF am 10. Juni 1971 ausgestrahlte Film von Pater Reinhold Iblacker "Noch 16 Tage ... Eine Sterbeklinik in London", der über das Leben im St. Christopher Hospz, London, berichtete. Die deutschen Filmproduzenten titulierten das Hospiz "Sterbeklinik", was zu vielen Irritationen geführt hat. Die eigentliche Grundidee des Hospizes wurde vielen Zuschauern nicht deutlich, vielmehr herrschte die Meinung vor, hier ginge es um die Kommerzialisierung und Institutionalisierung des Sterbens. Vgl.: Zielinski, H.R., Sterbeklinik – Ja oder Nein, in: Zielinski, H.R. (Hg.), Prüfsteine medizinischer Ethik I., 52–86 (Kath. Klinikseelsorge an den Medizinischen Einrichtungen der Universität Düsseldorf 1980) 70f.

435 So schrieb damals Anton Szekely zu diesem Film: "Schade, daß es ihn gibt. Er ist gestellt und zudringlich. Er hat den beigeschmack von Kommerzialisierung des Sterbens. Humanität beim Sterbenden als Job – eine unsympathische Vorstellung. Nun ist auch das Persönliche instituitionalisiert, die Verantwortung abgenommen, wir sind von einer Pflicht losgekauft. Der Sohn kann ruhig zum Fußballspiel gehen, während der Vater stirbt." Zielinski, Helmut Eeinhold, Prüfsteine medizinischer Ethik, (Grevenbroich 1980) 54.

versity of Cologne on April 7th, 1983. The success of this initial attempt gave rise to other groups in other parts of Germany. In the beginning of 1984 there was already in the Old peoples home and Nursing home in Stuttgart some elements of Hospice under the pastoral care of Diakonin Ursula Lesny. This existed under the name "Sitzwache in Pflegeheimen"

The first German Hospice movement was officially opened in Aachen in November, 1986. This house is called "Haus Hörn". It was founded by a catholic priest Dr. Paul Türks and his brother priests from the Congregation of St. Philip Neri. This House "Haus Hörn" was opened with 53 beds by this Congregation. This house admitted not only those patients whose days are numbered but also those who have a longer period to live unlike other Hospice Movements. After this period Hospice Movement spread like wide fire in Germany. For example in 1987 there was one Recklinghausen named after St. Francis with 8 beds near St. Elisabeth Hospital in a very small house. A section of this Hospice for Palliative Therapy existed in Malteser Hospital of Robert–Janker–Klinik in Bonn. Another in Munich by the Brothers of Mercy Hospital (*Barmherzigen Brüder Krankenhaus*) since 1991 with 10 beds which later increased to 25 beds.

Today is Hospice movement everywhere in the Federal Republic of Germany. It is interesting to note that since the past 8 years Hospice movements have spread almost every where in the Federal Republic of Germany.

Hospice movement is one of the principal ways of getting rid of the sick in the society and which also portrays european attitude towards Sickness and Death. The scope of hospice care is terminal illness.

As a practical matter hospice addresses itself to the care of those for whom the determination has been made that cure is not possible, that the disease will lead to the patient's death, and that efforts must be directed primarily as palliation.

In hospice care programs, the unit of care is not just the patient, but the patient and his or her family as already noted above. This section will not be complete without mentioning a renowned Swiss woman medical doctor who has done a several research in this area of human suffering and death. This aspect of her study has also African undertone especially in Igbo community. Dr. Elisabeth Kübler–Ross, had gathered alot of experience in this field. She has worked for over twenty years in the United States of America in Hospitals and also worked and taught in the Universities. Her wealth of experience will definitely be of immense help in this section.

In one of her Books titled "Interviews mit Sterbenden" Here she describes the human pains and the dying process in five phases. She sat several hours at the death–bed of many dying patients and had a deep rooted interview with them and came out with these five phase of human pains before death. These stages exposes a typical european reaction to Sickness and Death and to some extent Igbo people attitudes towards death.

First Phase: Denial of the truth: "No, it can not be myself" – Stage.[436] The person affected denies the fact of the forthcoming death and declines information which substantiates this fact.

Second Phase: Anger – Fury – Aggression, the "Why I"? Stage.[437] When one realises that the sickness is a reality, one becomes angry, aggressive, hostile, envious of the healthy people around. Then the big question "why me" At this stage is the dying aware of his loss which he or she is going to experience soon. At this moment visits of relatives and medical personnel is very important so that one should not die in lonliness and agony.

Third Phase: Negotiation – the "o.k, so I am the person, but ..." Stage.[438] This stage of dying process does not last long. One negotiates with fate. The dying tries at this stage to behave well and shows signs of charity by and makes amend of his or her mistakes in life. He or she starts making wishes of what he would like to experiece or witness before he or she dies. One said for example "I will like to witness the wedding ceremony of my daughter" Such wishes shows that the dying has alot to settle in life, quarells, fear or debts. It is important not to wave this stage of regrets away instead one should try to talk over it with the dying, for him or her to die peacefully.

Fourth Phase: Depression. The "Yes I am" – Stage.[439] At this Phase Kübler–Ross distinguishes between two forms of depression namely: the "reactive depression" and the "preparatory depression". Reactive depression: Here the dying regrets abouts lost of favourite places and things like place of work, as the 'bread winner' of the family and the subsequent consequent on the family. At this stage, the person concerned needs companion and words of encouragement.

The "Preparatory depression" is a very difficult stage for the Person helping the sick and especially for the relatives and friends of the dying. According to Kübler–Ross this stage is very important for the dying so that he or she can have internal peace and be prepared before dying.

Fifth Phase: Acceptance: the "It is all right" – Stage.[440] At this last phase he or she accepts death. Kübler–Ross described this dying–processes as successful.

---

436 1.Phase: Die Verleugnung und Isolierung, das "Nein, ich doch nicht" – Stadium. Vgl.: Kübler–Ross, Elisabeth, Interviews mit Sterbenden, (Stuttgart – Berlin 1971) 41ff.

437 2. Phase: Wut – Zorn – Aggression, das "Warum ich?" Stadium. Ibid. 50ff

438 3. Phase: Das Handeln, oder Verhandeln, das "O.k, also ich, aber ..." – Stadium. Ibid. 77ff

439 4. Phase: Depression. Das "Ja, ich" – Stadium. Ibid. 80ff

440 5. Phase: Das Annehmen. Das "Es ist in Ordnung" – Stadium. Ibid. 99ff

This stage should not be seen as a failure on the part of the dying but should be seen as a help to face the end peacefully.

The above dying–phases can be found also in African understanding of Death, especially in Igbo traditional society. One goes through this but there are no obvious records. But one must not go through these stages before one dies. In African context and especially in Igbo traditional society, the belief in life after death is very strong. That is why the Igbo people attitude towards sickness and death is some how different from European understanding where sickness and death should not be discussed publicly and therefore regarded as a taboo theme. People are afraid to discuss or face the consequences of sickness and death. This attitude towards sickness and especially death has something to do with religious faith of the people. The Igbo traditional religionists know that life continues after physical death and it shows more in their strong belief of life–after death. Igbo people sees death as a stepping stone to the next life which accords him or her the opportunity to make amends what he or she lost in the present life and to become what he or she wishes to be in life.

The adverbs – "everlasting", "perpetual", "constant", when used in reference to human life are synonymous with the noun 'immortality'. Immortality in Igbo language is "ndu–ebebe" or "ndirigaba"[441] which is the literary translation of 'everlasting life'.

Every culture recognises the fact that mortal beings do not live on earth everlastingly. This is clear from the experience of death of children, adolescents and the aged. In other words, death belongs to the history of human existence. However, the Igbo understanding of the transitory nature of this physical life and the eternal nature of the home beyond, is well brought out this much quoted Igbo song:

> Anyi biara afia n'uwaa,
> Azujuru abo, azujughi abo,
> Mgbe oge ruru, onye obuna eburu abo ya naa.
> We are on a market trip on earth,

441 Ezeogu, E., Ndu Uwa Ozo N'Echiche Ndi Igbo (B.A. thesis written in Igbo language, (Ikot Ekpene, Bigard Memorial Seminary, 1978). The word 'Ndirigaba' is unsed throughout this thesis to explain the Igbo concept of the after–life . See Daniel Nwafor Anih, Spiritual Care of the Family Among the Igbos of Nigeria after "Familiaris Consortio" of Pope John–Paul 11, Rome, May 30, 1991 p.75

Whether we fill our baskets or not,
Once the time is up, we go home.[442]

The European culture especially in German speaking countries recognises this fact but regards it as a topic that should not be discussed. Consequently when death occurs it becomes a disaster irrespective of the age of the person or persons concerned. Sherwin B. Nuland puts it this way: Today, we deny not only the thorn of death but also the power of Nature. We close our eyes with our hands to save us from the sight of this terrible Ordeal.[443]

Another concept that requires brief attention in this chapter is the Active euthanasia (aktiven Sterbehilfe) Hospics which we have already discussed in this section also takes care of patients in this category. The word "euthanasia" comes from the Greek – "eu" meaning "goodly or well" and "thanatos" meaning "death". So, euthanasia is literally the "good death". Euthanasia is generally classified as either "active" or "passive", and as either "voluntary" or "involuntary".

"Passive euthanasia" is usually defined as withdrawing medical treatment with the deliberate intention of causing the patient's death. For example, if a patient requires kidney dialysis to survive, and the doctors disconnect the dialysis machine, the patient will presumably die fairly soon. Perhaps the classic example of passive euthanasia is a "do not resuscitate order". Normally if a patient has a heart attack or similar sudden interruption in life functions, medical staff will attempt to revive them. If they make no such effort but simply stand and watch as the patient dies, this is passive euthanasia.

"Active euthanasia" is taking specific steps to cause the patient's death, such as injecting the patient with poison. In practice, this is usually an overdose of pain–killers or sleeping pills.

In other words, the difference between "active" and "passive" is that in active euthanasia, something is *done* to end the patient's life; in passive euthanasia, something is *not done* that would have preserved the patient's life.

The Netherlands is currently the only country in the world in which euthanasia is openly and legally practiced. There, euthansia and assisted suicide are defined by the State Commission on Euthanasia, Euthanasia is the intentional termination of life by somebody other than the person concerned at his or her request.

---

442 Vgl.: Nwokocha, C.C. op. Cit., pp 174 – 175, quoted, Obiego, c. o., op. Cit., p.196, Eboh, B., Man In African Religion: London: Geoffrey Chapman, 1981), p.139. Nwafor Anih , D. ibid. p. 79

443 "Wir können heute nicht nur den Stachel des Todes, sondern die Macht der Natur schlechthin leugnen. Wir legen die Hand vor die Augen, um uns den Anblick des Schrecklichen zu ersparen, ..." Nuland Sherwin, B., New Haven, Juni 1993 p.16

Euthanasia is a matter of contnuing controversy, a tinderbox for debate, an issue on which positions range widely and include enthusiastic advocacy of euthanasia, guarded acceptace of euthanasia, outright rejection of euthanasia, and vehement condemnation of euthansia, equating it with murder, genocide, or worse. But who knows? Euthanasia is an area in which honest people may still differ.

3.4 Conclusive Summary

In summary, this chapter has tried to present an analogical unfolding of the reflection on health and healing with the help of the concepts of suffering and sickness in the light of European culture. It calls attention to the fact that Christian suffering is to be thought anew in the framework of Salvation.

4. Chapter Four – Healing by Jesus and the Church

4.1 The Healing Ministry of Jesus Christ and the Healing Tradition of the Church; her concern for the Sick and Suffering

4.1.1 The Healing Ministry of Jesus Christ

From the history of the chosen people, God revealed himself as the healer of his people. Abraham the father of the nations experienced that revelation (Gen 17:15–20; 21:1–7), as well as Solomon the great king of the people (2 Chron. 6: 28–30). This revelation of God himself as the healer of all was not limited by time. God answered the prayer of all people and at all times and places.

The promises of healing are also very clear with the people of the new covenant. The Lord Jesus came to reveal God the Father fulfilling what was promised in the Old Testament. Hence Jesus said, "He that has seen me has seen the father". (Jn 14: 9) And He went about all Galilee, teaching in their synagogues and preaching the gospel of the kingdom, and healing every disease and every infirmity among the people. So his fame spread throughout all Syria and they brought him those who are sick and those afflicted with different types of diseases and pains, demoniacs, epileptics and paralytics and he healed them. (Mt 4:23–24; Mk.1:39; Lk. 4:14–15) And many people got attracted to him that they followed him wherever he went even to the mountains and across the seas and lakes. At times he had to slip away from the crowd to be in hiding, perhaps to have some rest but most often to have opportunity to pray. The people were astonished by the way he carried out his mission that they began to say that he taught not like the Scribes and the Pharisees but like one who has authority, that even the evil spirits obey his words. Even John the Baptist who was his forerunner had to send his own disciples to find out whether he was the awaited Messiah or not. Jesus answer to John was simple – "Go and tell John what you have heard and seen; the blind recover their sight, the cripples walk, lepers are cleansed, the deaf hear, the dead raised to life and the poor has the gospel preached to them." (Mt11:2–6)

So it was Jesus himself who began the Tradition of healing in the Church, and it was his own healing ministry that set the pattern for Christian healers who have been carrying on the ministry for nearly twenty centuries.[444]

There were no limits to the healing power of Jesus Christ. Jesus healed men physically, spiritually, emotionally and mentally. He healed men and women in all their relationships with one another and with God. That is to say that his healing was holistic. Jesus Christ was able to do this ministry in this way because of his unique relationship with the Father. He freely acknowledges that his father was the source of all power and all healing. "Truly I say to you, the son can do nothing of his own accord, but only what he sees the Father doing, for whatever he does, that the son likewise does" (Jn 5:19), and again "I can do nothing of my own authority" (Jn 5:30).[445]

In the ministry of Jesus, preaching, teaching, and healing went together and he sees each of them as an integral part of his message of salvation.

In offering men salvation, then Christ is saving men from a hopeless situation into a hopeful one: He saves them from sin into life of God. He saves men from illness into health.[446]

Hence the commissioning of Jesus did not regard sickness as normal order of life so everything that can make man sick was absolutely detested by Jesus. His healings confirm that the power of the kingdom of God had come and demonstrated Christ's victory over evil. Jesus' love for his people was so great, such that he had deep compassion on those who were sick. So his healing ministry was out of love and compassion and was a sign that he was the Son of God. "The work which the Father has granted me to accomplish, these very works which I am doing bear me witness that the Father has sent me."(Jn 5:36) Jesus did his ministry in obedience to the Father, never attributing any strength or powers to himself.

Jesus did not stop his healing ministry or his healing works with his own time. He saw the need to extend the ministry to other ages and to other nations of the world. Jesus transmitted the gift of healing to the Church, to equip her to be effective instrument of the witness of the kingdom. Hence the commissioning of the

444 R. Baldwin, The Healers, Indiana, 1986, p.10

445 Jesus Christ is the healer par excellence. It was Jesus who handed over the mission of healing to his disciples and then to the healers of today. He did all his healing in the name of God the fahter and never claimed any powers to himself, as is almost the case with most of the healing ministers of today. Healing ministers have to have Jesus as their model and master.

446 J.Turner, The Healing Church, Belfast, Ottawa, 1978, p.12

twelve who were his immediate and close followers to carry the gospel mission of preaching and healing the sick to the ends of the world. So the healing ministry was an endowment of the commissioned witness.

These are the signs that will be associated with believers; in my name they will cast out devils, they will have the gifts of tongues, they will pick up snakes, and if they drink any deadly thing, it will not hurt them; they will lay their hands on the sick and they will recover. (Mk 16:17–18)

And greater works than I have done shall they do so that the Father may be glorified. (cf Jn 14:12 &13) And He entrusted the Holy Spirit to remain with them and from then, He remains ever present and active in the Church.

4.2 Dimensions of the Healing Ministry of Jesus Christ

"Nothing is more certain about Jesus than, that He was viewed by his contemporaries as an exorcist and a healer".[447] During the lifetime of Jesus on earth, he healed all the sick who came to him or were brought to him in faith by their friends and relations. His life was a complete and total mission of reconciliation and healing. He healed through everything he said or did and through his presence. His healing was his life and message. Little wonder Buckley says,

His healing was ordinary to him in so far as this is what he came to do with his life. It was not extra – ordinary for him to make the blind see. He said that this was his mission the first time he stood up to preach in the Synagogue of the youth. (Lk 4:18)[448]

The healing of Jesus involves not only organic or physical healing of diseases but a complete healing or integral healing which concerns different dimensions of man. Since healing involves whatever is not functioning well in a man, Jesus heals whatever is sick in man whether physical, spiritual or emotional. As there are different kinds of sickness, so there are different dimensions of healing that Jesus wrought when he was on earth. Jesus healed the lepers, the paralytics and the epileptics of their sicknesses giving them the healing experiences of human love and divine presence. He rescued men and women who were declared social outcasts by the Jewish society, by healing them of their sicknesses that were the root of the high solid boundaries separating them from their brothers and sisters.

No two healing of Jesus are alike because no two people are the same. Every form of healing is subordinate and related to the person who is healed. The ten

447 J.Meier, Jesus, in "The New Jerome Biblical Commentary", London, 1991, p.1321
448 M.Buckley, His Healing Touch, Glasgow, 1997, p.48

lepers in the gospel were cleansed of the leprosy but nine were lacking in praise to God and gratitude to Jesus. By this they lack emotional healing. But the Samaritan leper who came back and threw himself on the ground at the feet of Jesus in gratitude received not only physical cleansing of his leprosy but "expressed an emotional healing of one man to another."[449] Towards the end of life of Jesus on earth, he continued his healing works.

> *As He hung dying upon the cross, he prayed for forgiveness for those who crucified him, promising paradise to the repentant thief, and comforted his grieving mother by bequeathing John to take his place. His life, whether in word or deed was a healing life. That is what he came on earth to do in order to obey his father's will.*[450]

This will of the Father he carried out perfectly well and in various dimensions. Considering therefore the various sick people that Jesus ministered to and the different forms of his healing, we classify his healing ministry under the following dimensions physical, spiritual, emotional and social.

4.1.2 The Physical Dimension of the Healing Works of Jesus

The importance of physical or organic healing has been played down or neglected by some people while upholding spiritual and emotional healing as more important and most accepted forms of healing.

> *But physical healing is so much an essential part of the Gospel ministry of Jesus Christ that to deny it in the Christian Church would be a betrayal of our Christian mission, responsibility and heritage. Many traditional Churches are extremely suspicious of most forms of physical healing and restrict them to special places of pilgrimage or as evidence of unique holiness in extraordinary people. Physical healing for them is often a challenge to their accepted norms of how God behaves with his Churches and people.*[451]

Jesus performed more of physical healings than any other kind of healings as recorded in the Gospels. Since physical dimension of man's health deals with his physical fitness viewed from the point of view of vitality and absence of pain, Jesus among his many healings, healed those kinds of illnesses that affect or have detrimental influence on man's physical vitality and soundness of his organs. And physical sufferings we know are painful and destructive to the body and sometimes prevent man from loving his God and living a truly human Christian life. But physical pain and its accompanying anguish have its own saving mission

---

449 M.Buckley, His Healing Touch, Op. Cit., p.181

450 Ibid., p.48 & 49

451 M.Buckley, His Healing Touch, p.179

which is sometimes difficult for the person suffering to understand. Hence Sandrin observes that,

The suffering (as the anguish that accompanies it) is ambiguous: It is a temptation to close up in one's self and abandon God, but it can become also avenue to him and opportunity to rediscover him closely. This of course is not innate in the suffering itself (and in the anguish that comes with it) but the fruit of the gratuitous love of God, of his "grace" to decipher "in faith" the proper experience of life.[452]

So Jesus healed the physical illness of the sick persons that came to him or were brought to him in faith by their friends and relations. Coming down from the mountain where he escaped to be alone in prayer, a crowd followed him. Among the crowd was a leper, who came up and bowed before him and said, "Sir if you want to, you can cure me. And Jesus stretched out his hand, touched him and said, Of course, 1 want to! Be cured: And the leprosy was cured at once." (Mt 8:1–4, Mk 1:40–45, Lk 5:12–16)

In the ancient world, leprosy was the most terrible of all diseases. It might begin with little nodules, which go on to ulcerate. The ulcers develop a foul discharge; the eye brows fall out; the eyes become staring; the vocal chords become ulcerated and the voice becomes hoarse, and the breath wheezes. The hands and feet always ulcerate. Slowly the sufferer becomes a mass of ulcerated growths. The average course of that kind of leprosy is nine years, and it ends in mental decay, coma and ultimately death.[453]

This was the sickness that Jesus cured restoring normal and healthy physical condition of the man, making him clean again. There were also cases of healing of the man with a withered hand (Mt 12: 9–14; Mk 3:1–6; Lk 6:6–1 1), and the deaf–mute (Mk 7.–31–37) and other healings of Jesus with physical dimensions.

At this junction, we must observe that most of the physical healings of Jesus are often linked with more profound spiritual healings and much desired social integration into the community. The story of the ten lepers takes into account the spiritual and emotional healing as well as the physical cleansing that took place on the road to Jerusalem. So the physical Dimension of the healings of Jesus deals with the putting to normal functioning, any sick organ of the body, making it functional and whole and in harmony with all the other organs of the body, since we know that every healing is of the whole person. Jesus, though, performed more of physical healings than any other kind of healing, does not per-

---

452 Luciano Sandrin, Introduzione, "Che cosa ho fitto male?" Una domanda che provoca, in L. Sandrin, (a cura di), "Che cosa ho fatto male?" Malattia e senso di colpa, Edizioni Camilliane, Torino, 1999, p.12

453 W. Barclay, The Daily Study Bible: The Gospel of Matthew, Vol 1, Edinburgh, 1975, p.295

form any physical healing for the sake of physical fitness alone. He heals the whole person giving the sick a total or integral cure.

4.2.1.1 Spiritual Dimension of the Healings of Jesus

We have already observed that healing involves more than mere physical healing of the body and the organs. It involves the person as a whole and no healing is wrought for it's own sake. Jesus approached each person that came to him for healing as an integral entity because he was able to see the influence of the body and the mind on each other.

> *Because healing is completeness, it has everything to do with all of man's relationships with those whom he loves and with those whom he loathes; it affects his attitudes to those whom he fears; those whom he resents and to those whom he is indifferent.*[454]

Healing also has something very significant to do with man's relationship with God, hence the spiritual Dimension of healing. Spiritual healing is often regarded as the most possible Dimension of healing since it is in God that man finds his completeness.

> *If such things as guilt, fear, jealousy and resentment lie at the root of some forms of illness and if we are still too proud to actually receive the gift of God's forgiveness or to ask for the forgiveness of others or what is even more difficult, to forgive ourselves, we may or can obstruct the healing energies of God. If we are to be healed, we must experience the force of God's healing power as something stronger than that which holds our spirit in it's grip.*[455]

There is therefore no wonder why Jesus often deals with the forgiveness of sins in most of his healing works. "Your sins are forgiven you" (Mt 9:2; Mk 2:5; Lk 5:20; Jn 5:14). He also talks often of faith. "Your faith has healed you"; "My daughter, your faith has restored you to health; go in peace." (Mk 5:34; Mt 9:22; Lk 8:48) While healing the Centurion's servant, Jesus said, "Nowhere in Israel have I found faith like this." (Mt 8:10; Lk 7: 10)

Spiritual healing is more important than physical healing and many people believe in praying for spiritual healing than for physical healing. Hence B. Heron in his work says,

---

454 J. Turner, The Healing Church, Op. Cit., p.8
455 Ibid., p.49

We should never pray for the healing of the body, without praying for the healing of the spirit and mind. The spirit, mind and body are inter–related. We find in practice that spiritual healing frequently over–flows into the healing of the mind and body.[456]

Jesus very often heals the spirit before any physical healing of the body. The healing of the paralyzed man in Capernaum, brought to him by friends comes to mind at this point. "And behold, they brought to him a paralytic, lying on his bed; and when Jesus saw their faith he said to the paralytic, "Take heart, my son; your sins are forgiven" (Mt 9:2). "The man's paralysis was obvious but Jesus saw a deeper need than physical healing."[457] It became therefore necessary to give a spiritual healing first to this man that was brought to Jesus on the faith of friends.

In this incident, the visible miracle is a sign pointing to the deeper miracle – the cure of the man's paralysis indicated that Jesus had removed the man's sins. This would be of the utmost importance for the beliefs of the first Christians, because they believed that sin could do them far more harm than any physical disability.[458]

4.2.1.2 Emotional or Psychological Dimension of the Healings of Jesus

Jesus healed not only physical and spiritual illnesses. He also healed those who were emotionally or psychologically tormented.

With all respect to recent psychological research, the development of new terminology and a heightened awareness of the importance of Psychiatric healing, it seems that Jesus – two thousand years ago–healed all forms of illness including emotional and psychological ills.[459]

Many writers in healing works often noticed these Psychological or emotional healings of Jesus, by the casting out of the evil spirits or exorcisms. Writing on the healings of Jesus which appear psychological in nature, Meehan says,

This includes some of the presumed exorcisms performed by Jesus where the spirit of God appeared to be in direct confrontation with evil spirits. At this time in which the Gospels were written, there was no category for mental illness. Neurosis and Psychoses as well as some physical illnesses were identified with the powers of evil that originated from unclean spirits. Hence some of these healings, originally perceived as exorcisms,

---

456 B.Heron, Praying for Healing, in Tom Coyle, ed, "Christian Ministry to the sick", London, 1986, p.93

457 J.Rhymer, The miracles of Jesus, Slough, United Kingdom, 1991, p.73

458 Ibid., p.74

459 B.M. Meehan, The healing power of prayer, Ligouri Publications, U.S.A., 1988, p.14

were quite probably healings in which Christ brought peace and stability to a troubled person.[460]

Such healings include the healing of the man in the synagogue in Capernaum (Mk 1:23–28; Lk 4:33–37). In their synagogue just then there was a man possessed by an unclean spirit, and it shouted, "What do you want of us Jesus of Nazareth? Have you come to destroy us? I know who you are, the holy one of God. But Jesus said sharply. 'Be quiet! Come out of him!' And the unclean spirit threw the man into convulsions and with a loud cry went out of him." (Mk 1: 23–26) Others of such healings include the healing of the man at Gerasa (Mt 8:28–34; Mk 5:1–20; Lk 8. 26–39), the healing of a dumb man (Mt 9:32–33; Lk 11:14) and the cure of the epileptic boy (Mt 17:14–17; Mk 9: 10–21; Lk 9: 37–43).

In the reconciliation of the woman who was a public sinner (Lk 7:36–50) and in the encounter with the Samaritan woman (Jn 4:1–42), Jesus showed a deep sensitivity to their emotional stress as well as to the physical realities of their life situations.[461]

We have already been observed that all healings of whatever nature or Dimension affects the person as a unit and is interactive. Hence the book of Proverbs said, "A glad heart is excellent medicine; a spirit depressed waists the bones away". (Prov 17:22) The emotional or mental states of man can therefore affect the physical body.

Because our mental states affect the functioning of our bodies, it is possible for us to stand in our own way of regaining health. Anger, malice, resentment, fear (other than that which is necessary for the protection of life), worry, anxiety, all have a detrimental influence on the functioning of the body, while love, kindness, peace, forgiveness (all the qualities we associate with Christian way of life), have a therapeutic influence. It is not surprising therefore that the bible stresses the importance of our mental outlook.[462]

It is now clear that some of our human illnesses whether emotional, physical or psychological can be caused because we sometimes fill ourselves with hatred and grudges coupled with unwillingness and or inability to forgive others and even forgiving ourselves. A very high percentage of the emotional illness he ministered to, remarked Buckley,

---

460 Ibid., p.13

461 B.M. Meehan, The Healing Pwoer of Prayer, p.14

462 G. Wright, Our Quest for healing, U.K., 1981, p.151

is caused by an awareness of being unloved in childhood, which breeds a sense of worthlessness of oneself and resentment of one's parents[463]

Only when we are able to empty or liberate ourselves, that the light of God's loving mercy flows into our lives and his healing Grace is released in our lives. That was what Jesus did in most of his healing works, during his healing mission on earth.

4.2.1.3 Social Dimension of the Healings of Jesus

Sickness whether physical or emotional can be aggravated or alleviated by social factors. During the healing mission of Jesus, he healed many people who were social outcasts or were socially marginalised or deprived in one way or the other. Under the Jewish laws, there were certain diseases that could make one ritually impure or unclean, which entailed the exclusion of the unfortunate victims, even from their biological families and communities, because of the fear that their sickness or disease was contagious. Leprosy was one such disease that deprived one of normal contact and relationship with the rest of his community members. Leprosy is described to cover a number of skin diseases believed to be contagious: itches, swellings, eruptions, or spots. (Lev. 14:54–56). The lepers were excluded from normal community life and had even to warn people to keep away from them when they were passing along the village streets. In their synagogues, the lepers had a special outlet in case they would want to receive communion during the celebrations. And in case any leper happened to be healed, he had to present himself to the priests, "the guardian of traditional knowledge who would examine him and certify whether he really were cured and could enter normal social life again."[464]

There were other illnesses or diseases, as promulgated by the Jewish religious leaders, that render one permanently or temporarily unclean and thus permanently or temporarily deprives one of normal social life of the Jews. Jesus cured a lot of these diseases and thus liberating a lot of people from this class of social outcasts. The healing of the woman with issue of blood was

one of the miracles which symbolized that Jesus could overcome conditions which made people outcasts or inferior, excluded from membership of privileged groups. This was of vital importance to the first Christians in the rigid social stratification of their times.[465]

---

463 M. Buckley, His Healing Touch, Op. Cit., p.167
464 J. Rhymer, The Miracles of Jesus, Op. Cit., p.85
465 Ibid., p.87

Portraying Jesus as the good shepherd and healer of his people, B. Haring writes,

Jesus the good shepherd takes upon himself the appalling suffering of the outcast whom the religious men set themselves as judges declare to be forsaken by God ... He heals the lepers, by touching them, giving them the healing experience of human love and divine presence. Similarly he rescues men and women who were social outcasts, scorned by those who did not feel their own need of healing and redemption. Jesus treats sinful women as persons gives them back a sense of dignity. He does the same with the class of tax–gatherers and others despised as "bad characters", "hopeless cases". He eats with the friends of Levi – Matthew, the tax gatherer, and even invites himself to the house of Zacchaeus one of those who were looked upon as traitors and exploiters.[466]

By contact with these social outcasts and particularly by healing them of their diseases, Jesus removed the cause of their exclusion from their communities and enabled them to become normal members of their communities again. "Jesus' Love even reached to the unlovable and did not fear sense contact with them."[467]

4.3 Methods of the Healing Works of Jesus Christ

Healing we know was a major part of the ministry of Jesus on earth. Jesus saw healing as an inseparable part of the proclamation of the Good news, such that, He "frequently emphasized that his healing ministry was a sign that the reign of God was breaking forth."[468] The fact that he healed was one major reason why people were attracted to him. The multitude surged to him wherever he went such that at times he looked for avenue to escape to the mountains or seashores to be alone for a while.

It is generally held that Jesus had no single method or uniform pattern in his healing ministry. He never restricted himself to any single method. Some he healed by his power of simple touch, as in the cases of the leper (Lk 5:12–14; Mt 8:3), Peter's mother in law (Mt 8:14–15), the two blind men (Mt 9:29–30) and Malchus (Lk 22:51). Some times he allowed people to touch him.

Other times people touch him without his notice and yet get healed as in the case of the woman with issue of blood (Lk 8:44). Some he healed by the power of his speech, as in the case of the ten lepers. He simply asked them to report

466 B. Haring, Healing and Reveling, Slough, England, 1984, p.11
467 B.T. Viviano, The Gospel of Matthew, in "The New Jerome Biblical Commentary", Op. Cit., Geoffrey Chapman, London, 1991, p.648
468 B. Meehan, The healing power of prayer, Op. Cit., p.7

themselves to the priests. (Lk 17:11–19) This they did and they were healed of their leprosy.

> *Sometimes Jesus encountered persons who were obsessed by fears and emotions that they could neither understand nor control – individuals who today, would be called mentally or emotionally ill. In Christ's time their obsessions and fears were seen as "unclean spirits". Jesus frequently freed such people from their fears and obsessions by commanding the spirits to depart.*[469]

It is obvious that Jesus met various people disturbed by various types of ailments during his ministry and he used different approaches to combat and set free those individuals harassed by the various ailments. His methods were often spontaneous.

> *This spontaneity that characterized the works of Jesus continued in the works of his followers. The Lord puts no restraint upon them as to the methods that they were to use. He left them free to act naturally, as He himself had done. But this freedom was in no way abused by them.*[470]

Jesus never used any medicines to obtain his cures but he never condemned the use of medicines or stopped people from using them. In fact Jesus emphasizes the importance of doctors and natural herbs and urged that they be given their rightful place and respect. Jesus never used any scientific means during his ministry, but he never condemned science. We now have a look at the two major approaches he used in bringing about healing to the sick.

4.2 Forms of Healing

4.2.1 Healing by Laying on of hands or his Power of Touch

The power of touch or laying on of hands has been one of the most usual items of healing services and has been on the increase in the recent years. The laying on of hands has been used right from the Old Testament. But in the Old Testament, "there is no account of the laying on of hands been giving for healing"[471]

It was usually used for blessing as in the case of Aaron raising his hand to bless the people (Lev 9:22) or by commissioning someone to an appointment as in the commissioning of Joshua by Moses (Num 27:16). In the New Testament

469 R. Baldwin, The Healers, Huntington, Indiana, 1986, p.11
470 G.Wright, Our Quest for healing, Op. Cit., p.111
471 J.Richards, The question of healing services, London, 1989, p.72

among other uses of the laying on of hands, it was used for healing. Cases of healing being wrought by both Jesus and the apostles abound. But little or no attention has been paid to the meaning, symbol and practice of the power of touch or laying on of hands. The laying on of hands says Gordon Wright

is a symbol of the transmission of divine power and life; a symbol, because it is not essential to the transmission of divine power and life. God often heals without the laying on of hands. But when practiced it suggests that the instrument is simply a channel through which God works.[472]

For J. Richards, "it is commonly held that laying on of hand is about some transfer of healing power by those who have an invisible form of healing or spiritual energy."[473] Both authors above see in the laying on of hands some sort of use of the divine strength to heal or work through the human person. Jesus used this power of touch during his ministry. The Church healing ministry still taps such forces for her use today. Whether the power of touch was used for blessing or healing or commissioning is not essential. God uses it as a channel to do his work. Any sick person who is blessed will hope that it results in healing.

Many of the people from the crowd that followed Jesus during his ministry came to him to be healed. He prayed for them, touched some of them and healed them. He healed in their synagogues, and in the streets and seashores. He was invited to the homes of the sick people and he touched them and healed them. Jesus went into the house of Peter's mother in law, took her by the hand and healed her. (Mk 1:31) Jesus touched and healed a leper (Mk 1:41; Lk 5:12–14; Mt 8:3). He also touched the affected sick part of the individual as he used mud to give sight to the blind man at the pool (Jn 9:6) He also used spittle at the eyes of the blind man at Bethsaida. "Nowhere is his power of touch better illustrated than in the cure of the blind man at Bethsaida."[474]

They came to Bethsaida, and some people brought to him a blind man whom they begged him to touch. He took the blind man by the hand and took him outside the village. Then putting spittle on his eyes and laying his hands on him, he asked, "can you see anything?" The man who was begging to see replied, "I can see people, they look like trees to me but they are walking about." Then he laid his hands on the man's eyes again and he saw clearly; he was cured, and he could see everything plainly and distinctly. (Mk 8:22–25)

The apostles themselves healed by the power of touch. Ananias laid hands on Paul that he might regain his sight. (Acts 9:12) and Paul healed the father of Pub-

472 G. Wright, Our Quest for Healing, Op.Cit., p.109
473 J. Richards, The question of healing services, Op. Cit., p.63
474 M. Buckley, His Healing Touch, Op. Cit., p.133

lius in Malta (Acts 28; 8). Peter healed the lame man at the beautiful gate. He took him by the hand and helped him to stand up (Acts 3:7).

At this juncture, we must note strictly that the laying on of hand was not Jesus most usual method of healing. More often, he healed by the spoken words. This stand is very much supported by McNutt's statement which says "It is clear that sometimes Jesus healed only through words or desire, as when he told the Canaanite woman who asked that her daughter be healed at a distance (Mt 6:28)"[475].

Though Jesus healed many times by spoken words, there is no debate whether he healed by the power of touch or laying on of hands. There are cases of people touching him and getting healed as in the case of woman with issue of blood (Lk 8:44). There are others who asked permission to touch him.

> *And when the men of that place recognized him, they sent round to all region and brought to him all that were sick and besought him that they might only touch the fringe of his garment, and as many as touched it were made whole (Mt 35:36)*

Jesus healed by mere laying on of hands without spoken words. The apostles did the same. It is still possible today, to heal the sick with the art of laying on of hands or through simple touch.

> God takes a hand wherever he can find it and just does what he likes with it. Sometimes, he takes a bishop's hand and lays it on a child's head in benediction; then he takes the hand of a doctor to relieve pain, the hand of a mother to guide her child and sometimes he takes the hand of an aul Craither like me to give comfort to a neighbour. But they are all hands touched by his spirit, and his spirit is everywhere looking for hands to use. Most of us offer our hands to Christ in the spirit in the work of healing; others seem to possess in their hands a quality of healing.[476]

4.2.2 Healing by the Power of Spoken Word

Jesus healing by the power of his words was evidently the main reason why people who sought after him were astonished by the way he carried out his ministry that they began to say that he taught like one who has authority; that even the evil spirits obey his words. That Jesus healed often by the spoken word is clear in the gospels. Even most of Jesus' healings by his power of touch were accompanied by his power of spoken word.

> *Of the individual healings recorded in the scripture, touch or laying on of hands accompanied only about a half of the healings by authoritative word. There is only one case*

475 F. McNutt, The power to heal, Op. Cit., p.36
476 J. Turner, The Healing Church, Op. Cit., pp.55 & 56

of touching to heal without accompanying words being recorded. That was the case of Malchus' ear (Lk 22:51) which was cut off at Gethsemane.[477]

This is to say that more of the healings of Jesus was by the power of his words. He commanded and it was done. He very often gave instructions that indicated healing. To the man sick of palsy, Jesus said, "Pick up your bed and go home" (Mt 9:6). To the man with withered hand, He said, "Stretch out your hand" (Mt 12:13). To the sick man at Bethzatha, "Rise, take up your pallet and walk" (Jn 5:8). And to the blind Bartimeus, He said, "Go your way; your faith has made you well" (Mk 10:52). There is also the classical case of the story of the Centurion's servant who was ill and was cured by Jesus at a distance.

This happened in Capernaum.

A Centurion there had a servant, a favourite of his who was sick and near death. Having heard about Jesus, he sent some Jewish elders to him to ask him to come and heal his servant. When they came to Jesus, they pleaded earnestly with him. 'He deserves this of you' they said, 'because he is friendly towards our people; infact he is the one who built our synagogue.' So Jesus went with them, and was not very far from the house when the centurion sent word to him by some friends: 'Sir' he said, do not put yourself to trouble; I did not presume to come to you myself; but give the word and let my servant be cured. (Lk 7:1–7; Mt 8: 5–13).

The Centurion knew the power of spoken word since he is one in authority. The multitude that was surging after Jesus during his ministry perhaps too, knew the power of words; hence they maintained he spoke like one with authority.

Jesus himself did not know less about the power of word. He cured and cast out devils by the commands of his words. The words of Christ are full of power. He has only to speak and we shall be healed. Any wonder, the Church took the words of the Centurion and made them her own "Lord 1 am not worthy to receive you, but say the word and my soul shall be healed.[478]

4.2.3 Places of the Healing Works of Jesus Christ

One fact about Jesus so widely and repeatedly upheld in the gospels is the fact that people crowded about him during his ministry. They brought to him wherever he was at whatever time, those who were sick or possessed and he healed them of their various ailments and drove out demons. Throughout Galilee and the cities, he went about preaching in their Synagogues and market places, healing

477 J. Richards, The question of healing services, Op. Cit., p.76

478 Cf, Communion Rite, Daily Roman Missal, Indiana, 1994, p.739

the sick among them. He carried his ministry even to the mountains in the lakes and throughout the countryside and they brought the sick in their stretchers to any place he was reported to be.

In the Synagogue of the Jews, he healed the man with a withered hand on the Sabbath (Mt 12:9–14; Mk 3: 1–6; Lk 6: 6–11). In the market places, they laid out the sick and he cured them (Mk 6:53–56; Mt 14:34–36). In their home, he cured Peter's mother in law of her fever Mt 8:14–15; Mk 1:29; Lk 4: 38–39).

On the seashore, he cured the woman with issue of blood (Mt 9–20–33; Mk 5: 25; Lk 8: 43). The Synoptics reported of mass healing in Capernaum by the lakeside (Mk 3: 10; Mt 4: 15; Lk 6:19). Even on the roadsides and hillsides, Jesus wrought many healing works. At a distance, he cured the son of the official at Capernaum (Jn 4:48–54), the centurion servant (Mt 8:5–13; Lk 7: 1–10) and the Canaanite's woman daughter (Mk 7:24–30) He healed the blind man of Bethsaida outside the village (Mk 8: 22–26).

So we can see that Jesus heals everywhere and at every time. He has no healing site or any miracle camp. There is no particular place for the numerous healing works of Jesus. Jesus therefore can heal you anywhere – during the Eucharistic celebration, in your homes, along the seashores when on board, and in the farms, villages or cities while you are working or trading in your stores.

4.3 The Aims of the Healing Works of Jesus Christ

There are no doubts that there are certain motivations, which gave meanings to the miracles of Jesus in general and consequently to his healing works. And since the gospel stories are full of many and different accounts of the healing miracles, they are bound to be many and various aims of the healing works. We shall therefore try to examine some of the significance or aims of the healing works while making use of some of the healing works of Jesus.

4.3.1 The Proclamation of the Kingdom of God

The healing works of Jesus involves much more than just ordinary healing of sicknesses. *They were also prophetic sings of his own identity and of the coming of the kingdom of God, and they very often cause a new spiritual awakening in the one who had been healed.*[479]

479 K.D. O'Rourke & P. Boyle, Medical ethics: Sources of Catholic teachings, C.H.A., St. Louis, 1989, p.134

O'Rourke and Boyle further stated that

The power that went out of Jesus when he cured remains in the life and prayer of the Church, a source of healing and reconciliation. Ever active, this power confirms the identity of the church today authenticates her proclamation of the kingdom of God and stands as a sign of triumph over evil.[480]

Hardly anything is more certain about the ministry of Jesus than the proclamation of the kingdom of God, that final saving act of God. Hence one of the primary and main significance of the healing works of Jesus is the establishment of the kingdom of God by the destruction of the kingdom of Satan. There have been facts in the Tradition and history of the Church that shows the real function of Jesus healing miracles as proofs of his divinity. His preaching and works initiated the coming of the kingdom of God among men. "After John had been arrested, Jesus went into Galilee. There he proclaimed the Good news from God. The time has come he said and the kingdom of God is close at hand. Repent and believe the Good News" (Mk 1: 14–15). Jesus himself saw the preaching of the gospel to be the climax of his miraculous works. Hence when John sent his disciples to Jesus to ask who he was, Jesus told them to go and tell John what they have heard and seen. "The blind see again, and the lame walk, lepers are cleansed and the deaf hear, and the dead are raised to life, and the Good News is proclaimed to the poor." (Mt 11:5) In line with the above facts, the Vatican documents state,

The economy of revelation is realised by deeds and words which are intrinsically bound up with each other. As a result the works performed by God in the history of Salvation show forth and bear out the doctrine and realities signified by words; the words for their part proclaim the work and bring to light the mystery they contain.[481]In the gospels, Jesus drove out Satan at various occasions especially during his healing ministry and some of the people accused him of doing that through the power of Beelzebul, the prince of devil. And Jesus invariably remarked,

Now if it is through Beelzebul that I cast out demons, through whom do your own experts cast them out? Let them be your judges, then. But if it is through the finger of God that I cast out devils, then know that the kingdom of God has overtaken you. (Lk 11: 14 – 20)

By this remark, Jesus establishes his superiority over the devil and initiates the coming of his kingdom and the extinction of the domain of Satan.

480 Ibid., p.134
481 The Second Vatican Document, Die Verbum, No 2

Very often before Jesus performs his healing works, He prepares himself by retiring into the desert place or to the mountains to be alone in prayer. Generally when Jesus retires to prayer to have a special time with the Father, the disciples normally presumes He had gone to prepare himself to do battle with the devil. This presumption was however because of the Jewish conception that sickness, diseases and death were signs of Satan's control over man. And this invariably made the evangelists recount many of the healings of Jesus as if they were exorcisms. We have to note that even the cure of Peter's mother in law was treated as if the fever were an evil spirit. "Leaning over her, Jesus rebuked the fever and it left her." (Lk 4: 38). But Jesus did not agree in the Jewish conception that associates sickness and diseases with sin. We earlier observed in this work that Jesus did not give room to the Old Testament religious problems of sickness which was associated with that of retribution originally conceived in temporal terms (Deut. 28:21), nor did he support the conception of disease as punishment due to sin (Ps. 38, 107). We remember when his disciples encountered him with the case of the blind man. They asked, "Rabbi, who sinned, this man or his parents for him to have been born blind? Jesus stated categorically, that neither the man nor his parents sinned. He added, "He was born blind so that the works of the Father might be displaced in him" (Jn 9:3).

Therefore, even the fact of Jesus doing most of his healing miracles on a Sabbath was not far from this fact of Jesus trying to displace the works of God in time and persons. Hence Jesus healed on the Sabbath primarily,

> *to emphasize his miraculous work as a new creation. In the old creation, God rested on the Sabbath, but now he has resumed his creative work to establish his dominion, save man from Satan and recreate him in his own image.*[482]

Jesus in his love for mankind does not wish man to perish to the force of the evil one. Goodness is always stronger and more powerful than evil. So Jesus with his goodness fought the power of evil in his healings. He fought the power of evil to establish his kingdom on earth. He sees in anything that militates against his mission as the intervention of Satan, the enemy. That was such that even when Peter started to remonstrate him, for announcing his passion he addressed Peter thus: "Get behind me Satan" (Mk 8:33). So nothing would stand between Jesus and establishing his kingdom on earth.

---

482 J. Kallas, The Significance of the Gospel miracles, London, 1961, p.64 in P. Daffy, Christ and Healing in "To heal the sick", Seminar papers, Bodija, Ibadan, 1970, p.15

4.3.2 The Compassion of Jesus Christ

The gospels present Jesus as having behaved and spoken in a manner that makes one conclude that he exercised his ministry in a deeply compassionate form. His willingness to violate the Tradition of his contemporaries shows the strength of his overwhelming love and compassion for the sick. He went to the extent of jeopardizing his life to show his concern such that he frequently healed on the Sabbath, a practice that defied the teachings of the Scribes and Pharisees. (Mk 6: 7) Jesus had compassion on so many people who followed him and were in need of his care and direction.

Jesus had compassion on those who were marginalised by the society of their day. When Jesus was at dinner in the house of Levi with a number of tax collectors and sinners, the scribes of the Pharisees party saw him and began to question his disciples why their master ate with tax collectors and sinners. Then Jesus gave this answer: "I did not come to call the virtuous but sinners" (Mk 2:17). So to the marginalised of the society, the lepers, men and women of bad reputations and many others confined to the margins of life either by the society or by religion, Jesus gave hope and life. To the poor of the society, he promised happiness and preached the kingdom to them. The compassion of Jesus is more than ordinary pity or sympathy.

> *It is the capacity to feel and suffer with the sick person – to experience something of the predicament of illness, its fears, anxieties, temptations, its assault on the whole person, the loss of freedom and dignity, the utter vulnerability, and the alienation every illness produces or portends.*[483]

We have earlier noted in this work the difficult plight of a sick man. Sickness of a serious type often isolates a man from others, makes him different, dependent and alone. Sickness often makes man lose sight of the goodness of God. All these problems Jesus combated by his healing works. He was deeply compassionate and one of the major significance of his healing works is seen in his compassion for the sick.

The word compassion comes from the Latin, which means, "to suffer with". According to Mackrell, "the essence of compassion is the sharing of the suffering not because 'a sorrow shared is a sorrow halved', but simply so that the sufferer is not alone."[484] Sharing of one's suffering does not mean that one literally shares the pain of the other but for the sick to know that others know that they are suf-

483 Edmund Pellegrino, Every sick person is my brother or sister, in Dolentium Hominum, Year III, no7, 1988, p.66
484 G. Mackrell, The Healing Miracles in Mark's gospel, Op. Cit., p.120

fering and that can offer a deep comfort. One does not need to contract Cancer or Aids to feel compassion for any person that suffers from any of the diseases. But a few good words and a few acts of care and concern can be very consoling to the sick person.

Einsamkeit ist für Jesus eine Grund Erfahrung und für ihn sehr wichtig.[485] Loneliness here does not just mean one being alone. It goes for him much deeper. "It is not the loneliness of a single sex; as happily married couples will testify. But it is not good for a man to be alone without God."[486] So Jesus had come to be with his people, to be a companion to his people especially those in need and then showed them his compassion. When Jesus withdrew to a lonely place with his apostles, the people saw them going and from every town they all hurried to the place on foot and reached it before them. So as he stepped ashore he saw a large crowd; and he took pity on them because they were like sheep without shepherd and he set himself to teach them at some length. (Mk 6: 30–34)During the earthly ministry of Jesus, he showed his compassion to many such as the Centurion's servant (Lk 7:1–10). To the widow of Nain who lost her only son, Jesus showed a deep compassion. This woman, already deprived of the support of her husband had her only son being carried out for burial, and Jesus felt sorry for her and said to the young man, "I tell you to get up." (Lk 7: 11–17)

And to the blind man at Bethsaida, Jesus banished his loneliness by taking him outside the village and then laid his hands on the man's eyes and he began to see clearly. (Mk 8:22–25) There are many other instances where Jesus compassion for those in distress drew near and he came to be with them and brought them wholeness.

True compassion as already mentioned is more than mere feelings of pity and sympathy, without adequate practical backing. The Christian must recognize this fact. Our brothers and sisters who are in need or are sick deserve our loving care and concern. They deserve our true compassion. And compassion for the Christian is an "obedient response to a loving Father", not "a noble act of self sacrifice."[487]

---

485 Ibid., p.120

486 Ibid., p.121

487 Donald P. Mcneill, Douglas A. Morrison and Henri Nouwen, Compassion, A Reflection on the Christian life, New York, Doubleday, 1982, p.42, in E. Pellegrino, Every sick person is my brother or sister, in Doletium Hominum, p.67

4.3.3 Arousing Faith in the Believers and Bearing Witness to God

The gospels made it clear that Jesus would not impose miracles of healing on people without their co–operation. Hence Alfons Weiser states:

In so many cases Faith is required before the miracle of Jesus takes place. This opinion is represented for example in Mark's gospel where he stated: Jesus could not perform any miracle in his village Nazareth because of their lack of faith. (6, 5)[488]Faith seems to be always a prerequisite in the miracles of Jesus. Many of the accounts of the gospels on the healing miracles of Jesus emphasize the faith of the people – faith of the sick people who benefited directly and/or faith of their friends and relations who accompanied the sick persons. Thus very frequently in the healings of Jesus, we find phrases such as: "Your faith has saved you" (Lk 8:48; 17: 19–1 18: 42–1 Mk 5: 34–1 Mt 9: 22). To the Centurion, he said, "I have never found a faith like this" (Mt 8: 5–13), and to the Canaanite woman whose daughter was sick, he said, "Woman you have great faith" (Mt 15–18). In the cure of the paralytic, it was the faith of the four friends that was upper most. "Seeing their faith, Jesus said to the paralytic, My child your sins are forgiven you" (Mk 2:5; Mt 9: 2; Lk 5:20). Other instances include the cure of the woman with issue of blood (Mtt9:20–22); the cure of the Blind Bartimeus of Jericho who insisted on calling out to Jesus to heal him (Mk 10–46). Many of these works of Jesus were meant to arouse faith on the people.

Unlike some miracle workers, Jesus never worked miracles for personal profits and self–praise. Among the aims of his healing works was to bear witness to God as the Messiah. His healing works, just like his entire ministry should be seen as a continuation of the creative work of God. This is clear in his testimony that "the work which my father has given me to carry out, these same works of mine testify that the father has sent me. Besides the father who sent me bears witness to me himself" (Jn 5:36–38), also when John heard of the works of Jesus from the prison, and sent his disciples to inquire about his identity and claims, Jesus referred them to his healing works to bear witness to God. "Go and tell John what you have heard and seen, the blind receive their sight and the lame walk, lepers are cleansed, and the deaf hear, and the dead are raised to life... "(Mt11:4–5) There are no doubts that a lot of the healings of Jesus was done to bear witness to God, that people may believe and have faith. "The work I do is the work of he who sends me" (Jn 14:10).

---

488 A. Weiser, Jesu Wunder – damals und heute, Verlag Katholisches Bibelwerk, Stuttgart, 1976, p.22. In manchen Fällen wird der Glaube ganz klar als Voraussetzung gefordert, dass überhaupt ein Wunder geschehen kann. So berichtet Markus zum Beispiel: Da Jesus in seiner Heimat Nazaret keinen Glauben fand, konnte er dort kein einziges Wunder vollbringen (6,5)

Over and over again, Jesus associated his miraculous deeds with his call to a faith which would believe in his power to forgive human sins and save people from the powers which afflicted them. No less than his preaching, his miracles manifested the reign of God and the divine promise to deliver them from the grips of evil."[489]

4.3.4 The Healing Miracles of Jesus Christ

Our brief examination of the healing works of Jesus Christ, the dimensions and methods of He used, instantly draws our attention to survey the healing miracles of Jesus as an important aspect of the life of Jesus on earth.

Next only to the crucifixion and resurrection, the miracles of Jesus are the most dramatic of all the events reported in the gospels and the most controversial. Many just dismiss them as fictions; others think they are exaggerated versions of more mundane events" some take them literally. For some people, they are the strongest evidence of their Christian beliefs, but the same stories cause others the strongest doubts.[490]

The different views of people on this all–important aspect of the events of the gospels give seemingly conflicting reports as well as conflicting questions. Different writers as well as theologians have put up various questions on the meaning and fact of the miracles of Jesus. Such scholars have put up doubts as to whether miracles happened actually. Some others denied out–rightly the possibility of miracles. There are however some scholars who believed strongly on the existence of miracles while there are some who believe miracles abounded but held that the age of miracles has passed.

From time to time, miracles have been seen as clear–cut proof of God's hand in history unambiguously underwriting the truths–claims of the faith. At such times apologists have taken the offensive, and have built miracles into the foundation of their apologetic systems, but at other times apologists have been pushed onto the defensive, and have appeared to some to be almost apologizing for their belief in miracles.[491]

But the apologists could not but hold firm in their belief in the miracles of Jesus and put up arguments to strengthen the faith of believers and to defend the truth of the Christian faith. Origen (ca.185 – ca.254) the greatest of the Apologists and the first Ecumenical Theologian says that,

489 G.O. Collins, Interpreting Jesus, Geoffrey Chapman, London, 1985, p.59
490 J. Rhymer, The miracles of Jesus, St. Paul's publications, Middlegreen, Slough, United Kingdom, 1991, p.9
491 C. Brown, Miracles and the Critical Mind, Eerdmans, Pater Noster Press, U.K., U.S.A., 1984, p.3

without miracles and wonders, the apostles would not have persuaded those who heard the doctrines and the new teaching to leave their traditional religion and to accept the apostles teaching at the risk of their lives.[492]

The rationalists of the 19th century began with the denials of the miracles of Jesus. They felt that the fact of the miracles was exaggerated or told to establish the Christian Church. Vielleicht einfügen: Sie waren zu fest davon überzeugt, dass die Naturgesetzte eheern seien und sie das sicher wüssten. Some of them held that the miracles were but claims of Jesus as a wonder worker and the disciples used that as a weapon for the conversion of the world to Christianity. Bultmann for example denies out rightly the miraculous power of Jesus Christ.

He explains the multiplication of the loaves and fishes as interior "miracles" – the large crowd shared out their food to one another so that all had enough. Such things as the transfiguration or the walking on the waters are for him clearly non–historical. The walking on the waters may well have been a view the disciples had of Jesus walking along the shore – because it was approaching down the light played tricks on the apostles who mistakenly believed that Jesus walked on the waters! This story is clearly theophanic revealing Jesus as the mighty God who treads down the waves.[493]

It is however not our intention to delve into these conflicting opinions and reports about the miracles of Jesus. We do not intend either to resolve the long debated questions on the facts of miracles. Individuals have rights to hold their different opinions about the mighty works of Jesus just as the evangelists who have recorded the events have different approaches to the healing miracles of Jesus. Each has his own view of Jesus and each recorded at different times within the life of the Church. It is therefore not out of place to have viewed slightly these conflicting opinions and ideas on the miracles, since the healings of Jesus are invariably miraculous. Even the most casual reader of the book of the gospels is struck by the dominance of Christ the healer and the healing miracles.

The miracles of Jesus are to be seen in the context of his life, teaching, healing and transforming work. The miracles constitute an integral part of his message, substantiating his claims to the agent of the kingdom of God. "But if it is through the finger of God that I cast out devils, then know that the kingdom of God has overtaken you" (Lk 11:20). This reveals that whenever we pray 'thy kingdom come', we are petitioning for the divine healing among other things. Jesus' use of the 'kingdom' shows that he does not only think in terms of an earthly reign but of dominion over everything as Lord. "Luke makes use of the miracle

492 Origen: Contra Celsum, Cambridge University Press, 195, p.42, quoted in C.Brown, "Miracles and the Critical mind", Op.Cit., p.4

493 R. Fuller, Interpreting the miracles, London, 1963, pp.21–22, in P. Daffy, "Christ and healing, in 'To heal the Sick' unpublished, Bodija, Ibadan, 1970, p.12

stories in the frame–work of his history of salvation and with missionary aim."[494] This view of miracles of Jesus comes over strikingly in the whole structure of Mark's gospel where Jesus is portrayed as the great exorcist, defeating the power of the devil by his healing miracles and by his casting out of demons. Hence the healing miracles of Jesus are a demonstration of Christ's victory over evils. Almost the whole of the first three chapters of Mark's gospel is entirely devoted to the accounts of the miracles and exorcisms. In Matthew, the account of the miracles "make known the servant of Yahweh who carries out God's will to show mercy on those oppressed by sickness and sin. Jesus is also the Lord who exercises his power."[495] While for John, "miracles are signs of the glory of God and a witness which the father bears to his son through the works he enables him to accomplish."[496] Here, it is of interest to note that

nearly one–fifth of the gospel record is taken up with either accounts of the Lord's healings or the reactions and debates arising from them and that there are forty one distinct occasions of healings mentioned in the four gospels.[497]

The reactions and debates arising from the miracles of Jesus have drawn some scholars into making distinctions between healings and miracles. Their primary reason for the distinction being that healing could be wrought through many means and miracles happen to be one of the major means of getting a healing. It is clear that all the miracles of Jesus are not on healing; hence we can talk of the healing miracles. Some of his miracles involve healing of the person while others are not.

A classical distinction is between miracles performed on persons (healing, exorcism, raising of the dead) and miracles performed on the natural elements (sea, wind, bread, wine, fishes).[498]

Jesus healing miracles therefore concern those miracles that are directly aimed at restoring health to the sick and the dying persons while nature miracles have to deal with Jesus exercising an extra–ordinary power over nature without aiming at the restoration of health. M. Kelsey recorded forty–one distinct occasions of healings mentioned in the four gospels, while R. Latourelle recorded twenty–eight miracle stories in all excluding doublets. J.Rhymer in his work 'the

---

494 Rene Latourelle, The miracles of Jesus and the theology of miracles, Paulist Press, New York, 1988, p.252

495 R. Latorelle, The miracles of Jesus and the Theology of Miracles, p.256

496 Ibid., p.256

497 M. Kelsey, Healing and Christianity, London SCM Press, 1973, Chapter 4, in B. Palmer, "Medicine and the Bible" Op. Cit., p.195.

498 R. Latorelle, The miracles of Jesus and the theology of miracles, Op. Cit., p.242

miracle of Jesus' struck a medium in the number of miracles in the four gospels. He notes that,

there are some thirty six descriptions of specific miracles in the four gospels, including a mention that Jesus had at sometime cast out devils from Mary Magdalene. Some describe Jesus casting out devils; some are miracles of healing without any mention of demonic possession – three are descriptions of Jesus bringing the dead back to life; and some show Jesus exercising an extra–ordinary power over nature.[499]

According to N. Onwu, scholars have categorised the miracles of Jesus into four groups, which include "healing miracles, exorcisms, nature miracles and resuscitation miracles"[500] But nature miracles are not among the healing miracles. It is therefore clear from this that we have three main types of Jesus' healing miracles namely healing, exorcism, and resuscitation. These three types of healings are included in the four groups of miracles of Jesus, and so they are called healing miracles. This then will lead us to the healing tradition of the church and her concern for the sick and suffering.

4.4 The Healing Tradition of the Church

4.4.1 Concern of the Church for the Sick and Suffering

During the life of Jesus on earth, the gospels have always presented him as being always in the midst of the sick and suffering, the lame, the blind, the dumb, the paralytics, the deaf, the bereaved, the insane, the lepers and outcasts. He travelled throughout Galilee and beyond, preaching and healing all kinds of diseases and infirmities. The people were filled with admiration that they began to say, "He has done all things well, he makes the deaf hear and the dumb speak"(Mk 7:37).

The deep interest which the Church has always demonstrated for the world of the suffering is well known. In this for that matter, she has done nothing more than follow the very eloquent example of her Founder and Master.

In the Apostolic Letter Salvifici Doloris of 11 February, 1984 Pope John Paul II emphasized that "in his messianic activity in the midst of Israel, Christ drew increasingly closer to the world of human suffering. 'He went about doing good', and his actions concerned primarily those who were suffering and seeking help" (no.16)

---

499 J. Rhymer, The miracles of Jesus, Op. Cit., p.25
500 N. Onwu, A critical introduction to the traditions of Jesus, CECTA, Enugu, 1991, p.181

The Jews always have a concept of man as a whole entity comprising both body and soul, so when they talk of healing, they talk of curing the whole person including the soul. They do not talk of the salvation of the soul in isolation.

In fact, over the course of the centuries the Church has felt strongly that service to the sick and suffering is an integral part of her mission, and not only has she encouraged among Christians the blossoming of various works of mercy, but she has also established many religious institutions within her with the specific aim to fostering, organizing, improving and increasing help to the sick.

This concept of the Jews is very clear in the healing ministry of Jesus. Jesus always gives a complete cure in his healings. In the cure of the paralytic, he first said to the man, "Courage my child your sins are forgiven you" (Mt 9:2; Mk 2:6; Lk 5:20) and later, "get up and pick your bed and go home" (Mt 9:6; Mk 2:12; Lk 5:24). So Jesus sees his mission from the father as that of healing, liberation and salvation. Hence when he unrolled the scroll at Nazareth he read the following passage,

The spirit of the Lord has been given to me, for he has anointed me. He has sent me to bring good news to the poor, to proclaim liberty to captives and to the blind new sight, to set the downtrodden free, to proclaim the Lord's year of favour. (Lk 4:18)

The core of Jesus life and ministry was the proclamation of the Kingdom and healing of the sick.

Both contain similar psychological and spiritual themes. Proclaiming God's kingdom brings it closer to others and this means healing. Healing others as Jesus did require knowledge of the inner spiritual realities and the capacity to mediate them to others.[501]

Jesus himself was aware that his miracles including his healings were evidence of the presence of the kingdom. Hence he says, "But if I with the finger of God cast out devils, no doubt, the Kingdom of God is come upon you" (Lk 11:20). Jesus' use of the word 'kingdom' reveals he did not only think in terms of earthly reign but of dominion over every heart that accepts him as saviour and Lord. So, "whenever we pray thy kingdom come, we are praying for divine healing."[502] Finally Jesus painted his healing works as the sign of his Messiah ship, when John the Baptist sent his disciples to inquire the identity of Jesus, whether he was the Messiah they were expecting. He answered, Go and tell John what you have heard and seen, (Mt 11:4–5; Lk 7:20–23). With this Jesus continued with his mission from the Father.

---

501 S. A. Galipeau, Transforming body and soul: therapeutic wisdom in the Gospel healing stories, New York, 1990, p.140

502 G. Wright, Our quest for healing, Op. Cit., p.21

Before he left the world to go back to the Father, Jesus entrusted to his disciples the same mission he received from his Father and gave them authority to preach the gospel and heal the sick.

He called the twelve together and gave them power and authority over all devils and to cure diseases, and he sent them out to proclaim the kingdom of God and to heal (Lk 9:1–2; Mt10: l–6–1 Mk 6:7).

Thus the mandate to the apostles or their commissioning to evangelization was enacted. Luke extended the commissioning further than Matthew and Mark by adding in his writing the commissioning of the seventy other disciples. To them, he said,

Wherever you go into a town where they make you welcome, eat what is set before you. Cure those in it who are sick and say, the kingdom of God is very near to you (Lk 10 1, 8–9.).

From the above one can easily observe that the evangelists placed the preaching of the kingdom and healing of the sick in the same plane.

The great attention given by the evangelists to Jesus healing is due to their realisation that this aspect of his ministry was of great importance for the life of the Christian Community.[503]

And ever since, the church has felt strongly the service to the sick and the suffering as an integral part of her mission.

This mission to the Church was not just an external mandate nor the message simply a mere doctrine. Hence, Haring says that, if we are to understand the full mission of the Church, her true nature and purpose, we must always bear in mind that it is infinitely more than an external institution. Above all, it is a wonderful sharing in the very mission of Christ and his mission from the father.[504]

A look at the mandate Jesus gave to the apostles (the church) helps one see the same concern at the centre of their mission. He sent them to towns and villages to announce his coming, to expel demons and to heal the sick. That was not all. He wanted them to be the leaven of the community by bringing to humanity the integrated vision of health as a wholeness of body and spirit in the service of the creator.

---

503 J. Helson and R. Wanjobi, Anointing and healing in Africa, Spearhead, No. 70, Gaba Publications, Kenya, 1982, p.7

504 B. Haring, Healing and revealing, St. Paul's Publications, Slough, England, 1984, p.26

Pope Paul VI addressing the sick on the problem of sickness for the Church said: This means that the Church, the Christian religion, is:

not an insurance company against ills of the present life, rather, if one looks carefully, it is a society in which suffering finds a special welcome. Certainly, the Church is wholly dedicated to the relief of the ills of mankind; sin primarily, also pain, misery, and death. It is compassionate towards every human weakness, and for precisely this reason there is between the Church and the one who suffers a profound understanding ... Charity gives urgency to the supreme precept of the Gospel to love whoever is weaker, lonelier, more needy, and afflicted with greater suffering.[505]

From the above citation, it is clear that the Church caters for the spiritual and bodily health of the sick. The Church has used and is using the sacraments and other rites (sacramentals), as well as medicine for the care of the sick.

All the sacraments have their healing effect. This is clearly seen in the sacramental ministry of the Church. The Church regards the sacraments as particularly chosen channels of God's saving power applied to every area of human life. By Baptism each Christian is initiated into this process of the saving power of the sacraments.[506]Today there are many organisms which directly engage Christians in the health care sector: over and above the religious congregations and institutions, with their social health care structures, there are organizations of Catholic doctors, associations of paramedics, nurses, pharmacists, volunteer works, diocesan and interdiocesan, national and international organisms which have sprung up to pursue the problems of medicine and health.

Health care is a tradition in the Church. The history of Christianity is in fact a record of service to the sick and of commitment to health. Baldwin testifies to it when he says:

Long before health care became a specific government concern, it already had been given a high place in the Church's list of priorities. Many of the hospitals the world over were church–sponsored.[507]

From the above assertion, one can see that much of the early Church commitment in health care was viewed as apostolic works of mercy and charity to the poor, the aged, the infirm and the dispossessed. The establishment of health programmes and facilities was to meet the needs of these persons. Most of the early hospitals were associated with cathedrals and monasteries in order to serve both

---

505 Pope Paul VI, "The Suffering Church as the True Church", Weekly Audience 3 Aug. 1966, in Herde Correspondence, Vol. 3, no. 12, Dec. 1966, p.375

506 Cf. Ad Gentes Divinitus 14

507 E. Baldwin, "Health Care and the Church", in Catholic Encylopedia, vol. 17 reprint 1981, p.247–248.

the spiritual and physical needs of the sick all at the same time. Later on religious orders of men and women were founded to nurse the sick. Examples abound: St. Catherine of Genoa (1477–1510) is considered a founder of modern hospital work. St. Vincent de Paul was born 21.4.1581 (Vincent Depaul, de Paul) Heilig gesprochen am 1737 gestorben am 27.9.1660 As Parish Priest of Chatillon–les–Dombes dort eine Confrerie des Dames de la Charite, founded an organisation of 'Bürgersfrauen' which took care of the poor and the lonely sick people of the parish. This organisation of Vincent has spread like wildfire all over the World. This Women Organisation of St. Vincent (Vinzentinerinnen) is today one of the biggest congregation in the Church with more than 45540 members in Deutschland under the name Elisabeth–Konferenzen and everywhere in the World.[508] Daughter of Charity of St. Vincent de Paul were intended to assist the conferences of charity. When these conferences were established at Paris (1629) the ladies who joined them readily brought their alms and were willing to visit the poor and the sick of the community. Besides the Daughters of Charity, Vincent de Paul secured for the poor the services of the Ladies of Charity, at the request of the Archbishop of Paris. He grouped (1634) under this name some pious women who were determined to nurse the sick poor entering the Hotel–Dieu to the number of 20,000 or 25,000 annually; they also visited the prisons.

The above illustrates the Church's commitment to the care of the sick. In Igboland, the missionaries also built hospitals very close to the parish churches and convents. An ample list of these can be made: Our Lady of Mount Carmel Parish church and Holy Rosary Hospital, Emekuku; St. Mary's Hospital and Immaculate Heart Covent, Amaigbo; St. Martin Parish and St. Vincent Hospital, Ihiala; Shanahan Hospital and St. Theresa's Parish, Nsukka; Mother of Christ Maternity Hospital and Holy Ghost Parish, Enugu; just to mention but a few.

The missionaries used medical services to attract possible converts to Christianity, as one author testifies: "Besides education, the missionaries tried to evangelize through medical services. It should be recalled that Father Lutz, the great pioneer missionary of Southern Nigeria won his first indigenous converts through the European medicine which he administered to children."[509] Today the provision of health care services is seen as an integral part of the Church's social ministry.

The Church strongly upholds the right to health care, long articulated as a basic human right. Pope John XXIII reaffirmed this when he writes:

---

508 Walter Kasper mit Konrad Baumgartner, Hörst Bürkle, Klaus Ganzer, Karl Kertelge, Wilhelm Korff, Peter Walter, Lexikon für Theologie und Kirche, zehnter Band,Herder – Freiburg.Basel.Rom.Wien, 2001, pp.799 – 800

509 Rose Njoku, The Advent of the Catholic Church in Nigeria, Ist Growth in Owerri Diocese, Owerri, Assumpta Press 1980, p.143

Beginning our discussion of the rights of man, we see that every man has the right to life, to bodily integrity, and the means which are necessary and suitable for proper development of life. These means are primarily food, clothing, shelter, rest, medical care and finally, the necessary social services. Therefore a human being also has the right to security in cases of sickness, inability to work, widowhood, old age, unemployment, or in any other case in which he is deprived of the means of subsistence through no fault of his own.[510]

In establishing Catholic hospitals the Church attempts to penetrate secular society. An important purpose of Catholic institutions as Vatican Council II puts it, is "to serve as a leaven und as a kind of soul for human society as it is renewed in Christ and transformed into God's family."[511] In this manner, the Catholic hospital seeks to be a place where the excellence of medical care, provided according to Christian principles will help the Gospel spirit permeate and improve the temporal order. A brief account of modern medical services and Christian hospitals in Nigeria here would not be out of place. Hence:

4.4.2 Medical Services of the Church/Congregational Hospitals in Nigeria

Western medicine was not formally introduced into Nigeria until the 1860s, when the Sacred Heart Hospital was established by Roman Catholic missionaries in Abeokuta. Throughout the ensuing colonial period, the religious missions played a major role in the supply of modern health care facilities in Nigeria. The Roman Catholic missions predominated, accounting for about 40 percent of the total number of mission–based hospital beds by 1965. By that time, mission hospitals somewhat exceeded government hospitals in number: 118 mission hospitals, compared with 101 government hospitals.

Mission–based facilities were concentrated in certain areas, depending on the religious and other activities of the missions. Roman Catholic hospitals in particular were concentrated in the southeaster and Midwestern areas. By 1954 almost all the hospitals in the Midwestern part of the country were operated by Roman Catholic missions. The Church in Nigeria played an important role in medical training and education, providing training for nurses and paramedical personnel and sponsoring basic education as well as advanced medical training, often in Europe, for many of the first generation of Western–educated Nigeria doctors. In addition, the general education provided by the Churches for many

510 John XXIII, Pacem in Terris, no. II, April 11, 1963; Cf. Pius XI, Divinis Redemptoris, AAS 29 (1937), p.78; Pius XII, Radio Broadcast on the Feast of Pentecost, AAS 33 (1941), pp.195–205

511 GS 40

Nigerians helped to lay the groundwork for a wider distribution and acceptance of modern medical care.

Ownership of health establishments was divided among the Federal Government and the Church. Among the prominent church–owned is the one in Ibo Tribe located in Abia state, near the large southern Nigerian city of Aba. This hospital is owned and managed by the Congregation of Immaculate Heart Sisters. Presently she has: 110 inpatient beds; 150 workers dominated by the sisters of the congregation; over 30,000 patients treated annually; seven full time physicians and 2 full time chaplains serving the sick. The motto of the Hospital is, "*We treat the wound; God heals it.*" The Hospital serves the community as a general hospital – complete with medical, surgical, paediatric, obstetrical and outpatient services. The Hospital continues to be a blessing to the sick especially those infested with HIV/AIDS and the poor while being a source for teaching and preaching the message of Jesus Christ. Countless people have become Christians because of the Hospital and its outreach.

Wit the new concepts of hospital and of medical care, there is more potential to heal and restore health, especially the HIV/AIDS patients, more opportunity to prevent disease. In conclusion we say with O'Rourke:

> *With all the changes, however, the purpose of Catholic hospitals remains in accord with the Church's mission to bring the person of the healing Christ to people, to penetrate society with Christian values, and to work for better society by striving for social justice in the field of health care.*[512]

4.4.3 The Mission in the Early Church or Apostolic Time

The early church of Christ beginning from the very first twelve apostles, the seventy, and all the other disciples of the Lord Jesus down to the apostle Paul, Stephen the martyr, Barnabas, Silas to mention, had the same injunction and power to preach and heal as Jesus had done. With Jesus, "the blind receive their sight, and the lame walk, the lepers are cleansed, and the deaf hear and the dead are raised to life and the good news preached to the poor" (Mt 11:5–6). The same thing those who believe in him have to accomplish both immediately after the resurrection and ascension into heaven and in the years to come. Hence he said,

> *I tell you most solemnly, whoever believes in me will perform the same work as I do myself, he will perform even greater works, because I am going to the father. Whatever*

512 K. O'Rourke, "Catholic Hospitals", in Catholic Encycl., vol. 17, U.S.A., 1981, pp.275–276

you ask for in my name I will do so that the father may be glorified in the son. (Jn 14: 12–13).

So as part of the mission and many works they will perform as Christ did is his healing works, the inspired account of which is found in the second book of the apostle Luke, the Acts. It is recorded that in the days immediately after the Pentecost, many healings took place at the hands of the apostles. Such include the cure of the lame man at the beautiful gate (Acts 3: 1–10), the cure of the paralytic at Lydda (Acts 9: 32–35), the raising of a woman to life at Jaffa (Acts 9:36–43), and the raising of a dead man at Troas (Acts 20: 7–1 1) etc.

At this juncture, it is pertinent to note that Scholars have divergent views about the healing works of the apostles in the early Church. There are scholars who believe ardently in the healing miracles, some believe miracles existed at the time of Jesus and ceased soon after, while some others agreed that healing continued till the time of the apostles and the early church and ceased with them. There are also those who held that miracles are no more prominent after Jesus while others still reduced all things to Psychology. Writing on the healing works, J. Redford says,

We must realise that the healing miracles of Jesus – and, after the resurrection of Jesus, the healing miracles of the apostles (Acts 3: 1 –1 0) were but signs of a new beginning. This does not mean that miracles entirely ceased after that beginning had itself come to an end. But they have never assumed the central place in the life of the Church which they had at those special times of the first announcement of the Good News. This is because the 'sign' the miraculous has given way to the 'reality'; the death and resurrection of Christ.[513]

The above stand of Redford seems to get a support from Galipeau who holds that though the apostles continued with the healing works of Jesus, it never took any importance place in their mission.

While healing has never totally disappeared from the practice of the Church, it has never again flourished as it did in the gospels. Part of the reason has to do with the later evangelists. By elaborating their healing stories to paint a picture of Jesus as more divine, they unwittingly led their readers away from the original dynamics of Jesus healing. Belief in Jesus became more important than carrying on his life and work.[514]

Some other scholars hold that the apostles had limited success in the fulfilment of the mandate of Jesus. They healed certain sicknesses and cast off demons

513 J. Redford, The healing word: Scripture and the pastoral ministry to the sick, in "Christian ministry to the sick", ed, Tom Coyle, Chapman, London, 1986, p.62

514 S.A. Galipeau, Transforming body and soul, Op. Cit., p.140

but failed in some areas like in the case of the epileptic demoniac (Lk 9: 37–43). In order to prove further that the disciples did not meet up completely with the injunction, Galipeau quotes the gospel of John 16:7 as an evidence to show the disciples lack some power that should only be given to them with the coming of the Holy Spirit. "I tell you the truth: it is to your advantage that I go away for if I do not go away, the counsellor will not come to you."[515]

Having given these divergent views of scholars, we still have our own evidence from the bible and other scholars to show that the apostles carried out the mission of healing entrusted to them by their master. MacNutt holds that

the Jerusalem Church (Peter) and the gentile Churches (Paul) all carry on the same preaching and healing as Jesus himself did because Jesus is the one who is still doing it... Just as Jesus connected preaching and healing in his presentation of the gospel the early apostles carried on that Tradition with no diminution of power.[516]

The early Church especially in the apostles Peter and Paul proclaimed the kingdom and cured the sick. The first healing that Peter recorded was the cure of the crippled at the beautiful gate (Acts 3: 1–10), while Paul himself cured the man born blind at Lystra (Acts 14:8). Other healings of the apostles include: the cure of the paralytic at Lydda (Acts 9:32–35), the raising of the woman to life at Jaffa (Acts):36–43), the raising of the dead Eutychus to life at Troas (Acts 20:7–1 1) and the laying of hand and cure of the father of Publius who was sick of fever and dysentery (Acts 28:7).

The bible recorded other instances of miraculous healings by the other disciples apart from Paul and Peter. As the number of the disciples in Jerusalem increased, Stephen one of the deacons, a man full of the Holy spirit, who was appointed by the early Church worked miracles and great signs among the people (cf Acts 6: 5–8). it was also known that after Saul persecuted the Christians and scattered them, many of them, who escaped, went from place to place preaching the good news and working miracles. One of them Philip preached in a Samaritan town proclaiming the gospel and unclean spirits were cast out and several paralytics and cripples were cured. And there were great rejoicing in the town (cf Acts 8:38). Even Simon the magician was astonished for the wonders and great miracles that took place when he went around with Philip (Acts 8:13). Also in Samaria the apostles Peter and John laid hands on the people and they received the Holy Spirit (Acts 8: 14–17). A good number of the other disciples in the early Church preached and healed as Jesus did and the healing mission of Jesus continues throughout the ages.

515 Jn 16:7 quoted in S.A. Galipeau, "Transforming body and soul", p.142
516 F. MacNutt, Healing, Op. Cit., pp.55 & 56

It is interesting at this point to note that out of all the followers of Jesus to whom he delegated his power to heal, only a few out of the number recorded in the early church belonged to the original twelve. This goes a long way to portray that the power to heal was not to be restricted to the twelve or the seventy. His mission for healing was for all nations and generations. But one fact is obvious. The authority and power to heal must be obtained only in his name.

> *There are the signs that will be associated with the believers; in my name they will cast out devils; they will have the gift of tongues, they will pick up snakes in their hands, and be unharmed should they drink deadly poison; they will lay their hands on the sick who will recover. (Mk 16; 1 7–18)*

The followers of Jesus actually used his name in healing. Peter for example was very emphatic on this when he healed the crippled at the gate called beautiful. "It is the name of Jesus which through faith in it, has brought back the strength of this man whom you see here and who is well known to you" (Acts 3:16). These early disciples of Jesus were extremely happy as they discovered for themselves this power of Jesus in their ministry. They came back rejoicing, saying, "Lord even the devils submit to us when we use your name" (Lk 10:17). But at this point, Jesus warned them against pride and against self–aggrandizement, a vice that we see creeping in, and is gradually taking root in the healing ministry of our time. He said to the disciples in response to their happy discovery that the devils submit to them.

> *I watched the Satan fall like lightening from heaven. Yes I have given you power to tread underfoot serpents and scorpions and the whole strength of the enemy; nothing shall ever hurt you. But you do not rejoice that the spirits submit to you: rejoice rather that your names are written in heaven. (Lk 10:18–20)*

Here, we conclude this section of the inquiry into Our Lord's mission to the early Church by posing this all important question, namely; was the power to heal the sick given to all members of the early Church? In response to this question, we hold that Our Lord gave a special mission to the twelve and the seventy, and later to Stephen, Paul and Philip and to some others as directed by the Holy Spirit. The power was not given to all individual Christians of the time, neither was it given to all who were surging after Jesus and later after the apostles and the disciples. We noted that one Simon the Magician from Samaria followed Philip and his disciples for a long time in a bid to get the power from them but to no avail. "Give me the same power, he said so that anyone I lay my hands on will have the Holy Spirit" (Acts 8: 13–19). While writing to the Church at Corinth, Paul very well emphasized that the power to heal was not given to all Christians but to those whom the spirit wills. He made it clear that all in Christ's body are of different parts, differently gifted, to work with different gifts as apostles, prophets, teachers, helpers, and good leaders and still aspiring to the higher gift, the gift of Love (cf 1Cor 12: 27 – 13).

4.4.4 The Mission and the Early Christian Writers/the Fathers of the Church

The first Christians after Jesus and the apostles lived in intense fear of persecution from within the Jewish community and later from the Roman emperors. It was such that it was dangerous to be a Christian then. Historical facts had it that after fire destroyed much of Rome in the year 64, Nero made a scapegoat of the Christian community. "He fastened the guilt and inflicted the most exquisite tortures on a class hated for their abominations, called Christians by the populace.[517] This hatred and persecution persisted that the Church had to thrive underground but strong in faith and rich in the gifts of the Holy Spirit and the gift of healing. Many healing works were wrought during the period. But unfortunately not much record was kept of the healing ministry. Most of what we know of this time came from the writings of the fathers of the Church.

According to Carlo Cremona, "the fathers of the church were an expression of the continuity and authentic interpretation of the message of Christ and the doctrine of the Church "[518]

> *These were theologians who sought to continue the teachings of the apostles and to resolve theological problems that arose as the Church expanded. But they were not historians. They wrote for the Christians of their time, not ours. It was their expectation that Jesus would return soon, so they were not concerned about preserving records for the benefit of future generations. As a result, they left no detailed descriptions of the healing ministry as it existed in the early church. When they wrote about healing, it was in almost casual way, as it were simply an accepted part of the ordinary Christian experience.*[519]

However, one fact is obvious – that the healing gifts existed and healing works were wrought during this period in the name of Jesus Christ.

> *Of the methods employed to effect this healing, one rebuked the evil spirit in the name of Jesus. Other methods involved laying of hands on, touching, or breathing on the men-*

517 R. Baldwin, The Healers, Huntington, Indiana, 1986, p.37

518 C.Cremona, Care of the sick and the fathers of the church, in "Dolentium Hominum", No 31, 1996, p.39

519 R.Baldwin, The Healers, Op. Cit., pp.38&39

tally ill person. Sometimes during the ceremony the accounts of Jesus healing actions were related and holy water was utilized.[520]

As the Church lived on, the account of the healing action of the Church did not continue to grow great. Some of the great theologians and writers did not address the question of healing gifts in the Church. Some stated that the period in which miracles or healings happened was of special dispensation meant perhaps for the institution and growth of the church. Some believed the age of miracles has passed. Others maintained that healings were reserved to special places and times. But there were no such things in the Bible or teaching of the church. God had never withdrawn his healing gifts from the church at any time nor had Jesus ever thought of the healing as a temporary service to humanity. Instead Our Lord intended that this ministry, rather than diminish should continue to wax stronger. Hence he said, "He that believes in me, the works I do, he shall also do and even greater works" (Jn 14: 12–13). We shall now see some of the Church fathers and early writers who in their writings made mention of healing and the related ministry of exorcism or ministry of deliverance as is popularly used by this age.

4.4.5 Justin the Martyr (100–165)

Justin was born at Nablus, Palestine about the year 100. He was from a Pagan and Greeco–Roman background, well–educated man whose interest in Philosophy led him to study the teachings of the Jewish prophets and of Jesus Christ. He was later converted to Christianity. Though he retained the garb of a philosopher, he is the most important Christian Apologist of the second Century and the first of whom we possess written works. These are the two apologies of which the first was addressed to Emperor Antonius and the second to the Roman Senate, setting forth the moral values of Christianity. In the sixth chapter of the second apology, he writes,

> *Even now, your own eyes will teach you the truth of this last statement. For many demoniacs throughout the entire world, even in your own city, were exorcised by many of our Christians in the name of Jesus Christ, who was crucified under Pontius Pilate; and our men cured them, and they still cure others by rendering helpless and dispelling the demons who had taken possession of these men, even when they could not be cured by all the other exorcists, and exploiters of incantations and drugs.*[521]

---

520 B.M. Meehan, The healing power of prayer, Op. Cit. p.22
521 Justin Martyr, 2nd Apology: To the Roman Senate, 6, in "The Ante – Nicene Fathers", Grand Rapids, Michigan, Various dates.

4.4.6 Irenaeus, Bishop and Martyr (130–202 A.D.)

He was born in Asia Minor, was one of the most important theologians of the Second Century. He gave testimonies to a wide variety of healings during the early periods of the Church. His writings did much to combat the heresies that were rampart in the time particularly those of the Gnostics and Valentinians. In his treatise against heresies, he identified the fact that the heretics were not able to perform the miracles that Christians accomplished. He saw healing as a natural activity of Christians that channels the creative power of God through prayer.

He says about the Christians,

> *For they are able to give sight to the blind, hearing to the deaf, to put all demons to flight ... The infirm, the lame, or those paralyzed or those disturbed in other parts of the body, are cured –, it often happens that those who have contracted some bodily illness or have had some kind of accident, are restored in this way to good.*[522]

Also in his discourse on healing he says,

> *Yea, more over as I have said, the dead even have been raised up, and remained among us for many years. And what shall I say more? It is not possible to name the numbers of gifts, which the church scattered throughout the whole world, has received from God, in the name of Jesus Christ, and which she exercises day by day for the benefits of the Gentiles, neither practising deception upon any, nor taking any reward from them... For as she has received freely from God, freely also she Ministers to others.*[523]

4.4.7 Tertullian (160–230 A.D.)

He was one of the early Christian writers. He was converted at Carthage in North Africa. In his writings, he revealed the power of Christ working in the Christians to heal the sick and raise the dead to life. About the beginning of the third century he wrote a protest letter to Scapula, a local Roman official who was bitterly persecuting the Christians. In the letter, he noted that some Roman officials who publicly oppose the Christians were privately seeking prayers for healing from the same Christians.

> *All these things you may learn from the officials in your staff, from the same advocates who themselves have benefited from the Christians, although in Court they vote as they like. For the secretary of a certain Gentleman, when he was suffering from falling sickness caused by demons, was freed from it –, so also were a relative of some of the*

522 Cf. B.M. Meehan, The Healing power of prayer, p.21

523 Irenaeus, Discourse on healing, in "Against Heresies" 11,6.2, 31.2, 32, 4–5

others and a certain little boy. And heaven knows how many distinguished men, to say nothing of common people, have been cured either of devils or of their sickness. Even Severus himself (the Emperor Septimus Severus), the father of Antonius, graciously remembered the Christians. He searched for Proculus – a Christian whose surname was Torpacion, a manager in the employ of Euhodia – who had cured him once by means of Oil, and kept him in his pace until his death.[524]

4.4.8 Origen (85–254 A.D.)

Origen is another scholar of the early Church, who witnessed and acknowledged the healing gifts of the church. Writing on the effects of healing prayers, he said the name of Jesus could cause a total healing in a person's life. He cited the examples in which the Greeks and Barbarians who accepted Jesus Christ and who invoked the name of Jesus in prayer also shared the gift of healing.

> *For by these men, we too have seen many persons freed from grievous calamities, and from distractions of mind, and madness and countless other ills which could be cured neither by men or devils.*[525]

While the writers mentioned above testified to the many miraculous cures during the period in question, we take note of the observations of R. Baldwin concerning the veneration of relics. He says,

> *Many of the church fathers – including Saint Jerome, Saint Gregory of Nyasa and Saint John Chrysostom – took the veneration of relics for granted – some including Saint Augustine, Saint Ambrose and Pope Leo 1, attributed miraculous cures to such practices*[526]

We have to make mention of the veneration of relics here since

> *from the fourth century through the middle ages, Catholics sought healing primarily through sacramental anointing or through visits to shrines where bones or other relics of the saints and martyrs were kept.*[527]

The Christian community of Smyrna (Izmir today), where Saint Polycarp was burnt at the stake around the year 156, made this important and all revealing remark as they preserved and revered his remains.

---

524 Tertullian, To Scapula 4, "Anti Nicene Fathers",
525 Origen, Against Celsus, 1, 46 & 67
526 R.Baldwin, The Healers, Op. Cit., p.62
527 Ibid., p.59

We took up his bones, which are more valuable than precious stones and finer than refined gold and laid them in a suitable place, where the Lord will permit us to gather ourselves together, as we are able, in gladness and joy, and to celebrate the birthday of his martyrdom.[528]

4.4.9 Saint Augustine of Hippo (354–430)

Augustine, a convert to Christianity, and a bishop was recognized as one of the greatest theologians of any era and one of the shapers of the Christian theology. Among his early writings were his thoughts on healing gifts of the church, where he warned Christians not to expect and seek miraculous healings as they occurred during the time of the apostles. However before the end of his priestly life he witnessed a number of miraculous cures in his own Cathedral at Hippo. By then adult baptism were very common and after baptism, the newly baptized, all clad in white, emerged from the Cathedral, receiving greetings with kisses and handshakes from their friends and relations. At these occasions many sick people were noticed to have been cured of their illnesses and diseases of various types on touching the newly baptized. From there a healing Tradition grew up in the Cathedral on adult baptism days. Reversing his earlier position about healing miracles, he humbly admitted he had been wrong. In one of the final sections of his great work the City of God, he wrote of the miracles that occurred in his own diocese of Hippo:

I realised how many miracles were occurring in our own day and which were so like the miracles of old and also how wrong it would be to allow the memory of these marvels of divine power to perish from among our people. It is only two years ago that the keeping of records was begun here in Hippo, and already, at this writing, we have nearly seventy attested miracles.[529]

Also having witnessed many more miraculous healings wrought at different occasions by various individuals he notes, "it is a simple fact that there is no lack of miracles even in our day. And the God who works the miracles we read in the Scripture use any means and manner he chooses."[530] Among the many miracles that happened in his own Church where the relics of the Martyr Saint Stephen were placed, he witnessed two of the healings himself – the healing of a young man named Paul and that of her sister named Palladia, both of whom suffered from convulsions. They went to the Church every day to pray before the shrine of

528 R. Baldwin, The Healers, p.59
529 Saint Augustine, The City of God, XXII, 8,
530 Saint Augustine, The City of God, as in R. Baldwin, The "Healers", pp.63 & 64

the martyr Saint Stephen, asking God to forgive their sins and bring them back to health. They both regained their good health before the shrine of the martyr in the Cathedral in Hippo. Augustine himself told the stories of how they were cured.

In Augustine's thinking, the world is sustained by the immanent power of God. When humankind began to take this marvellous reality of God for granted, however, God broke through in a more unusual manner, using healings and miracles to draw people's attention to God's presence in the world.[531]

4.4.10 Saint Gregory, Bishop of Tours (573–594)

Saint Gregory who was bishop of Tours (573–594) where Saint Martin also bishop of Tours (316–397) had acquired his reputation as a healer, wrote of his own healings at the tomb of Saint Martin. He narrated how he was carried critically ill to Martin's tomb where he was restored to health. He also told of healings that resulted when people were anointed with oil from the various shrines of Martin and the cures of pilgrims who slept in the shrines of Saint Martin and the martyrs.

4.4.11 Saint Gregory the Great, Bishop of Rome (590–604)

Gregory was apparently one of the last fathers of the Church to give testimony to the healing gifts of the Church. He saw the healing gifts as a fore taste of heaven and as the perfect human kind with God that we could experience there.

In his view, miraculous healings pointed towards the conclusion of time, making the world the "ante chamber" of heaven. He included the power of the saints in his approach to healing and urged people to see how they had "friends at court" who would intercede for them in their needs and difficulties.[532]

Though in spite of this view of Gregory and many other good things he wrote about miraculous healings including his own healing through the prayers of a monk, Gregory emphasized the value of suffering. In his work on the Pastoral Care of the sick he wrote, "The sick are to be admonished that they feel themselves to be sons of God in that the scourge of discipline chastises them".[533]

---

531 B.M. Meehan, The healing power of prayer, Op. Cit., p.23

532 Ibid., p.24

533 Gregory the Great, Book on Pastoral Care, in R. Baldwin, "The Healers", Op. Cit., p.69

4.5 The Healing Mission in the Church Today

We have now seen that the healing mission of Jesus is not a reserve of the early Church or the Apostolic age or any particular time or age. We have also noted that healing has never totally disappeared from the practice of the Church in any time of the history of the Church and that the followers of Jesus and faithful believers in his teachings have been commissioned to preach and heal as Jesus did. This practice is not absent in the same Church of Christ today. The Church of Jesus in our age continues in the same mission of Jesus. The reason for the continuation of this mission is that Jesus promised his believers the advocate while giving them the mandate.

I tell you most solemnly, whoever believes in me will perform the same works as I do myself, he will perform even greater works because I am going to the father... I shall ask the father, and he will give you an advocate to be with you forever." (Jn 14: 12 – 16).

Jesus is still with the Father in heaven and since he is still there, we can expect the fulfilment of his promises, which includes the healing of the sick. So the healing works of Jesus has continued after his departure from the earth, and the Church today is ever active in the healing works through various means.

One of the avenues strongly employed by the church today in the commission given by Jesus is the establishment of hospitals. She has established many religious institutions within her, with the specific aim of fostering, organising and providing help to the sick.

It is on record that, from the year 313 A.D. onwards, the church could organise care for the poor and the sick on a very large scale indeed. Institutions bearing a whole variety of names sprang up everywhere and with increasing frequency. Their names reflected the kind of people they cared for: "hospitals" for the sick; "homes" for the elderly –, "hospices" for pilgrims and "Orphanages".[534]

In fact the establishment of the first hospitals in many countries of the world has been attributed to the church through the religious institutions. According to J. Mally, "Many catholic hospitals were founded as extension of religious communities that ministered to the sick and the dying and were largely staffed by women religious."[535] He further states that,

534 Jesus Alvarez Gomez, The care of the Sick in the history of the Church, in "Dolentium Hominum", No 31, 1996, p.45

535 E.J. Malley, Healthcare Handbook, CHA, St. Louis, 1986, p.1

Catholic hospitals and healthcare institutions frequently describe themselves in religious terms, as an apostolate or ministry, an extension of Jesus healing mission and part of the Church's ministry of mercy and wholeness.[536]

Some of these hospitals established by the Church began as centres for the poor. An example is the hospital erected by saint Ephremus in 373 A.D.

During a period of famine in Odessa, Saint Ephremus berated the rich for their indifference and with the donations he received created an "emergency hospital" with three hundred beds. This hospital took in the poor and the sick drawn from the city and the surrounding country side.[537]

And up till today the Church has not in any way been less involved in this commission by Jesus through their establishment of hospitals and other healthcare institutions.

On February 11, 1985 the Holy Father John Paul II, through the 'Dolentium Hominum' created the Pontifical commission for Apostolate of Healthcare workers, which serves as the co–ordinating organism for all the Catholic institutions, religious and lay, committed in the apostolate of the sick. By means of the commission, the Pope invited all the episcopacy of the world to be a sign of the profound concern the Church has for the world of the suffering and the sick. Many of the bishops have heeded to this invitation. In most places however, the call was not anything new, though it still served as a reminder or an invigorating force for what was already there.

In Nigeria, the first general hospital that opened its door to the populace, the sacred Heart Hospital Abeokuta was built by a Catholic French priest Jean Conguard in1895.[538]

In Igboland of Nigeria, the Church also established the first hospitals. The first missionaries landed at the bank of the River Niger in Onitsha, on a Saturday, in December 5, 1885 with Fathers Lutz and Horne to begin the mission. It is on record that

a dispensary was opened as a vital point of contact with the people who came for treatment ... This initial move was so successful that day after day, parents crowded the Catholic mission where Fr Lutz provided medication for their children's ailments.[539]

---

536 Ibid., p.1

537 Jesus Alvarez Gomez, The care of the sick in the history of the Church, Op. Cit., pp.45 &46

538 G. Sofoluwe &F.J. Bennett, Principles and Practice of Community Health in Africa, Ibadan, 1985, p.82

Today there are many healthcare institutions established by the catholic Church in Nigeria as an avenue for the continuation of the healing mission, which Jesus entrusted to his Church.

The healing ministry through prayer and faith – healing was not in the lime-light in the Catholic Church in Nigeria until recently. "Before the 10th of May 1973, no priest was fully involved in the healing ministry."[540] That is to say that that an important aspect of the mission to heal was not much the prerogative of priests or was forgotten or not considered as part of the mission. Pastors so to say were either not aware that the healing of the sick in body and spirit was an essential part of their ministry or they were so engrossed in the preaching of the word to the suffocation of the twin sister of the mandate of Jesus. "Wherever you enter a town where they make you welcome, eat what is set before you. Cure those in it who are sick, and say 'The kingdom of God' is very near to you" (Lk 10: 8–9). This command until recently was not forcefully carried out. The priests were satisfied with ordinary and routine visit to the sick and the anointing with oil of the sick.

Today, it is a renewal and a revival. The Charismatic dimension of the Church in Nigeria is now active, healing the sick and casting out the devils through prayers and laying on of hands. A good number of the priests and even lay men and women are engaging in the healing ministry of Jesus. Many of the priests are becoming more disposed to the healing ministry by prayers and many more are discovering their charisms in this area of the apostolate. The only thing left is the correct application and use of these charisms, which is giving much concern to the Church in our age.

4.5.1 Forms of Healing in the Church

The mission of the Church to be a mediation of healing in the world flows from its task of proclaiming the reign of God. Jesus went about his mission of preaching and healing the sick and his fame spread throughout Galilee and beyond. Those who were suffering from diseases and painful complaints of one kind or the other were brought to him and he cured them. Large crowds followed him, coming from Galilee, the Decapolis, Jerusalem, Judea and Transjordan. Later, before he left the world to go back to his Father, he entrusted the mission to the

539 C.A. Obi, Background to the planting of Catholic Christianity in the Lower Niger in a "Hundred years of the Catholic church in Eastern Nigeria, ed, C.AObi, Onitsha, 1985, pp24 – 25.

540 G.C. Ikeobi, "What I think God is doing in and through me", a paper presented at the National Pastoral seminar on Healing Ministry, Enugu, 1992, p.23

community that was built up from the crowd and they continued the work of making present the reign of God, bringing relief to the sick and the afflicted. Hence,

Divine healing is simply the healing of Christ through his Church, as instituted by Our Lord himself, as carried on by the apostles and for several centuries more by the ministry of the Church.[541]

This power given to the Church had been used by the Church and is still available and being used by the church in various forms. Christ categorically stated that healing power would be associated with believers who in his name will cast out demons and cure the sick. Throughout the history of the Church, this ministry has never ceased. Organic diseases or even functional disorders have been healed without resorting to the skills of experts in medicine. Laying on of hands or anointing with oil or simple prayer have brought about some radical changes in the body and spirit.

The perduring phenomenon of pilgrimages to shrines like Lourdes manifests the faith of the Christian people in the power of God to grant physical, emotional and spiritual healing.[542]

The importance placed by the Church on the Visitation and pastoral care of the sick contributed greatly to the founding of hospices and hospitals in the early days of the Church which persisted till today. All these ways by which the Church has carried out her ministry to the sick throughout her history can be narrowed down to three major forms, namely:

1. Ordinary form through gifts and services (Charisms); (1cor 12:7–9; Acts 6: 1–2; 2 Cor 5–6; Col 1:24)
2. Extraordinary form through cures that were usually believed to be miraculous (Acts 3: 1–6).
3. Sacramental form, through prayer and anointing (Jn 5–13–16)[543]

4.5.1.1 The Ordinary Form of Healing

The ordinary form of healing is one of the major forms of healings in the Church, experienced or manifested through the use of the various gifts (charisms) of the Father to various individuals in the church, as the Holy spirit sees fit, and of

541 E.H. Cobb, Christ Healing, London, 1964, p.2

542 R. Ryan, Healing and the mission of the Church, in C. Stuhlmueller, ed, "The collegeville Pastoral dictionary of Biblical Theology", Minnesota, 1996, p.421

543 Cf Catholic Bishops' Conference of Nigeria, Guidelines for the healing ministry in the Catholic church in Nigeria, Lagos, 1997, pp.5&6

which no two are the same. (1 Cor 12: 4–11; Rom 12: 6–8; Eph 4: 1–12) The purpose is to serve and build up Christ's body, the church. This form of healing is not a prerogative of any group as some people think but it is the whole Church that is called to this service. The clergy as well as the laity are called by Jesus Christ to use the gifts within their respective reach for the service of one another particularly the sick and the weak members of His Body.

4.5.1.2 Charisms

The word Charism though found only in the New Testament comes from the Greek word "Charisma" often translated "gift" or from the root "Chairo" meaning "I rejoice" and "Charis" meaning "thanks, grace or favour". The term though does not occur in the Old Testament but the concept of Charism can be related to powerful effect of the divinely given spirit of the Lord as manifested in some powerful kings or Charismatic leaders like Samson (Judg 14: 6), Samuel (1 Sam 11:6), Gideon (Judg 3:39).

> *In the New Testament, the term Charism appears mainly in the Pauline literature, as individual spiritual gifts to believers by the spirit meant to be exercised for the edification of the community, and each is motivated by love which is the greatest of the gifts.*[544]

And according to the church document 'Christi fidelis Laici',

> *The Charisms are graces of the Holy Spirit that have directly or indirectly ausefulness for the ecclesial community, ordered as they are to the building up of the Church to the well–being of humanity and to the needs of the world.*[545]

These various gifts of the Holy Spirit are classified into variety of spiritual gifts. According to L. Thomas and J. Alkire,

> *They are natural gifts that are raised to a supernatural level by the power of the Holy Spirit. They are not things, like wrapped presents from God; instead, they are ways of doing an activity, namely serving the people of God lovingly.*[546]

In his letter to the Church in Corinth Paul writes,

> *Now there are varieties of gifts, but the same spirit –, and there are varieties of service but the same Lord –, and there are varieties of working, but it is the same God who*

544 J.L. Gillman, Charism, in "Collegeville Pastoral Dictionary of Biblical Theolgy", Op. Cit., p.128

545 John Paul II, Apostolic Exhotation, Christi Fidelis Laici, 30 Dec 1998, p.59

546 L. Thomas & J. Alkire, Healing Ministry: A practical guide, Sheed and Ward, Kansas, 1994, p.202–208

inspires them all in everyone. To each is given the manifestation of the spirit for the common good. To one is given through the spirit the utterance of wisdom and to another the utterance of knowledge according to the same spirit, to another faith by the same spirit, to another gifts of healing by the one spirit, to another the working of miracles, to another the ability to distinguish between spirits, to another various kinds of tongues. All these are inspired by one and the same spirit, who apportions to each one individually as he wills.

(1 Cor 12: 4–11) It is in the passage above that Paul made the most extensive and comprehensive discussion about the gifts of the Holy Spirit. Paul's response to the concerns of the Corinthian Church brought to his attention the richly blessed manifestations of the spirit within the Church, such that he said, "You are not lacking in any spiritual gift"

(1 Cor 1: 7). However the proper exercise and evaluation of these gifts by the Corinthians was problematic and required Paul's lengthy instruction about the purpose and proper exercise of the gifts.[547]

In the then Corinthian Church, there was the problem of some members of the Church claiming monopoly of the gifts of the Holy Spirit. They consider themselves more Charismatic and more important than the others. But none in the Church is a passive member. None is more important. None is more charismatic than the other. The whole Church is Charismatic in its members, each with his own gift for the good of the community. Therefore, using the image of the human body, an organic unity of diverse parts, Paul argues that each member of the body has its function to perform, and the exercise of gifts cannot lead to divisions in the body, but that parts should have the same concern for one another (cf. 1 Cor 12–. 25). Any wonder the council of the Church speaks of the ministries and charisms "as gifts of the Holy Spirit which are given for the building of the body of Christ and for its mission of salvation in the world."[548]

The Charisms are received in gratitude both on the part of the one who receives then, and also on the part of the entire Church. They are infact a singularly rich source of grace for the vitality of the apostolate and for holiness of the whole body of Christ, provided that they be gifts that come from the spirit and are exercised in full conformity with the authentic prompting of the spirit, gifts exercised for the growth of the whole church,[549] *gifts given for service (1 Cor 12: 5); and for the edification of the community*

547 J.L. Gillman, Charism, in "The Collegeville Pastoral Dictionary of Biblical Theology", Op. Cit., p.120

548 The second Vatican Ecumenical Council, Lumen Gentium, 4.

549 John Paul II, Apostolic Exhortation, Christi Fidelis Laici, p.60

(I Cor 12: 7); and "not for self aggrandizement or boasting,"[550] *"nor for self enrichment,"*[551] *or for any type of abuse.*

4.5.1.3 Love or Charity – The Greatest of the Gifts

The beneficial exercise of all the spiritual gifts is determined according to Paul ultimately by the one who follows the "more excellent way" (I Cor 12: 3), that of love ... Love is the foundation, the more basic, pervasive, and enduring value that gives all other charisms their effectiveness.[552]

The terms 'Love' and 'Charity' are synonymous. Love, the greatest of all the spiritual gifts is best expressed by the Greek term 'agape'' Agape is total dedication to the welfare of others, regardless of personal cost. It is en–rooted in service. This is natural only to God but he gives us a share to it at the time of our baptism. It first unites us to God and then directed to other human beings.

As a theoretical conception, charity has meant both possessive and selfless love, as well as favour, grace, mercy, kindness, righteousness and liberality. In it's practical application, Charity denotes the distribution of goods to the poor and the establishment and endowment of such social–welfare institutions as hospitals, homes for the aged, orphanages and reformatory institutions.[553]

In ancient Egypt, Charity was perceived as an inner disposition toward fellow beings and as a means of propitiating the gods for the purpose of achieving immortality, but it also meant, as the book of Going Forth by Day indicates, giving bread to the hungry, water to the thirsty, clothes to the naked, and even a boat to the one who had none.[554]

The above conceptions of Charity shows that love principally has to do with service, service to others, expressed in different ways, formal or informal for the growth of the community of people – the people of God. So the whole Church as such is directly called to the service of Charity.

In the very early days the Church added the agape to the Eucharistic supper, and thus showed herself to be wholly united around Christ by the bond of Charity. So too, in all ages, she is recognised by this sign of love, and while she rejoices in the undertakings of others, she claims works of Charity as her own inalienable duty and right. For this

---

550 J.L. Gillman, Charism, in "The Collegeville Pastoral Dictionary of Biblical Theology" Op. Cit., p.129

551 The Catholic Bishops Conference of Nigeria, "Guidelines for the healing ministry in the Catholic Church in Nigeria", p.8

552 J.L. Gillman, Charism, in "The Collegeville Pastoral Dictionary of Biblical Theology" Op.Cit., p.130

553 D.J. Constantelos, Charity, in Mircea Eliade, ed, "The Encyclopedia of Religion, Vol 3", Macmillan, London, 1987, p.222

554 D.J.Constantelos, Charity, "The Encyclopaedia of Religion"., p.223

reason, mercy to the poor and the sick, works of charity and mutual aid intended to relieve human needs of every kind, are held in special honour in the church.[555]

The Church therefore made Charity a major concern of her ministry and established numerous institutions for the sick, orphans, widows, indigent and others in need of rehabilitation and assistance. This concern is still very much alive in the church till date. The church continues not only the work of rehabilitation and assistance but extends to other areas of social services, peace commission and justice. It is therefore not just enough to give alms but

Wherever men are to be found who are in want of food and drink, of clothing, housing, medicine, work, education, the means necessary for leading a truly human life, wherever there are men racked by misfortune or illness, men suffering exile or imprisonment, Christian charity should go in search of them and find them out, comfort them with devoted care and give them the helps that will relieve their needs. This obligation binds first and foremost the more affluent individuals and nations.[556]

The Christian service of Charity therefore calls first and foremost on the more affluent members of Christ's Body

to help the poor rehabilitate themselves by lending them money, taking them into partnership, or employing them, for in this way, the desired end is achieved without loss of self–respect for the recipient. This is regarded as the highest form of Charity in the medieval Judaism, particularly in Momes Maimonides.[557]

And for today this should be regarded not only as the highest form of charity but should also be known as the highest and clearest form of healing of the body and the spirit.

Creating employment opportunities and teaching technical competence for self–employment could be the new forms of the healing ministry. When people have work to do, they create zest for life.[558]

The leading team of missionaries that set their feet in Igboland did that. At the creation of Onitsha into a prefecture, Father Lutz became the first Prefect of Onitsha Prefecture.

---

555 Second Vatican Ecumenical Council, Decree on the Apostolate of Lay people, Apostolicam Actuositatem, 18 Nov. 1965, (hereafter as A.A.), No.8

556 A.A. No 8

557 D.J. Constantelos, Charity, in Mircea Eliade, ed, "The encyclopedia of Religion, Vol 3", Op. Cit., p.223

558 L. Mbefo, Priests and the Healing Ministry in the Nigerian Church; Op. Cit., p.10

He introduced the missionary policies and methods which characterized the Catholic Mission in Igboland up to 1900. Besides the usual direct means of winning converts (preaching, catechization, religious worship and rituals), he inaugurated a series of indirect means of evangelization. He introduced the use of the school (for boys and girls), charitable work (dispensaries, hospitals orphanages and asylums), trade and industrial institutions (for carpentry, masonry, tailoring, shoe–making etc), farming and gardening, as means of attracting and retaining converts to the Catholic religion.[559]

Where are the trade and industrial institutions now? Does not the Church in Igboland today need them, to retain her Christians too?

Love must be the primary motive for all ministries because ministry is service to others on behalf of the body of Christ, for the sake of the reign of God. Thus the priest in particular is called to this ministry of charity, the greatest of the spiritual gifts which in practical terms is very effective in the healing ministry of Christ, needed to build and protect the body of Christ (1 Cor 13:13), and for the good of humanity.

The whole formation imparted to the candidates to the priesthood aims at preparing them to enter into communion with the Charity of Christ, the good shepherd. Hence their formation in different aspects must have a fundamentally pastoral character.[560]

And not only that,

By virtue of the sacramental consecration brought about by the outpouring of the spirit in the sacrament of Holy Orders, the spiritual life of the priest is marked, moulded and characterised by the way of thinking and acting proper to Jesus Christ, head and shepherd of the church, and which are summed up in his pastoral charity.[561]

The life of Jesus is a continual manifestation of his pastoral charity or rather daily enactment of it. He feels compassion for the crowds because they were harassed and helpless like sheep without shepherd (Mt 9: 35–36). He goes in search of the straying and scattered sheep (Mt 18: 12–14), and joyfully celebrates their return. He gathers and protects them. He knows them and calls each one by name (Jn 10: 3). He leads them to green pastures and still waters (Ps 22–23), and spreads a table for them, nourishing them with his own life. The good shepherd offers his life through his own death and resurrection, as the church sings out in the Roman liturgy: "The good shepherd is risen! He who laid down his life for his sheep, who died for his flock, he is risen alleluia."

559 I.R.A Ozigbo, Igbo Catholicism: The Onitsha Connection 1976–1984, Africana Publishers, Onitsha, 1985, p.6&7.
560 John Paul II, Apostolic Exhortation, Pastores Dabo Vobis, p.108
561 John Paul II, Pastores Dabo Vobis, p.41

The entire Church is called to the service of Charity. The entire faithful is called to evangelization at their reception of the sacrament of initiation and by the gifts of the Holy Spirit immanent in the Church. They are called to "confess their faith in full adherence to the word of God, which is celebrated in the sacraments and lived in charity, the principle of Christian moral existence."

The greatest of the commandments is to love God with all your heart and your neighbour as yourself (cf. Mt 22: 37–40). Christ made this love of the neighbour his personal commandment and enriched it with a new meaning when he said, "In so far as you did this to one of the least of these brothers of mine, you did it to me" (Mt 25:40). He therefore made charity the distinguishing mark of his disciples, as he also said "By this will all men know you are my disciples, by the love you bear one another" (Jn 13:35). The clergy as well as the Laity are all called to live out this commandment of love thereby giving healing to many who are down in spirit, who are victims to malnutrition and hunger and who are victims to societal marginalisation.

The Laity have even better avenues to live out this commandment of love in their lives. In our societies, especially in the urban cities, people live very near to their neighbours; very often in the same building. The urban co–habitation and nearness of residential buildings give room for the practice of this command, which Jesus solemnly entrusted to the Church because one is aware of the joys and agonies of the other member. What happens to one member of the Church happens to the other members too. When one is happy, the other rejoices with him and when one is in sorrow, together they suffer.

> *That is why mercy to the poor and the sick and charitable works and works of mutual aid for the alleviation of all kinds of human needs, are held in special honour in the Church.*[562]

This responsibility is always before us not only in our places of residence but also in our places of work and in our Christian communities, especially with regard to the care of our sick brothers and sisters. We care for them both spiritually and physically. We should always carve out time to visit the sick members of our parish communities and even outside our own communities. We pray with them, chat with them and help the indigent ones with some material gifts. This gives a great sense of belonging to most of the sick who are not able to join their own communities in their celebrations because of sickness. By this practice, the friends and families of the sick and all those who take care of them have a special share in the healing ministry of Jesus. Hence the rite of Pastoral care of the sick states that,

---

562 The second Vatican Ecumenical Council, Apostolicam Actuositatem, 8.

Every Scientific effort to prolong life and every act of care for the sick, on the part of any person, may be considered a preparation for the Gospel and a sharing in Christ's healing ministry.[563]

In addition to these visits to the sick, those who care for the sick both in the houses and in the hospitals, including the doctors and nurses should, in addition, to their normal duty of physical health caring, always arrange for necessary sacraments for the sick at the appropriate times. Pastors of souls, particularly the parish priests should always show interest in the pastoral care to the sick by constant personal visits and other acts of charity. They should also arrange for regular communion visits to the sick and the aged. This brings the Church's love and consolation of faith to the sick members of the fold. The communion visit to the sick should not however be left for the priests alone. The creation of more lay ministers of communion should be encouraged to help in communion Visitation to the sick.

The use of special or lay ministers of communion will help to ensure that the sick members of the parish receive communion regularly and particularly on Sundays. Hence the Vatican document states,

Pastors of souls will take every care to make it possible for the sick and the aged to receive the Eucharist frequently, even if they are not gravely ill or in danger of death. In fact if possible, this could be done every day, and should be done in paschal time especially. Communion may be taken to these people at any time of the day[564].

4.5.1.4 Extra–Ordinary Form of Healing

By extra–ordinary form of healing, we shall be dealing with that type of healing that normally comes to the mind of many today at the mention of the word healing. That type of healing that generates what may be called a type of fanatic appeal and excitement among people. It is that form of healing through cures that are normally believed to be miraculous in nature. "This has gone on quietly in the church over the centuries"[565] and can be traced to both the Old and New Testament of the history of the people of God. This brings us therefore to the core of this research.

The ancient world believed that only God could control and manipulate nature. So "any human being who seemed to heal a sick person was normally

563 Cf. Rite of the Pastoral care of the sick, No.32

564 Instruction on the Worship of the Eucharistic Mystery, Eucharisticum Mysterium, 25, May 1967, No. 40

565 The Catholic Bishops' Conference of Nigeria, Guidelines for the healing ministry in the catholic church in Nigeria, Op. Cit., p.6

viewed as empowered by God to do so."[566] The healing of Naaman's leprosy by bathing in the sea of Jordan at the instruction of Elisha the prophet was one such example of God working through human instrumentality. His healing made Naaman exclaim, "Now I know that there is no God in all the earth except in Israel" (2Kgs 5:15). There are other instances where miraculous cures are mentioned such as in the case of the son of the widow at Sarephta called back to life by Elia (1 Kg 17:17–24); and that of Elisha raising the son of the Sunamite woman (2Kg 4:18–37). Tobias also restored sight to his father (Tob 11:7–15).

In the New Testament, miraculous healing of the sick was wrought not only by Jesus but also by his apostles. In the nascent Church, the charism of healing shows itself in the miraculous cures wrought by the apostles. Peter and John cured the lame man who was always laid at the beautiful gate of the temple, at the hour of prayer. (Acts 3:1–10) The Acts also tells of how people carried their sick into the streets on cots and mattresses, hoping that when Peter passed by, his shadow might fall on the sick and make them well.

Healing in the Church was also attested to in the miraculous cures affected by the Saints. Miraculous cures have been viewed by the church as signs of sanctity of the departed heroes to whom they were attributed. Part of the norms for official process of beatification and canonization of the saints as fixed by the Benedict XIV, includes the authentication of cures or miracles attributed to such a saint. "The church, in–fact has recorded and documented many more healings of that kind than healings attributed to the prayers of the living."[567]

Blasiussegen

An eloquent example of such Saint in our day especially here in Deutschland is St. Blasé (Blasiussegen). In Germany Blasiussegen – the annual blessing of throats is a traditional sign of the struggle against illness in the life of the Christian. This blessing is ordinarily given during Mass or a celebration of the word of God on February 3, the memorial of St. Blasé. 1625 Saint Blasé was the bishop of Sebaste in Armenia during the fourth century. Very little is known about his life. According to various accounts he was a physician before becoming a bishop. His cult spread throughout the entire Church in the middle Ages because he was reputed to have miraculously cured a little boy who nearly died because of a fishbone in his throat. From the eighth century he has been invoked on behalf of the sick, especially those afflicted with illnesses of the throat.

---

566 J.J. Pilich, Healing, in "Collegeville Pastoral Dictionary of Biblical Theology", Op. Cit., p.414

567 R. Baldwin, The Healers, Op. Cit., p.151

Another category of miraculous cures is the ones that occur at places of pilgrimages like in the shrines of Saints or places of reservation of their relics. For example, the early Christians valued handkerchiefs and cloths which had been in contact with Saint Paul's skin, and used them as instruments for healing (cf Acts 19–. 12).

In fact the most widely accepted and most popular manifestation of healing in the Catholic Church in modern times are the thousands of cures reported at the grotto of Lourdes, France, visited by millions of Pilgrims since apparitions of the Blessed Virgin Mary were reported there in 1858. Several dozens of the healings have been investigated by medical authorities and authenticated by the church as miraculous.[568]

This form of healing as we have traced through both Testaments of the bible and through the history of the Church is almost often experienced as the supplicants have exhausted all that is possible within human reach and the only thing left for them is a supernatural intervention of God, There is no wonder therefore, the catholic Bishops of Nigeria affirm,

It embraces prayers being offered for the physically and mentally ill, who may or may not have exhausted the medical resources at their disposal. It goes on to embrace exorcism of the spiritually impaired following the guidelines laid down by the competent ecclesiastical authority (Canon 1172). In more recent times however, this form of healing ministry of the Church has assumed a more public profile, particularly within the Catholic Charismatic Renewal.[569]

The practice of praying for recovery from sickness in private or liturgical prayer is found throughout the Christian Centuries. God heals in answer to prayers. Praying for one's own needs or the needs of others can be the beginning of a process of healing or becoming whole from impairment. "Pray all the time, asking for what you need, praying in the spirit on every possible occasion. Never get tired of staying awake to pray for all the saints" (Eph 6 18). Prayer is primarily communion with God. It is not a means of persuading a reluctant God to do what he would not have done. It is neither a means of obtaining what we happen to want nor something, which we turn to as a last resort.

Some ministers get themselves locked into a type of message. 'The only thing we can do is pray'. In so doing, they miss exploring other options or avenues of care.[570]

---

568 R. Baldwin, The Healers, p.60

569 Catholic Bishops' Conference of Nigeria, Guidelines for the healing ministry in the Catholic Church in Nigeria, Op. Cit., pp.6&7

570 L. Thomas & Alkire, Healing as a Parish ministry, Op. Cit., p.42

Such healers, Thomas calls "Religious Mechanics".[571] What the minister should do is to seek healing in prayer because healing sought in prayer is something more profound than mere physical cure.

Ever since God took on a human nature 2000 years ago, He has been calling us – and empowering us – to share in his work. We share in this mission when we become fully present to the Supplicant. In deep worship, God's power flows through us. Healing occurs.[572]

Healing does not occur just by self–minded prayer, filled with the thoughts of our needs, sickness and fears. But if in the midst of prayer, particularly thanksgiving praise, we concentrate upon Jesus Christ who is the healer, we think about his great love for people and how he went about doing good, we are at one with God in the sense of completeness which makes us whole. Here "healing ministry becomes worship which helps one to meet God in the most loving way possible. "Any wonder Turner extensively asserts:

That a congregation meets at all in the name of Christ means that something already has happened. In every service, there is a healing of some kind in someone – it may be a healing of their loneliness as they meet in fellowship with others. It may be a healing of sorrows as through the preaching of the word of God new hope is born in their hearts. It may be the healing of burning memory when they simply receive the gift of God's forgiveness. It may be the healing of an embittered spirit when they, because forgiven, are able to forgive. It may be a healing of some anxiety as they realise that God is great enough to cope with the tiny details of their lives. It may be a healing of self despising when they realize how much they matter to God and to others. It may be a healing of their obsession with money when, through worship, they discover again the things that are of true worth. If these inner fears, conflicts, emotional disturbance and faulty attitudes lies at the root of much illness then we need not be surprised when people say they felt sometimes in a service, a warm glow go through their body and they have found themselves spiritually and physically made whole.[573]

The practice of healing through the centuries was not only found through cures affected through prayers and through pilgrimages to shrines of Saints and places of reservation of their relics. Within the twentieth century, renewal of the healing ministry has been growing rapidly. The power of healing was evident not only in the most popular Ministers but also in vast numbers of the members of the Church. And even before this, the Pentecostals and some related Protestant groups "were experiencing what has been described as a renewal of the various gifts of the Holy Spirit including the gift of healing. No one could deny the heal-

571 L. Thomas & J. Alkire, Healing as a parish ministry, p.42
572 Ibid., p.82
573 J. Turner, The Healing Church, Op. Cit., pp.71&72

ings and miracles that God wrought through some of these Pentecostals and the force with which they preach their convictions. No one either – will deny the force and conviction too, with which they draw the members of the Catholic Church and the mainline Protestant groups such as the Church Missionary society (C.M.S).

Though some of these Pentecostal services are often dominated by flamboyant ministers who showed little regard for the dignity or spiritual value of suffering, implying that suffering was something that need be endured only by those who lack sufficient faith in God's healing power. Most Catholics had little use for that brand of 'faith healing.'[574]

With the appearance of the Charismatic Movement in the Church in the late 1960's and early 1970's, thousands of Catholics all over the world became more interested in the gift of healing. It is on record that

the first time Catholics participated in a big way in the Charismatic revival was in 1967, in a retreat at Duquesne University, in which many participants were said to have experienced speaking in tongues and baptism of the spirit. In 1973 and 1975, a Church official in the person of Joseph Cardinal Suenens attended the conference organised by the Charismatics. The conference of 1975 was greeted by Pope Paul VI.[575]

Within this period, many Catholic prayer groups began to be formed within the Catholic Charismatic renewal, a name which was given "to reflect the fact that baptism in the spirit and Glossolalia are understood within the frame work of the Sacramental life of the church."[576]

Prayer for healing later became a regular part of the Catholic Charismatic prayer meeting. Reports for spiritual and physical healings were frequently given, and individual members of catholic prayer groups began to acquire reputations as healers. With these developments and the recommendation of the second Vatican council, the establishment of healing ministries in the church became common and was widely accepted in the church. The Vatican document stated:

It is not only through the Sacraments and the ministrations of the Church that the holy Spirit makes holy the people, leads them and enriches them with his virtues. Allotting his gifts according as he wills, he distributes also special graces among the faithful of every rank. By these gifts, he makes fit and ready to undertake various tasks and offices for the renewal and building up of the Church ... Whether these Charisms be remarkable or more simple and widely diffused, they are to be received with thanksgiving and consolation since they are fitting and useful for the needs of the Church. Extra–ordinary gifts

574 R. Baldwin, The Healers, pp.148 & 149

575 M.B. Agnew, Charismatic Movement, in "Modern Catholic Encyclopedia", 1995, pp.157 – 159

576 M.B. Agnew, Charismatic Movement, in "Modern Catholic Encycloepedia", p.158

are not to be rashly desired, nor is it from them that the fruits of apostolic labours are to be presumptuously expected. Those who have charge over the Church should judge the genuineness and proper use of these gifts, through their office not indeed to extinguish the spirit but to test all things and hold fast to that which is good (1 Thess 5:12, 19–21).[577]

4.6 The Sacramental Form of Healing

4.6.1 Introduction

Sacraments are simply defined as signs of inward grace. That is to say, as we have been often taught, that the sacraments are channels of God's saving and healing grace.

The grace of God communicated in the celebration of the sacraments is a source of healing for both the body and the spirit.

The seven sacrament of the church and all the other signs and symbols of salvation are directed to the continuing event of salvation history. If we want to penetrate more deeply into the synthesis of proclamation celebration of the mystery of salvation and the healing ministry, we must pay much attention to this vision of sacramentality and faith witness. It is a saddening fact that, during past centuries, Moral theology and Catechisms dealt with the sacraments only after the commandments, and with a very legalistic casuistry. The result was to a great extent, a sterilizing blindness to the healing power of the sacraments and of the Church at large.[578]

We cannot therefore meaningfully discuss the healing ministry of the Church without the sacramental form, which is clearly evident in the anointing of the sick. The Church herself teaches that the other sacraments too, notably the Sacrament of Reconciliation and the Eucharist, have a healing value of their own. The pride of place in this regard is the sacrament of the Holy Eucharist, which the Second Vatican Council described as the "source and summit (fons and culmen) of the whole Christian life".[579]

577 Second Vatican Ecumenical Council, Lumen Gentium, 21 Nov. 1964, No 12
578 B. Haring, Healing and revealing, Op. Cit., pp.5&7
579 L.G. no 11

4.6.2 The Sacrament of Anointing of the Sick

It is part of God's plan that we should combat all illness and should prudently seek the Messing of good health. We will thus be able to play our part in the secular society and in the church.[580]

The rite of the anointing of the sick is one of the Sacraments entrusted to the church by Our Lord Jesus Christ, to bring relief to the sick in mind and body. It is

the prolongation of the concern which as the gospels teil us, Our Lord himself showed for the bodily and spiritual welfare of the sick and which he commended to his followers.[581]

The anointing of the sick first appeared in Christian Tradition in the sixth chapter of the gospel of Mark where Jesus sent out the twelve apostles into the countryside to preach and to heal.

And He called them to him, the twelve, and began to send them out by two and he gave them authority over unclean spirits. ... So they went out and preached that men should repent. And they cast out many demons and anointed with oil many that were sick and healed them (Mk 6: 7–13).

The Sacramental anointing of the Church's ministry to the sick was based on the above passage of Mark and on the epistle of James, where the author urged the elders of the Church to pray for the sick and anoint them with oil in the name of the Lord. (Jm 5: 13–15)

In the early Church, anointing does not appear to be part of the clerical ministry. According to the Apostolic Tradition of Hypolytus, people had and used their own oil, blessed by the bishop at the end of the Eucharistic prayer. The faithful anointed themselves and their neighbours with the oil. The rite of anointing was not restricted to the dying or in danger of death. Rather it was used for all sorts of conditions – blindness, boils, cuts etc.

In the fifth century, Pope Saint Innocent 1, wrote to one of his bishops that when the Christians were sick, they not only had a right to be anointed by the clergy with holy oil, but to use it themselves for anointing in their own need, or the need of members of their households.[582]

Sacramental anointing of the sick with the intention to heal appears to have remained a constant Tradition for the first eight hundred years of the Church. It

580 Hominum Dolores, Introduction to the rite of Anointing and Pastoral care of the sick, Vatican city, 7 Dec. 1972, No. 1

581 Hominum Dolores, Introduction to the rite of Anointing and Pastoral care, No 5

582 R. Baldwin, The Healers, Op. Cit., p.67

was not until the Carolingian reform at the close of the eight century that we found some significant change in the practice of the early church. Quite suddenly within the century, the anointing of the sick that has been repeatedly practiced by the lay people to restore people to health disappeared and was replaced with the "extreme unction", then exclusively celebrated by the clergy alone. "Greater emphasis was placed on the forgiveness of sin and other spiritual effects of the sacrament, and the rite became more associated with the dying."[583] Much of what is done in the ministry of anointing seems to be in fact to the dying instead of the sick. The anointing had become 'extreme', the 'last sacrament' in every sense.

In this system Reconciliation was available only once in a life time" it is not therefore surprising people put off all recourse to anointing until death was certain and imminent. The application of oil very soon developed elaborate variations. The simplest practice was to anoint just the head, representing the whole person, or else extremities, so that the effects could radiate through the whole body.[584]

The sacrament of anointing was so characterized a death–bed reconciliation that one early medieval Spanish treatise on the Sacraments says that,

if the patient should recover after anointing, he may not return to his earlier way of life 'since once anointed, he is dead to the world'. The anointed were considered to be 'consecrated' for death. 'If they recovered, they could not soil occupation (Master Simon), if married, they needed their spouse's permission to be anointed at all. Thank God some rejected these extreme ideas of 'consecration' but the notion of unrepeatability did take root and influence attitudes till this day[585]

Even the great scholastics of the 13th and 14th century such as Albert the Great and Thomas Aquinas elaborated their theology of extreme unction as the sacrament of the dying, a preparation for after–life and for glory. The Council of Trent did not approve the scholastic view, though it however opened a narrower door to the recovery of the discipline. The necessary changes in attitude and practice were very slow. The Theologians, Canonists and Catechisms in the 16th and 17th centuries continued to insist on the danger of death.

Not only until 1753 that Pope Benedict XIV appealed to the ancient 'custom of the Church', to justify a repeated reception of the sacrament, and a couple of years later, he wrote that the sacrament was instituted by the Church as heavenly medicine, not only for

---

583 R. Ryan, Healing and the mission of the Church, in "The Collegeville Pastoral Dictionary of Biblical theology", Op. Cit., p.421

584 C. J. Walsh, The history of the rites, in T.Coyle, (ed), Christian Ministry to the sick, Op. Cit., p.12

585 Ibid., p.13

the salvation of the soul but for the health of the body and should therefore be given to people, at a time when they are conscious and aware of what they are doing.[586]

In spite of all the efforts, people continued to speak of the anointing as the 'last rites' or 'last sacraments' even till the eve of the assembly of the second Vatican council in 1961.

On the reformation of the ritual for anointing the sick, the fathers of the Second Vatican Council said,

Extreme unction which may also and more properly be called 'anointing the sick' is not a sacrament for those only who are at the point of death. Hence as soon as any one of the faithful begins to be in danger of death from sickness or old age, the fitting time for that person to receive this sacrament has certainly already arrived.[587]

This marked a turning point in the history of the rite of anointing. The anointing is no longer to be referred to as the "last anointing" or "extreme unction". It is a sacrament of the church for any seriously sick person and not for the dying. The new name 'anointing of the sick', means exactly what it says, and it has developed very strong overtones of healing in keeping with the practice of the early Church as interpreted in the epistle of James (cf Jm 5:13).

Administered to any Christian who is in a life threatening condition this sacrament is a remedy for the body and spirit, relief and strength for the patient in his corporeal–spiritual integrity, casting light on the mystery of suffering and death and bringing a hope which opens the human present to the future of God.[588]

Hence the anointing of the sick helps the Christian to combat both physical and spiritual sickness.

It should be no surprise to us, therefore, when we find that in the prayers and texts of the rite of anointing, there is not a single reference to death. On the contrary, the whole thrust of the rite is that the sick person should struggle against the sickness and desire the blessing of good health once again. This is expressed best of all perhaps in one of the blessings of the oil, that the sick person will be freed from pain and illness and made well again in body, mind and spirit.[589]

586 Ex quo Primum 1756, in T.Coyle, ed, Christian Ministry to the sick, Op. Cit., p.15

587 Sacro Sanctum Concilium, No. 73

588 Pontifical Council for Pastoral Assistance, Charter for Healthcare workers, St. Paul's, Boston, 1994, p.96

589 A.Boylon, The new rite of anointing and Viaticum, in T. Coyle, ed, "Christian Ministry to the sick", Op. Cit., p.34

The whole person receives help from it for his salvation; he feels strengthened in his trust in God and he receives reinforcement against the temptations of the devil and the fear of death.[590]

Anybody who is seriously sick is encouraged to receive the sacrament of anointing. The effect of the sacrament is oriented towards the whole health of the person towards saving him and raising him up as seen in the prayer of the rite of anointing. "May the Lord in his mercy save you and raise you up."[591] The prayer also brings out the communal aspect of the celebration, which we know is strongly emphasized by the biblical text of James, "Is any sick among you? Let him call for the elders of the Church and let them pray over him. ... the prayer of faith will save the sick man and the Lord will raise him up" (Jm 5:14–15). The prayer of faith in this rite involves not only just the prayer of the priest visiting the sick person, but the prayer of all the faithful people around the sick. But in some places in the Church today, you notice that the communal sense of the anointing has not yet been properly understood. Hence we note that,

The full meaning of the sacrament would be expressed if the sick person being visited is fully conscious and still in a condition to take part in the prayers and if friends and family members are around to join in the prayers. Very often, you notice that in some hospitals, the nurses ask the relations of the sick to go out of the ward when the priest is coming– to visit the sick person. Sometimes they get the curtains drawn round the bed of the sick. That is not the best approach. It is good to have somebody friendly around the sick, at least to sit beside, hold his hand and pray with him while he suffers the agony of his sickness.[592]

In many places in the church however, the loving and healing celebration of the sacrament of anointing is not only celebrated communally but also celebrated sometimes within the context of the Eucharistic celebration, This is liturgically sound and recommended.

This should be done from time to time. The sacrament will more often be a family celebration when the sacraments are given to bed–ridden or dying persons, though even on these occasions the basic community may be represented. Whether they are sick or healthy, Christians should be carefully prepared to participate in the celebration of the

590 Congregation for Divine Worship, Sacrament of Anointing and Pastoral care of the sick, Nov. 17, 1972, No 6, Vatican Polyglot Press, 1972, p.81

591 Cf. Ritual for sacrament of anointing of the sick.

592 M.C. Obiagwu, Moral/Spritual Care of the terminally Sick Person, a paper presented at a conference organised as part of the celebration of the third World day of the sick, Onitsha, 6th Feb. 1995, p.12

sacrament, either as sick recipients of the sacrament or as healthy co–organisers, giving prayerful expression to their compassion and concern.[593]

By this participation in the communal celebration of the anointing, a good number of the Christ's faithful share in the healing ministry of Jesus.

4.6.3 The Sacrament of the Holy Eucharist

We have earlier seen that the sacraments are the channels of God's saving and healing grace and that the grace of Christ communicated in the celebration of the sacraments is a source of healing for the body and spirit. The Holy Eucharist being the source and the summit of the whole Christian life is,

the central and most fruitful sacrament of the healing grace of God, a principal sign of 'forgiveness of sins', of healing hurt memories, a source of peace and an energizing resource for the peace mission of all Christians.[594]

The other sacraments as well as every ministry of the Church are linked with the Holy Eucharist and are directed towards it, for the Eucharist contains the Church's entire spiritual wealth, Christ himself, who is our Passover and living bread. The Eucharistic worship itself is directed towards God the father, through Jesus Christ in the Holy spirit who "loved the world so much that he gave up his only son, so that everyone who believes in him may not be lost but may have life eternal."(Jn 3:16)

On the night in which he was betrayed, Jesus instituted the Eucharistic sacrifice of his body and blood in order to perpetuate the sacrifice of the cross through out the centuries and so to entrust to his beloved Spouse, the Church, a memorial of his death and resurrection, a sacrament of love, a sign of unity, a bond of charity, a paschal banquet in which Christ is consumed, the mind is filled with grace, and a pledge of future glory is given to us.[595]

"The Eucharistic bread and wine are material things but they are not raw materials. They are offerings, which earth has given and human hands have made."[596] They represent human work and productivity and all concerns, sufferings achievements and failures that people bring when they offer themselves at

---

593 A. Shorter, Jesus and the Witch Doctor: An approach to healing and wholeness, London New York, 1985, p.223

594 B. Haring, Healing and Revealing, Op.Cit., p.58

595 Second Vatican Council, The Constitution on the sacred Liturgy, No. 47

596 Cf. Offertory Prayer, Order of the Mass

the Eucharistic celebrations. In the Eucharistic celebration are prayers and responses for mercy and forgiveness, hymns and prayers of praise and thanksgiving, prayers of intercession and petition, time for silent adoration and contemplation. All these prayers and responses make the Eucharistic celebration a worship. And we know that healing comes within the realm of worship. Also in the Eucharistic Liturgy of the Word, listening meditatively to the word of God opens our minds and hearts to the healing which the Eucharist offers. Here we remember once again the words of the Centurion, "Say the word and I shall be healed".[597] It is therefore fitting that all ministers of the Church should carry out their ministry of healing within the context of the Eucharistic worship, for we pray for healing in many parts of the Eucharistic celebration. If we examine the post communion prayers of the Roman Missal, we find out that several of the prayers explicitly envisage health of mind and body.

> *They address Jesus as the author of all healing. They acclaim the body of Christ as a food 'which can heal forever'. They ask that it may 'make them well' or 'restore their health' and that it may 'turn our anxiety for them into joy'.*[598]

The prayer before Holy Communion explains this fact better. It shows that none is worthy or healthy enough to partake of that meal. Hence the Communion prayer, "Lord I am not worthy to receive you but say the word and I shall be healed."[599]

4.6.4 The Sacrament of Reconciliation

When Jesus appeared to his disciples after his resurrection, he breathed on them, and said, "Receive the Holy Spirit. For those whose sins you forgive, they are forgiven; for those whose sins you retain, they are retained" (Jn 20:22–23). By the virtue of the above command of Jesus Christ, the Church has the power to forgive sins and erase people's faults. This as it were became the Lord's resurrection gift to His Church. This Lord's resurrection gift to the Church, namely the power to forgive sins through the Holy Spirit remains with the church specifically in the sacrament of reconciliation. The practice of one receiving reconciliation with God through 'going to confession', an experience that brings great peace to the soul is one of the deepest desires of the sinful heart and a peculiar characteristic of the Catholic Church.

---

597 Cf. Communion prayer of the Mass.
598 A. Shorter, Jesus and the Witch doctor, Op. Cit., p.205
599 Cf. Communion prayer of the Mass.

The biblical concept of peace is amazingly comprehensive. It includes salvation, wholeness, integrity, healthy and healing inter–personal relationships, cultural, economical and social relationships and transformations which serve the cause of peace and of wholeness and integrity.[600]

God's gift of peace is lost through serious sin. In the sacrament of reconciliation, believers celebrate the healing power of Christ's forgiveness. Those who are alienated from God, others and themselves through sin are enabled to know pardon and peace offered them by the risen Christ and be reconciled to both God and to the Christian community. This experience of being forgiven in the confession gives peace to the soul and brings healing not only to the soul but also to the body. According to A. Shorter,

this unburdening of oneself to another in confession is immensely strengthening and healing. Not only are the individual sinners healed but also the wounds which their sins have inflicted on the society and their contribution to the phenomenon of social sin.[601]

Jesus himself linked the Absolution of sin with the physical healing of the sick, as is shown in the healing of the Paralytic who was lowered down to him through the roof of the house. "But that you may know that the son of man has authority to forgive sins while on earth, he said to the man who was paralysed, I say to you, rise, take up your bed and go home"(Lk 5:24). It is obvious that we have not realised the intensity of healing that flows from this sacrament of reconciliation, hence we have not focused on the healing power of this sacrament. This, Buckley says, "is because of the impersonal nature in which this sacrament is administered and because it deals mainly with the matters of the soul and not with the healing of the whole person."[602] He therefore emphasizes,

It is the whole person who is reconciled and healed through this sacrament. Whenever in our healing services we emphasize the healing needed for conversion, it is quite amazing to discover how many people who wish to receive the sacrament of reconciliation in order to start a 'new life' or have a fresh beginning.[603]

While emphasizing the usefulness and necessity of this sacrament, the Vatican Council in turn says,

The wounds inflicted by sins on the individual and the community are many and varied. In the same way, the remedies offered by penance are varied. Those who depart from

600 B. Haring, in J. McManus, Healing in the spirit, Op. Cit., p.117
601 A. Shorter, Jesus and the Witch Doctor, Op. Cit. p.209
602 M. Buckley, His Healing Touch, p.207
603 Ibid., p.207

the fellowship of the love of God through grave sin are recalled through the sacrament of Penance to life which they had lost.[604]

We recognize two effects of sin: sin as an offence against God, causing an alienation between God and self – and the wound of sin that is the inner hurt caused in a person by the sinful actions or words. The sin itself will be manifested in a cold, deliberate malicious act of one kind or another –, the wound of sin will reveal itself through some kind of reaction. Just as a person in pain may cry out, so a person with the wound of sin may very well 'strike out'. For the sin itself we need the Lord's healing. Both are signified in the words of Absolution: 'Through the ministry of the Church, May God give you pardon and peace' Pardon is for the sin, and peace is for the wound of sin."[605]

In this chapter, we discussed extensively the healing ministry of Jesus and how the church in her tradition carried this noble intention of Christ to the four corners of the earth; hence the healing tradition of the church vis–à–vis her concern and care for the sick and the suffering. The next section shall take care of the basis and challenges for an inculturated pastoral care of the sick and the healing ministry in Igboland.

604 The Second Vatican Document, Misericordiam Suam, 7 Feb., 1974, 11, 7.
605 J.McManus, Healing in the Spirit, Op. Cit., pp.117 – 118

5. Chapter Five – Incultaration of Healing

5.1 Basis and Challenges for an Inculturated Pastoral Care for the Sick and the Healing Ministry in Igbo Land

5.1.0 Introductory Remarks

There is no doubt that the Catholic prayer–healing ministry, as part and parcel of the Church's ministry in the Contemporary Igbo society has some pastoral contributions to make to Christianity in the area and to the society in general. We know too that it has also generated a lot of anxieties, tensions and excitements for the Church to contend with. The Hierarchy, the Clergy and the Lay Faithful are all concerned, and all hands are on deck to welcome the contributions and proffer responses to the challenges.

The Church in Igboland understands well that the Igbo is naturally religious and very eager to get to the Supernatural and therefore, he is easily attracted to whatever seems to be providing a response to this quest of his. She knows too, that, the traditional religious nature of the Igbo, such as his belief in the Supreme Being, his attitude to Sacrifice and prayer and some of his natural qualities provided a fertile soil for the implantation of the Christian religion in the area. He has also a strong attachment to any course that can guarantee his security and the sense of the sacred. The sense of the sacred so much sustained his firmness in his traditional religion. He believes so much he is protected by the gods and the ancestors from the attacks of the evil spirits, so he makes recourse to the traditional oracles and the traditional medicine men and the diviners. However, we saw in our study of the Anthropological component of the Care of the sick, that in as much as he goes to the 'dibia' for the care of his various sicknesses, he still knows that God is the ultimate healer.

With the advent of Christianity in the area, the Igbo resorted very much to the Church to fulfil these needs and aspirations. Though the structure and the practices of the established Churches seem not to have adequately met the needs. The monotony and formality in the celebration of the liturgy of the Church do not animate the Igbo enough.

> *Africans especially the young people love active participation in Worship and prayers, singing and body movement. They like the use of instruments at worship and free*

atmosphere in which people can worship according to the prompting of the Holy Spirit.[606]

So the Igbo like all the other Africans love sensational participation and celebration in worship that can animate the spirit in him. One can then understand why in spite of the fact that a good percentage of the Ibos have professed Christianity, some still find succour outside the Church. Many still turn back to the traditional religion and practices, a lot of which practices are sensational and overtly psychological and appeal to the Igbo soul. Some believe strongly in the use of charms and amulets to solve their many problems of life. The same is also observed of many African Christians.

Hence one Zairean poet depicts the African Christians in these phrases:

OH UNHAPPY CHRISTIAN
MASS IN THE MORNING
WITCH DOCTOR IN THE EVENING
AMULET IN THE POCKET
SCAPULAR AROUND THE NECK[607]

However, today the situation is changing rapidly. The Igbo Christian prefers to take succour in the prayer/healing ministry. The healing ministry though loaded with its own challenges and abuses seems to be providing answers to some of these quests, orthodoxly or otherwise to the teaching authority of the Church. Acknowledging the contributions of the healing ministry so far, Chris U. Manus has this to say,

Nigeria Faith healers and miracle workers have become agents of the mission of Christ who came to liberate oppressed humanity by their super human feats in arresting all manners of afflictions and by their pacification of all kinds of Spiritual torments, they appeal to the common folks and the cream of the society.[608]

Having gone so much in introducing the Pastoral Contributions of the healing ministry in Igbo society, we shall have a look at some positive aspects of the healing ministry before we get into exploring the various abuses and their implied challenges to the Church in Igbo land.

606 N.Ndiokwere, The African Church Today and Tomorrow, Vol.1,Op.Cit., p.41
607 Cf. N. Ndiokwere, The African Church today and Tomorrow, Vol. 1, Op.Cit., p.53
608 Chris. U. Manus, Miracle Workers/Healers as divine men: their role in Nigerian Church and Society, Asian Journal of Theology, Vol. 3, No.2, p.658

5.2 Positive Contributions of the Healing Ministry

5.2.1 Inculturation

One of the major contributions of the healing ministry in the Church in Igbo society of Nigeria is its effort to inculturation. As says M. Dhavamony,

> *Inculturation is a theological term currently used both by the Magisterium and by the theologians in order to take seriously the identity and internal coherence of the Christian faith and of other cultures and religions in the evangelising mission of the Church. The process of inculturation realised on the model of the redemptive incarnation, situates Christianity as an essentially sacramental reality at the heart of man and his culture.*[609]

The Igbo is fundamentally and deeply a religious being (Homo Religiosus). The Igbo traditional religion as we have earlier seen cannot in earnest be separated from the culture of the people. We need therefore a good knowledge of the term culture to have clear approach and understanding of inculturation and its practice in the context of the healing ministry in Igbo society of Nigeria.

Culture, we know, is part of human phenomenon, which with its concomitant world view, arises out of human efforts to come to terms with their environment – social, religious, moral, political and so on. The term has several meanings and usages. It can be defined as "that complex whole which includes knowledge, belief, art, morals, law, custom and any other capabilities and habits acquired by man as a member of society".[610] According to Julian Saldanha,

> *Culture designates the peculiar manner of behaving of a particular community or social group, its typical way of thinking and judging, of feeling and of perceiving itself and others: every group has its attitudes and scale of values.*[611]

These attitudes and values, rich in their contents, constitute their meanings and views of the world, and make up ideal and behavioural pattern or the way of life of a group of people. It is a mirror through which a living human society sees its experiences from different spheres of life. The most important element being the invisible, underlying system of values, meanings and view of the world (Weltanschauung). The vehicles of this invisible element in a culture are manifold: symbols, rituals, art, literature, philosophy and all that is comprised under the rubric of "oral culture" (proverbs, riddles, songs, stories, myths legends, epic

---

609 M. Dhavamony, Christian Theology of Inculturation, Editrice Pontificia Universita Gregoriana, Roma, 1997, p.89.

610 E.B. Taylor, Primitive Culture, 1, London, 1913, p.1, in M. Dhavamony, Christian Theology of Inculturation, Roma, 1997, p.41

611 J.Saldanha, Inculturation, St. Paul's Publication, Bandra, Mumbai, 1997, p.11

poems and ballads). All this is shared with a group, so that culture is essentially communitarian.[612]

The term culture therefore embraces much. For A. Shorter,

> *It embraces the whole context of life and is as relevant to modernity and modern problems, as it is to traditional beliefs and values... Culture is a mental world, a web of meanings clothed in images and behavioural norms. It is a pattern of human thought and behaviour. It is a prism through which a human society views the whole of its experience, domestic, political, social, economic, religious. Culture is learned by the human being in infancy and developed throughout life. It enables the individual to relate cognitively, emotionally and behaviourally to the world and to communicate this understanding to others. It gives identity to groups of individuals; Culture is therefore an essential aspect of the human phenomenon, indeed a human right.*[613]

No wonder therefore, the Vatican Document observes that "Only through culture can human beings achieve true and full humanity that is through the cultivation of the goods and values of nature".[614]

Igbo culture as we have earlier seen in this work is the pivotal point of the people's life and it is in a dynamic process of growth. This is because of its contact with other cultures. Cultures borrow from one another and that makes them grow and alive. The Christian religious culture has deeply affected Igbo traditional religion and culture. You cannot strictly speaking, dissociate Igbo religion from the culture since it is clear that the Igbo is deeply a religious being and religion permeates every aspect of his life. Religion occupies a central position in his social and cultural life such that it can be seen when he eats and drinks, as he baths and dresses, in the way he rules and settles cases and in marriages and marriage ceremonies. In fact his religion is his life and it is his culture.

Inculturation as we know it today is a household word in the Church. It is also a term officially introduced by the Magisterium of the Universal Church only in the late seventies. "After its use by the thirty – Second General Congregation of the Jesuits (1974 – 1975) and the 1977 Synod of Bishops, it has found its way into every day language, where it is now an accepted term"[615]

---

612 J.Saldanha, Inculturaion, Op. Cit., p.12

613 A.Shorter, Christianity and the African Imagination: After the African Synod. Resources for Inculturation, Nairobi: Pauline Publications, 1996, p.16, in E. Hillman, the Gospel as Good News for African Cultures, C U E A Publication, Nairobi, Kenya, 1999, p.130

614 G.S. no.53

615 Metena M'nteba, Inculturation in the 'Third Church': God's Pentecost or Cultural Revenge?, in G. Alberigo and A.N. Mushete, eds, Concilium, Towards the African Synod, SCM Press, London, 1991, p.129

"Inculturation" appeared for the first time in an official Church document in the "Message to the People of God" delivered by the Synod of Bishops of 1977. The message refers to Catechesis as an "instrument of Inculturation". Pope John Paul II has since used the word several times, for example in his apostolic exhortations on Catechesis (1979) and on the Christian family (1981).[616]

Today, much is being said about inculturation of the gospel and various aspects of evangelisation to the way and life of the various people within which the Church is established.

In order that a people be Christian, it is necessary that Christianity becomes incarnate in its culture, and as such, given the universal exigency of the Church it is necessary that Christianity be inserted in all cultures of humanity.[617]

Many terms however have been originally used to designate the term inculturation such as adaptation, accommodation, indigenisation, acculturation etc. So Inculturation is still a new term in the Christian Theology and is still under development. It is not just a technique of evangelisation or a tactic of communications. It "is popularly described in Roman Catholic official and non official documents as the incarnation of the Christian message in cultures."[618] The term signifies "planting the seed of the faith in a culture and allowing it to blossom to express itself according to the resources and genius of that culture"[619] It can also be understood as

an approach in mission evangelisation and involves evangelising a culture from within, that is to say proclaiming the Good News to people from within the perspective of their culture.[620]

Speaking on Catechesis and Inculturation in the Synod of Catechesis in October 1977, Pedro Arrupe observes,

Inculturation is a solution to the problem of real influence of faith on culture. The absence of inculturation is one of the main obstacles to evangelisation. Catechesis presupposes the inculturation of the faith. The theological principle is that Christ is the one and only Saviour and saves only what he assumes to himself. Hence Christ must assume his body (Church) all cultures, purifying them and removing everything which is contrary to

616 J.Saldanha, The teaching of John Paul II on Evangelisation, IMR, 1985, No. 4, pp.358–369, in J.Saldanha, Inculturation, Op.Cit., p.15

617 M.Dhavamony, Christian Theology of Inculturaion, Op.Cit., p.90

618 E.E.Uzukwu, A listening Church: Autonomy and Communion in African Churches, Orbis Book, Mary Knoll, New York, 1996, p.6

619 Y.Congar, Christianisme come foi et come Culture, Roma, 1976, in M. Dhavamony, Chrisstian Theology of Inculturation, Rome, 1997, p.91

620 J.Ukpong, Christology and Inculturation: A New Testament perspective, in R. Gibellini (ed) Paths of African Theology, SCM Press, London, 1994, p.40

his spirit, thus saving them without destroying them. It means faith reaching man in his most profound experience of life, even to the extent of influencing his way of thinking, feeling and acting under the inspiration of the spirit of God. It makes possible the widespread contribution of all cultural values in the service of the Gospel. Inculturation leads to a continued sharing between the Word of God and the rich varieties of human expressions.[621]

Inculturation therefore involves a dialogue between culture and the Gospel. Dialogue is a conversation, a discussion, a give and take between two or more persons or issues. It involves a two–way process and therefore, so is inculturation. Little wonder John Paul II says that,

Inculturation includes two dimensions: on the one hand, the ultimate transformation of authentic cultural values through their integration in Christianity, and on the other hand, the insertion of Christianity in the various human cultures.[622]

Three things characterize this approach in Christian mission. First is the utilization of the resources of the culture being evangelised in expressing the Christian faith. Second is that the Good News of Jesus is pronounced to challenge and animate the culture. Third is that all this is done from the perspective of the culture and through the agency of an insider or insiders in the culture.[623]

This therefore goes to say that inculturation has to deal with the expression of the Christian message in its various aspects to the Christians of a particular area or cultural ambient taking into consideration the culturally rhythmical pattern of the entire life of the people. Hence,

When the Church enters into contract with cultures, she must welcome what is compatible in these traditions in order to bring the riches of Christ to them and to be enriched by the wisdom of the nations.[624]

This approach to the gospel message is meant to help the Good News permeate the life of a particular people and bear the desired fruit of salvation.

---

621 P. Arrupe, Other Apostolates Today, Selected letters and addresses III, Gujarat Sahitya, Prakash, Anand, 1981, in M. Dhavamony, Christian Theology of Inculturation, p.91

622 John Paul II, Encylical Letter, Redemptoris Missio, (hereafter as R.M.), 7 December, 1990, 52 AAS 83 (1991), p.229

623 J.Ukpong, Christology and Inculturation: A New Testament perspective, in R. Gibellini, Op. Cit., p.41

624 R.M. No.54

The healing ministry of the Church in Igbo society of Nigeria no doubt, through the structure and mode of operation of the ministry has in one way or another helped in inculturation in Igboland. One prominent area is in the liturgy of the Mass particularly in the format of the celebration of Mass for the sick and needy or what some call "Hẹaling Mass". The liturgy of the Mass is so well adapted to suit the religious quest of the Igbo. Talking on the inculturation of the Igbo liturgy, E. Uzukwu observes,

Despite the room for adaptation of the Roman Liturgy to local situations, (SC 37–38), very little has been done apart from translating latin liturgical texts and permitting dancing during the offertory procession. Among the predominantly Roman Catholic Igbo, the liturgical texts have not been completely translated, gestural behaviours such as clapping or dancing are unknown in the Eucharistic liturgy except during special fund raising masses such as harvest festivals and bazaars. However popular Charismatic movements and healing ministries are gradually introducing into the Roman Catholic Church symbolic objects and gestures that characterise the spiritual Churches.[625]

Today in Igbo society of Nigeria, the liturgy of the Mass is celebrated in almost all the parishes in pomp and ceremony. The Mass is sung in the local language of the people from the beginning to the end accompanied by locally made musical instruments. Hymns are locally composed expressing the people's faith and sentiments. The local music invariably attracts a lot of people to the Church particularly the youth. A lot of people who would not have ordinarily attended the Sunday Masses now attend the celebrations to listen to the music and also to dance especially during the offertory procession. The situation is such that some people visit the Altar premises for offertory up to two or three times on a Sunday dancing, clapping and singing praises to God. So here is one area where the healing ministry has very much helped in bringing the ministry of Jesus home to the Igbo people. Beating of drums within Mass and the subsequent dancing and clapping is no more only during festivals and offertory but today it constitutes a vital part of the Eucharistic celebration from the introductory part to the end of the Mass. Thanks to the Charismatic Renewal and the healing/prayer ministries.

Also the abundant use of holy water during the celebration of masses particularly on Sundays and Saturdays' blessing of articles and children in the parishes is a normal and regular practice in the Church today. It is no more a reserve of any Pentecostal or the independent Churches or the named "Uka mmili" (the Water Churches) or the "Uka akura aka" (the clapping Churches), but also of the Catholics. Some charismatic and ecstatic experiences are also observed within the celebrations. Today while people dance bringing their offering during offer-

625 E. Uzukwu, Inculturation and Liturgy (Eucharist), in R. Gibellini (ed), Paths of African Theology, Op. Cit., p.95.

tory, the average Igbo Catholic like to be bathed with holy water no matter how expensive the clothes he or she is putting on. He is said to believe that the Holy water poured on him takes control of all his problems and drives away all evil spirits. But not only this. In Igbo Tradition and culture, it is believed that rain or water brings good tidings. The Igbo believes that any journey preceded or interrupted by rain is a successful one 'ije mmili'. Rain is also said to bring fertility to the earth. One will not therefore be surprised why the Igbo Christian gets home today satisfied, with his dress soaked in water after Mass.

The healing ministry has also taught the people how to pray better and how to pray for themselves without waiting for the priests to lead them or to pray for them. In the liturgy of the Mass today, particularly during the prayer of the faithful, one notices a marked difference in the prayers, compared with what used to be in the past years. During the prayer of the faithful, the faithful render beautiful spontaneous and inspiring prayers garnished with beautiful proverbs and idiomatic expressions. One really sees a good number of the faithful taken up in the prayers. They are no more ashamed to participate fully in the liturgical celebrations. A good organised healing ministry has been known to instruct the faithful on the importance of prayers and how to say the prayers well and by themselves.

5.2.2 Strengthening of the people' faith and Confidence in God

It appears that the African converts to Christianity operate on a conceptual framework, very different from that of their pastors and theologians. This is a great challenge for the Church, calling for re–evangelisation and a critical examination of the content and method of Catholic evangelism in Africa.[626]

This call for an examination of the content and method of evangelising the African Catholics is not only necessary but also urgent. And in a particular sense, this has a more urgent call in Igbo society of Nigeria. Thanks to the emergence of the healing ministry, which is bent towards providing responses to this call if the boat is well steered by the sailors. Hence Don Dei Ibekwem in his usual manner remarks,

626 G.Enusani, Healing and Deliverande ministry: What is really happeing?, Seminar Paper on Healing ministry, Emene, Enugu, 11th – 14th Febrary, 1992, p.2

If the true shepherd does not tend the flock the wrong ones or even the wolf may devour the flock what will I tell God? You see women Catholic and non Catholic healing and blessing water, oil, drugs, food etc –, with some apparent efficacy.[627]

The prayer–healing session is one avenue that has contributed and is still contributing in the building and solidification of the faith of many Igbo Catholics. Many Catholic Christians, who left the church to one hand clapping Church or the other, are coming back every day, with the emergence of the healing ministry in the Catholic Church. People using charms and other types of magical powers reject them for a true faith and trust in Christ Jesus. We remember that, the first Catholic healing ministry in Igbo society was conducted as a means of controlling Catholics who were drifting away to the independent churches and prayer centres. Since then, the ministry has continued to strengthen the faith of the Christians who frequent it. It has made not only the Christians to seek holiness but also the ministers. The idea of Christians visiting the traditional oracles and shrines under the cover of darkness in search of security and health has been minimised and replaced with visits to healing and prayer centres. Even non–Christians and non–Catholics frequent the Catholic healing ministries today to seek answers to their misfortunes and problems. Though the question of incessant presence of evil spirits and their malevolent activities seem to be over–exaggerated by some of the Christians who visit the healing centres.

Jesus came to free mankind from fear both real and imaginary, because he came to give life in abundance. His healing activities began with the casting out of the evil spirits, so one does not doubt the existence of evil spirits in the world. The prayers of deliverance and healing of the Church's rituals show that there are powers of the devil that should be attacked and subdued, but only in the name of Jesus. There is therefore no known factor that places the people nearer to God and to the Church than a healing/prayer session well organised. Hence most of the people who attend organised prayer sessions behave well and practise their faith well, not minding the rotes of the fanatics and over–enthusiastic ones among them. The pastoral advantages of a well–organised prayer session cannot be over–emphasised. Hence we can affirm that,

There is no more willing audience than the group gathered for healing prayers described above. The consequent growth in their faith is strikingly shown in the way they behave ... Action usually follows knowledge. They now know more and better, and so they relate better in life. One person's problem is the problem of all; the joy of one is that of all. The terms "Brother" and "Sister" come to them spontaneously for that is what they

627 Don Die Ibekwem, Testimony, Seminar Paper on Healing Ministry, Emene, Enugu, 11th – 14th Februar, 1992, p.1.

are to themselves and to others...One is very much reminded of the life of the early Christians.[628]

5.3 Some Pastoral Abuses in the Healing Ministry

5.3.0 The Situation

From our study so far, it is clear that the healing ministry of Jesus Christ has come to stay in Igbo society of Nigeria. It is also clear that the healing ministry has added a new vigour to the work of evangelisation in the area. Many who were lured away from the Church in one way or the other are being brought back, and new converts are made to the Catholic Church. There are countless good aspects of the prayer/healing ministry but the ministry however has many abuses and challenges for the Catholic Church in Igbo society to look into. Most of the abuses are not in the ministry 'per se' but the manner and mode of operation of the ministry by some ministers, particularly the nature of promises made by the ministers and the rites performed in some of the Catholic prayer ministries. Some of the ministers do a lot of things that have raised some serious questions unfamiliar to the traditional teaching and beliefs of the Church, all in the name of the healing ministry. Some of the priest–healers are even competing with the traditional medicine men and healers in some of their methods of healing. Some other Catholic healers and priests have taken completely after the pastors of the Pentecostal and independent Churches. The Catholic Church in Igboland is therefore concerned about these aberrations and abuses inherent in the loving ministry of the Church.

We have mentioned earlier that what makes the average Igbo to frequent many of these healing/prayer centres are various misfortunes and problems of life and the search for security.

An average Nigerian Christian wants an immediate positive response from God to take away misfortunes. A quick and instant recovery indicates for him the presence of God. Where and when this instant result is delayed, the Christian God is pronounced impotent and no right thinking fellow can be reckless to the point of hanging unto such a

628 G.Ikeobi, Catholic Response to the Challenge of Prayer Houses: The origin of Tuesday Prayer in Onitsha, in V.A. Nwosu, "The Catholic Church in Onitsha, people, places, and events (1885 – 1985), pp.273&274

useless God. Exploiting this sentiment, some of our priests create the impression that nobody comes to them without instant positive answer to his problems.[629]

The above citation so to say gives the basis and foundation of most of the abuses found in the healing ministry in Igbo society. Some of the healing ministers create the impression that a child of God is not supposed to suffer hardship of any type, such as sickness, poverty, lack of issues, backwardness in the business world, delay in marriage, to mention but a few. And any thing contrary to this, the client is declared to be without faith. Some of these ideas given to the Christians by the healers push some of the healing ministers to use both orthodox and unorthodox means and practices to obtain their promises and solutions to different kinds of misfortunes, thereby confusing the simple Christians who are very often vulnerable in their faith. Some of the people are very much at home with anything said or done that brings them nearer to the Igbo traditional religious approach rejected by Christianity. And unfortunately too, a good number are confused into believing that these priests that provide them with the seemingly new and different approach to Christianity are the authentic pastors of the people. What a misconception! Hence Osy Anike observes,

It is interesting to see how our Christians rush to these healing homes with the same vigour with which they rushed to the traditional medicine men and how they change from one healing home to another which, in their reckoning, is more "result oriented". This mad rush has so much blind folded them to such an extent that they can hardly discern between genuine miracle and magic. A quick examination of some of the nefarious and dubious activities going in some healing homes will cast doubts on the genuineness of some of the healing centres.[630]

Some of the unorthodox and unfamiliar doctrines and practices found within some of the prayer/healing ministries include, less recognition of suffering as part of Christian life, demanding heavy amount of money for Mass or Consultation, Pride and Intransigence on the part of some of the ministers, exclusive claim of the Holy spirit by members, de–emphasis of the role of medicine and medical care, use of Indian incense, inappropriate use of the sacramentals such as burying of the crucifixes on the ground as charms and other practices and methods of healing contrary to the Church's teaching.

---

629 G.Ikeobi, Priests, Healing and Prayer ministry, in A.N.O Ekwunife & co (eds), "The Renewal of Christian life and Ministry: The Nigerian experience". Snaap Press, Enugu. 1995, p.217

630 Osy Anike, Miracle or Magic?, Misunderstanding and Aberration in the healing ministries, in "Torch Magazine", Enugu, April–June 1993, p.38

5.3.1 Less recognition of suffering as part of Christian life

Healing is as essential to the Christian gospel as much as suffering is, to the same gospel. The gospel preached by Jesus Christ looks on sickness as an evil to be eradicated especially when it damages the quality of life, but that does not endorse the attitude that neglects suffering or omits the cross of Christ. That is to say that the gospel does not approve of any attitudes that overemphasise the importance of health and healing, nor does it exaggerate in any way the spiritual importance of suffering. Christians have to understand the meaning of suffering in Christian life and the acceptance of the salvific value of suffering in the journey of Christian faith. But very often some healing ministers and attendants of the healing ministries tend to forget this basic fact of Christian life in their excessive desire to get rid of discomfort and acquire good health and other good things of life. Such people look upon all crosses and sufferings of life as evils that must be avoided at all costs. This is a wrong attitude to the Christian life of suffering and the Christian theology of the cross. One notices today, a good number of our Christians changing from one priest–healer to another in a bid to wipe away all problems of life. And some of our priest healers give the impression that attending their particular prayer session or ministry signifies an end to all earthly misfortunes and discomforts, instead of educating the people, "to avoid a one dimensional conception of prayer– ministry namely, solely as a place where the impossible becomes possible, where miracles are performed and cures take place."[631] It is not possible to avoid crosses, pains and suffering in the Christian life as in ordinary life.

In Christianity, crosses and trials in life are not absolute evils but can lead one to God with right understanding and attitude towards them. Suffering in Christianity teaches salutary lessons, and in some way, not always known to us, manifests God's glory.[632]

Our priests and theologians need to know this and always have it behind their skulls while they minister to the people of God. Priest healers should centre their Catechesis on the saving power of the cross by exposing the theology of the cross to their adherents.

Suffering is the badge of our race. It is everywhere and seems indeed to belong to the very texture of the human project. Not to know this and the inability

631 B.C.Okolo, Healing ministry in the Nigeria Church:Dangers next door, in "B.T.S", Op. Cit., pp.89–90

632 Ibid.,p.90

and unwillingness to accept this datum of the cumulative experience of our human history results in added suffering.[633]

Jesus' own life was a most perfect example. He is the servant of Yahweh predestined to suffer and die. He rejected the Devil's plea to work a miracle for his own advantage and comfort. (Lk. 4:1–13; Mtt 4:1–11; Mk 1:12–13) He made the prophecy of his passion himself, about how he will be mocked and scourged unto death. (Mtt 20:17–19; Mk 10:28–30; Lk 18:31–34) He allowed himself to be mocked and beaten by the Jews, heaping insults on him. (Lk 22:63–65; Mtt 26: 67–68; Mk 14: 65) And instead of evading all these sufferings by using his position as the Son of God, he gave up himself to death, death on the cross, in a place called the skull. (Lk 23:33–34; Mtt 27: 35–38; Mk 15: 24–28; Jn 19: 17–24) After his death and resurrection, he appeared to his apostles and instructed them, opening their minds and said,

So you see how it is written that the Christ would suffer and on the third day rise from the dead, and that, in his name, repentance for the forgiveness of sins would be preached to all nations." (Lk 24: 45–47, Acts 10:40)

By this Jesus shows the cross as an integral part of his life and mission. So, the healing that we need is that good docile disposition of the mind that helps us to stand our ground and suffer well.

When we remain open to God's saving power, these afflictions, deprivations of any kind and even death itself will have a complete, new and different meaning to us. This new, different and accepted dimension is HEALING IN THE ULTIMATE. It is the REAL MIRACLE. That is what Christ did that made it possible for him to destroy our death by dying and raised us to life by rising from the dead. We have to accept and teach our people that all those manifestations of instant cures that form the pastoral goal of many priests now and which in turn is becoming the yard–stick with which the faithful measure the pastoral relevant of their priests, are not the only, nor even a reliable way of identifying God's presence in our Church. We and the faithful should therefore not hang our faith on those outward manifestations. We should know, understand and teach that even in real prolonged sufferings, our omnipotent God is ever present in full, helping and sustaining the invalid. Sincere souls generally find him there and the resultant relationship defies description. It is the prayer which brings us to this level of living faith that heals.[634]

633 Cf. L.Mbefo, Priests and Healing Ministry in the Nigerian Church, Op. Cit., p.1

634 G.Ikeobi, Priest, Healing and Prayer ministry, in A.N.O. Ekwunife & co. (eds), "The renewal of Priestly life and ministry: The Nigerian experience", Op. Cit., p.221–222

5.3.2 Exclusive claim of the Holy Spirit, pride and neglect of Constituted Authority

As we have earlier observed in this work, the healing ministry was first initiated by Jesus Christ himself. It has been central to the ministry of the early and Apostolic Church and has continued to the Church of today. Charism as gift of the Holy Spirit has also been well exercised in the early Church and they have been given for the good of the community and not for personal gains or self–aggrandisement.

Today, in the Church in Igbo society of Nigeria, the exercise of the gift of the Holy Spirit by some priests and charismatic lay people leads to chaos and confusion in the local Church. Some of the priest–healers do not want any longer to remain under the guidance of their local Ordinaries. Many want to have uncontrollable independence of their actions and even of the priestly ministry, all in the name of possession of the gift of the Holy Spirit. Some behave as if they have never had the Spirit all the other days of their life as Christians and more so as priests. Many behave as if the Holy Spirit is a spirit of confrontation and disobedience. Many are even convinced that the Holy Spirit has convicted them such that they do not see any reason working in understanding with their Superiors and Ordinaries. They abhor all directions from authorities and see such as a sign of jealousy on their acclaimed gift of the Holy Spirit. Similar actions are found among some lay individuals who are said to possess one gift or the other. Many of them find it difficult to accept the leadership of their various parish priests or chaplains especially when the said priests are not of the "charismatic" type. We must understand that,

> *we are not those leading the Spirit which the Authorities also have... There must be always somebody to moderate what is happening around us. When anybody refuses this, the person may be thinking of his or her own Church. This is how many Churches sprang up in the name of ministries. Disobedience and pride are behind it.*[635]

A good number of the priests in Igboland have seen the healing ministry almost as a full time assignment, not always from their Ordinaries or Superiors but as a claim from the Holy Spirit forgetting that it is only a part of Christ's whole earthly mission or ministry. Sometimes, a good lot of the Priest–healers abandon their legitimate assignments, in order to have time to carry out duties pertaining to their healing ministry. Sometimes they are quietly disobedient and stubborn even when their Ordinaries or Superiors call them for dialogue. They may have very little to discuss with whoever calls them to take precaution of what they are

635 T.Onoyinma, Attention Please No. 1, Snaap Press, Enugu, 1996, p.29

doing and consider such an individual to lack the faith and deliverance that the Holy Spirit has bestowed on them. But as the Second Vatican Council clearly puts down,

the validity and usefulness of any Charism including healing and prayer Charism are to be judged by those who preside over the Church and to whose special competence it belongs, not indeed to extinguish the spirit, but to test all things and hold fast to that which is good.[636]

But this has not always been the case. In some places, including the Igbo land of Nigeria, the validity and the use of charims in the Church have been misconceived and misinterpreted particularly by those who are said to possess some of the charisms, especially the charism of healing.

According to E. Uzukwu,

In Port Harcourt, Onitsha, Enugu, Orlu, Aba dioceses to name a few, our Bishops find it difficult at times to exercise their supervisory ministry over the powerful "priest healers". The Charismatic priests appear to be very conscious of their power which is often times maintained through the exploitation of the superstitious and the irrational, of which distressed faithful are easy victims. The orderly exercise of Charisms for the benefit of the community appears not to be uppermost in the minds of some healers.[637]

Any ministry in the Church is for the benefit of the entire Church and for the building up of community and not just for any selfish interest. Any healing minister should try as much as possible to avoid the danger of self–fascination and uncontrollable independence. In this Generation of ours, particularly in our own part of the world, where good living and health of the body are highly prized, there is the tendency to generate some sort of power and independence on any priest or individual who is attributed with the gift of healing of sickness or the ability to control any type of misfortunes. The priest healers therefore, need to make humility their watchword and always pray for it. For without humility, it is difficult to progress in holiness, it is difficult to lead the people of God to heaven, no matter how gifted one may be. Priests should always work in understanding with the Constituted Authorities of the Church to always be the light, which they are meant to be from their Ordination to the priesthood.

636 L.G. 12

637 E.E. Uzukwu, A listening Church: Autonomy and Communion in African Churches, Orbis Book, Mary Knoll, New York, 1996, p.123

5.3.3 The Danger of Commercialisation of the ministry

One of the major areas of abuses of the healing ministry today is the Commercialisation of the ministry. We are only too aware of the effects of too much money and material wealth on human beings. We are also aware of how easily our people worship money and idolise those that have the money. It is all money everywhere. "Everyone is possessed with such greed nowadays; they are all so overwhelmed by the idea of money that they seem to have gone mad.[638]

Selfless service and non–profit oriented service is under the crucible of extinction. Charitable services are moving unto the valley of death. Nothing is done for nothing. This is an unfortunate situation of a people. People do a lot of funny things to get money. Some can even kill in order to get money. Some are said to have killed their mothers in order to make money. What an abomination! Money becomes everything and serves for everything. Consequently, it would be an ideal for any priest "to avoid being directly associated with so much money or material possession or their love under any pretext whatsoever."[639] To associate any priest with money does not tell any good about him and his priestly ministry. And to associate any priest–healer with any demand of money to render his services makes a mess of the whole loving ministry of the Church.

The association of the prayer ministry, faith healing cures of sorts, etc. with lots of money and material property does not appear healthy and to call a spade a spade, it is counter witness to the gospel.[640]

The healing ministry is a free gift of Jesus Christ to his Church. You do not charge money for dispensing what is not yours – the gift of God, which was given to the Church for the good of the community. "Freely you have received, freely you should give" (Mtt 10:8). But unfortunately, the attitudes of some of our healers sometimes lack much to be appreciated. It is said that some request fantastic amount, sometimes up to ten thousand Naira[641] for the celebration of what they call "Healing Mass", as if there is any mass that is not healing in nature and character. Some also collect money for consultation. This sounds uncomplimentary and unreal, but it is true. According to K. Chigbo,

> *They charge money for dispensing the gift of God. Some pastors boldly charge for healing. Others rename such charges thus – consultation fee, thanksgiving levy, Appre-*

---

638 F.Foster, Money, Sex and Power (reprinted), Nigeria, Wellspring Publications, 1992, p.13, in K.Chigbo, "Catholic Healing Ministry on Fire", Enugu, 1997, p.56
639 B.C.Okolo, Healing Ministry in the Nigerian Church: Dangers next door, Op.Cit., p.88
640 Ibid., p.88
641 Naira is Nigeria's currency

ciation fee, "One out of ten" and so on. And charges of course vary according to cases or problems.[642]

What a commercialisation and a negation of this loving ministry of Jesus Christ! Jesus never collected any money from anybody that came to him for healing.

We also never heard or read of any of the apostles who collected money from those they prayed for healing. Elisha the prophet found it unnecessary to accept Gold and Silver from Naaman whom he cured of his leprosy. (2 Kgs 5:15–19) It is, in an attempt to forestall this commercialisation of the ministry that the Catholic Bishops Conference of Nigeria decreed,

> *Trading in any form is forbidden. Consequently, the charging of fees for ministries, the practice of producing articles for sales – such as clothing, soaps, cosmetics, jewellery, etc., – to which miraculous powers are ascribed should be discontinued.*[643]

But incidentally some of the priests who engage in the healing ministry do not only charge fees and impose levies. Some have turned the prayer centres into business centres. Sales of objects of various types and sizes abound in these healing and prayer centres. Sometimes the sales form part of the ministry. Some special objects with special trademarks or labels of some of these healers are made mandatory to those who attend the prayer sessions. Attendants are occasionally asked to discard objects like water bottles or bottles of olive oil they brought from their homes to buy the miraculous ones sold in the centres. Stickers and products like pomades and ointments are also advertised to possess miraculous powers. Hence some of the ministers have turned into big commercial giants and many more are warming up for similar status.

However, we are not in any way saying that healing ministers should not receive any gifts or offerings from the faithful, neither are we saying that they should discourage them from expressing gratitude to God for the various gifts or favours they might have received from God. What we are emphasising is the danger of commercialisation or extraction of money from the faithful in the name of the ministry or even excessive accumulation of money and material wealth on the part of the priest.

Accumulation of money or wealth has a way of confusing or distracting even the virtuous. In sending the apostles out, the master ordered the apostles not to

642 K.Chigbo, Healing Ministry on Fire, Op. Cit., p.40

643 The Catholic Bishops Conference of Nigeria, Guidelines for the healing Ministry, Lagos, 1997, p.24

carry money or belongings. Authentic healers always maintain a safe distance from money and what money can purchase.[644]

Not only that. We add that authentic healers should also know how to use and where to direct the money and material wealth that accrue to them through the ministry. They should also know whether the food items and other material wealth that accrue to them, should be allowed to rot and be thrown away while others die in need and want. They should know whether the money they get is private or Church money and so know how to disburse the wealth, whether to embark on personal projects or Church projects with the money. This I believe is very important since I have seen or personally encountered not just a priest but more who after having accumulated enough wealth and material properties, have on the other hand accumulated enough sad moments and discontentedness for themselves and their priestly ministry. This is particularly very common among priests who after having got enough money began to construct what we may call private prayer centres or quasi–private Churches or what they themselves call pilgrimage centres. The moment they are transferred from such centres to other places or given other assignments by their Bishops, or even when they are asked to go and further their education or lecture in the Seminary or University, you see how attached they are and how sad they become. Some see it that the Church or their Bishop is snatching away their properties from them. A good number of them see the new assignment or posting as stifling of the Holy Spirit by their Ordinaries. Many of them become very antagonistic with their brother priests whom they believe are jealous of them and might have instigated their movements or transfers. What a misplacement of priority! After all, neither Christ nor his Apostles were reported to have set up a healing centre or a miracle camp. Priest–healers who are not large hearted enough to construct prayer centres for their diocesan or congregational uses and for the entire Church should not embark on them at all.

The ministry is for the benefit of the members of the Church and not just for the fascination of some. Priests in Nigeria who parade gifts to fascinate the lay or to make money are compared to the Ofeke dibia (foolish and ignorant Medicine men) of the Igbo Tradition. It is pertinent that those whom the Tradition refers to as Ofeke dibia or Charlatans are those who make real money from traditional medicine. They constitute danger to the community because they could practise sorcery or poisoning to make money.[645]

644 G.Ikeobi, Healing and Exorcism: The Nigeria Experience, Op. Cit., p.74
645 E.Uzukwu, A listening Church, Op. Cit., p.126

5.3.4 Unnecessary Emphasis on the influence of demons

There have been certain illusions to the effect that the African continent appears to have some extra of 'agents of the powers of darkness and of evil' and therefore, does seem to have a more urgent need for the special ministry of deliverance (through miracles and spiritual healing). This position sounds far fetched and unacceptable.[646]

Similar impression that the evil spirit is everywhere, infesting food and drinks, and pursuing people about is being given of the Igbo society today by many people especially the regular clients of the numerous prayer/healing ministries in Igboland and some of the pastors and ministers of these healing centres. This is also noticed in the numerous newly introduced and sometimes ill chanted Charismatic songs, which have taken over the place of Sacred and other Church music. Most of the songs either accuse the devil or evil spirits of one problem or the other or/and tell the devil that he has no power over the children of God. Some chant songs of war or defeat over the strength of the wicked and evil spirits as if life is all an attack of the demons and evil spirits – "Zogbue Ekwensu n'ukwu" (March the devil to death), "Ekwensu ifechaa fechaa izulu ike" (Devil after flying about you rest ...) "Ekwensu onweghi ihe ipulu ime" (Devil you can't do anything) etc. These songs are not bad in themselves, but their uses seem not to be in order and 'ad rem'. They are sung at any place and at any occasion and at any time. These invariably over exaggerate the existence and the influence of these demons and evil spirits on the society. Sometimes one begins to wonder if those who misuse these songs are not themselves possessed or influenced by the evil or bad spirits.

That there exist demons and evil spirits, we do not argue. That God allows some powers to the demons over human beings and the material universe we do not debate. But that this power of the evil spirits is unlimited and uncontrollable stands to be contested. That evil spirit possession and the attack of demonic forces are widely presumed to be the root cause of most of the sickness and misfortunes that people suffer today also needs to be discussed.

This is precisely why the Catholic Bishops of Nigeria uphold

> ***that demon exists and has power over people and the material universe. But this power is limited by divine providence even though the sin of mankind gives wider scope to it. (See L. J. Elneer "Exorcism" in the New Catholic Encyclopaedia. Vol.5, Washington, 1981). Christian faith believes in this divine providence, as well as in the omnipotence and omnipresence of God. Christian faith teaches too the basic goodness of the universe, and the***

646 C.Ejizu, Cosmological Perspective on Exorcism and Prayer–Healing in Contemporary Nigeria, Op. Cit., p.17

fact that if God permits evil, He does it for a good purpose. God knows how to turn everything including evil to the good of those who love him.[647]

Nigeria priests and healing ministers, like their counter–parts all over the world grapple with human problems of diverse kinds and complex natures. Anybody who is acquainted with the theological debates on the problem of evil knows that the Nigerian situation, nay, the situation in Igboland, is not unique. For the people to see evil spirits in everything in life is not healthy. And for the priest healerts in their attempt to help the simple faithful out, sympathetically as it is, trying to reach out to as many forms of evil spirits and demons as possible lacks much to be allowed and encouraged in the Church of Christ.

Seeing demons where there are none, blaming them for all troubles, having obsessive fear of them and preaching about them excessively, are marks of a superstitious trend that does not find support in Christian Tradition. instead the Church cautions against such undue preoccupations and counsels reservation and prudence about diabolical intervention and miracles.[648]

What we experience in some of the prayer/healing centres or gatherings in Igbo society is not very encouraging. It is somehow far from the teaching of the Church on the existence of the demons and evil spirits.

A careful observer notices that most of the prophets and Charismatic leaders of the independent Churches and healing houses often share and identify with our people in most underlying traditional understanding and beliefs that fan and highlight the influence of the evil spirits. Catholic priest–healers, especially the most recent ones, have in some aspects taken after these pastors of the independent Churches, such that all forms of sickness and misfortunes including barrenness, mental illness, epilepsy, premature deaths, failure in the business world, failure of farm crops and even the most clinically dictated cases of diabetes and hypertension are explained away by the activities of ubiquitous evil spirits, angry gods and the demons, operating through man and nature.

They do not for a moment deny the presence of spirits to be cast out, Witchcraft spells to be housed, but faced with them they assert the power of God to free and to restore. In practice there seems to be a wide range of response at one end clearly controlled by a Christian sense of God and Christ; at the other it is still rather deeply embedded in the religious metaphysic underlying traditional treatment.[649]

---

647 Catholic Bishops Conference, Guidelines on Healing ministry, Op. Cit., p.10

648 Sacred Congregation for Divine Worship (S.C.D.W.), Les Formes Multiples de la Superstition, Christian faith and demonology, Vatican City, 1975, Chapters 1&4

649 A. Hastings, African Christianity, London, 1976, p.72, in C. Ejizu, Cosmological Perspective on Exorcism and Prayer, Op. Cit., p.16

This is not all.

Before now, only human beings suspected the presence of the evil spirits. Now it is science – the computer, which states definitely that evil spirits are at work and declares with finality that the only remedy is spiritual healing, which in effect means exorcisms. Let us hope that the formula for exorcism will also be provided by the computer.[650]

We know Homeopathic doctors to be popular with the use of computers in detecting the presence of the evil spirits and diseases but this issue is no more the prerogative of Homeopathic doctors as one would imagine but also a priority of some of our priest–healers. It is really unfortunate that some of our priests began to pay regular visits to some of these doctors and are learning their method of exorcisms and inserting it into the healing ministry of the Church. Some of them have forgotten that the Church has her own rites of exorcisms. And moreover, there are priests appointed specially in each diocese for the service of exorcisms.

All these developments remind me of B. Haring writing about the incessant invasion of the evil spirits and witchcraft in the traditionalist cultures where all serious afflictions in forms of sickness, miscarriage, death of a beloved one and other calamities are attributed to the attacks of the evil spirits. This Haring says,

aggravates their anguish, destroys relationships and creates a pestilent atmosphere of suspicion leading to all kinds of persecution. Innocent people are suspected, persecuted, treated to diabolical abuse and tortured, and forced into making false confessions in a world full of evil cruelty. This is surely an atmosphere in which the "princes of darkness" can use their weaponry of deception and hatred.[651]

The situation in Igboland is therefore crying for a check. It is crying for a re–orientation and intensive education of the Christians on the existence of these spirits in the universe. That evil spirits exist is a fact. But, that evil spirits are infesting everything including foods and drinks is not a fact. People do all sorts of things these days all in the name of getting rid of the said evil spirits. There are a lot of funny practices in the Church today in a bid to ward off the spirits. In gatherings today, both liturgical and social, the mode of prayers one experiences is occasionally long and flamboyant flow of commands and shouting at God to get rid of the powers of the evil spirits as if everyone in the gathering is possessed and needs exorcisms. In short, many of the abuses within the healing ministry emanate from the belief in the invasion of the evil spirits and the attempt to get rid of them. Today almost everybody claims to discern the presence of the evil

---

650 G.Ikeobi, Healing and Exorcism: The Nigerian Pastoral Experience, Op. Cit., p.66

651 B.Haring, Healing and Revealing, St. Paul's Publication, Middlegreen, England, 1984, pp.65–66.

spirits and have his or her own ritual for casting them away. Let us see J. Nwosu in his reply to my questionnaire. He writes,

Four out of the twelve priests here at Holy trinity Compound, claim that they deliver the people possessed or being attacked by the "evil forces" under consideration. Their stories about such phenomenon are, at worst, frightening and, at best, embarrassing. Since their operations do not seem to be amenable to empirical data, it becomes difficult for one to rush into conclusions. There is certainly "something" that sometimes makes an otherwise normal person so abnormal that his/her humanness becomes questionable. The task on hand, I think, is to find out the cause of such 'abnormality' and proffer the cure. Until that is done, no one, I think, can provide an answer that can convince anyone that those "evil forces" actually exist and affect some people or that they do not exist, and do not affect some people.[652]

Let us also see the observation of a lay man and an Engineer, Mr Chukwukaelo Nweke in a personal letter to the researcher. He writes,

We want new Generation of priests. We need priests that will revolutionise the current thinking in Nigeria. Every priest whether Catholic or Protestant is trying to out–do one another in casting out the devil. The priests have turned to NATIVE DOCTORS. Every priest now is a seer, he casts out devils, he destroys witches, he uses "OMU NKWU" to detect where juju is buried. They all try to overtake Rev. Fr. M. P, Edeh of Elele. Most of them have turned the Catholic Church into something else. Any good thing that gets into the hands of a black man is turned into something else ...[653]

The healing ministry of Jesus Christ is an integral part of his mission entrusted to his Church. And this mission entails the driving out of the evil spirits or demons. Christ himself contested against the evil spirits and the demons. He did not allow the devil to destroy his beloved ones. But he did not exaggerate their existence and power. With mere power of the words he sent them away. The same power, He gave to his disciples. He also taught people to avoid evil and live in a closer union with him. He taught people to avoid evil of violence, consumerism, jealousy, greed, money mania, insatiability, bitterness, enmity and vindictiveness and such other vices fostered against their brothers and neighbours. All these vices greatly aggravate pain and anguish, destroy relationships and create a negative and ungodly atmosphere, which leads to all kinds of sickness, ill luck and misfortunes. We do not deny the existence of the evil spirits but priest–healers should not encourage the impression that the evil spirits are present in everything that happens to people. A prudent and experienced priest should not

652 P. Okonkwo, Personal letter, Holy Ghost Cathedral Compound, Enugu, 26 August, 1999, p.1&2

653 Chukwukaelo Nweke, Personal letter, Umungasi, Aba, 28/10/99, p.1

always jump into exorcism like some members of the Charismatic society, commanding the evil spirits to go out 'IN THE NAME OF JESUS, AMEN'.

5.3.5 Inappropriate use of the Sacramentals

The question of indiscriminate and inappropriate use of sacramentals in the Catholic Church in Igbo society of Nigeria cannot be ignored. In short, that is dangerously stepping towards the destruction of the much cherished Catholic doctrines and rubrics on the celebration of the sacramentals in the area. We have earlier in this work seen that the sacraments as signs, are the channels of God's saving and healing grace and the grace so communicated in the celebration of the sacraments is a source of healing for the body and spirit. So the "main aim of the sacraments is to sanctify men, to build up the Body of Christ, and finally to give worship to God.[654] And because they are signs, they presuppose, nourish and strengthen faith by words and objects. In the same vein,

> *Sacramentals are sacred signs, which bear a resemblance to the Sacraments. They signify effects, particularly of a spiritual nature, which are obtained through the Church's intercession. By them, men are disposed to receive the chief effects of the Sacraments, and various occasions in life are rendered holy.*[655]

The Church therefore allows many types of Sacramentals in order to sanctify the world and her members at various times and occasions in life. Sacramentals could either be sacred persons, images or things or elements like the medals. It can be the oil of the sick, crucifix, holy water or any such objects. The power of God communicated on the sacramentals can act as a source of healing for the faithful.

> *Thus for well disposed members of the faithful the liturgy of the sacraments and sacramentals sanctify almost every event of their lives with the divine grace which flows from the Paschal mystery of the passion, death and Resurrection of Christ. From this source all Sacraments and Sacramentals draw their power.*[656]

So we can use a lot of material objects which the Church has left at our disposal for the healing and sanctification of men and for the praise and worship of God. But only "proper use of these materials"[657]can thus affect this purpose.

---

654 Vatican Council II, The Constituion on Sacred Liturgy, Sacro Sanctum Concilium, 4 December, 1963, 56 (1964), (hereafter as S.C.), No. 59

655 S.C. no. 60

656 S.C. no. 61

657 Cf. S.C. No. 61

The Catholic healing ministry in Igbo Society of Nigeria is making abundant use of these Sacramentals, sometimes to a point that calls for attention and concern. There is over enthusiastic use of these sacramentals. There are adulteration and faking and many other inappropriate uses of the sacramentals difficult to be properly fixed within the correct Church rubrics or pastoral ambient. Some of the Sacramentals are sometimes used to represent or act as magical powers. K. Chigbo says some of the practices, border on Neo–Paganism. According to him,

> *Our people have old ways peculiar to them through which, they believed demons were exorcised or expelled and through which sickness were cured. They offered sacrifices to spirits believed to be responsible for cases of ailments, infliction and misfortunes. The role of traditional medicine men, herbalists and priests was to offer the appeasement and expiatory sacrifices... Today for some Christians, crucifixes, candles, portraits, relics and holy water have become Charms and amulets.*[658]

This should not spring up much surprise. The use of the sacramentals seems to have taken a more prominent place than the sacraments. Little wonder the average Igbo Christian seems to misunderstand the difference between the sacraments and sacramentals.

> *The Sacramentals evoke the notion of things seen to be happening, while the Sacrament doesn't seem to have much to do with the present realities of earthly life. It specialises in preparing people for some distant life in the world to come, while a Sacramental tackles the human problems of hostile environment, of evil spirits and other known and unknown forces ubiquitous in the cosmos.*[659]

One can therefore understand why there are some practices found today within the Church in Igbo Society that keep the Church Hierarchy uncomfortable, such as the issue of burying of the crucifix on the ground at the four corners of the house or compound to ward off the entrance of the demons or the evil spirits. There are other uses of the Sacramentals that call for review and Catechesis such as the issue of hanging bottles of holy water in farmlands or on trees to act as charm or watchmen. It is also said that some bury not only the crucifixes on the ground but also blessed candles, salt and holy water in an attempt to get rid of the evil spirits, sickness or one misfortune or the other. They invariably invent their own rituals for these activities provided their clients believe that something extraordinary is going on. People fall in love with novelties.

It has also been observed that some use the candles in a way that encourages certain basic attitudes and values that clearly stem from the Igbo traditional per-

---

658 K.C. Chigbo, Healing Ministry on Fire, Op. Cit., p.42

659 G.Ikeobi, Priest, Healing and Prayer ministry, in A.N.O. Ekwunife, "The renewal of Priestly Life and ministry", Op.Cit., p.223

ception of reality, such as the traditional Sacrifice (ichu aja), usually offered in a junction pathway. Today it is not only the traditional medicine man that asks his client to carry their sacrifices to a four–junctioned pathway, 'ebe uzo gbara ino'. To this category also belong the priests or healers who recommend "the positioning of seven or more lighted candles on seven pathways as an attempt to check any calamity befalling any family."[660]

At this junction, it is important to acknowledge that some Nigerian Scholars and theologians are of the opinion that the cosmic spheres of Nigeria and their compenetrability suggest a more sober appreciation of these novel pastoral practices. One of such Scholars, L. Madubuko says,

> *The fact is that the triumph of resurrection which is the principal message of the crucifix has nothing to fear from the dirt of the earth. Building an edifice on the top of the crucifix would in my own sensitivity be an eloquent way of building on the victory of Christ over all forces. "Christ is my rock" is not meant to be only an abstraction.*[661]

On praying with lighted Candles in form of a cross and the client lying to sleep within such a cross, Madubuko again says, "With adequate catechesis" I believe this is a legitimate expression of faith in the power of the event of the cross."[662] Looking at the two proposals, his arguments at the first instance look so sound and plausible. But I believe Madubuko might not have been well informed on all the practices surrounding the two issues and the aims of burying the crucifix on the ground and of lying to sleep in midst of lighted candles.

On praying with Candles lighted in form of a cross and the client lying to sleep within such a cross, we refer to the findings of K. Chigbo. He says,

> *The patient is forced to lie flat with a cross drawn on the floor according to his/her height. The patient does not rise from that position, even to ease himself, until one set of candles burns out. The candles are placed at the 12corners of the cross. The victim often lies there on a bare floor without clothes, except pants or wrappers at the waist: gross indecency and torture.*[663]

The ministers concerned in this practice ask their clients to lie to sleep in midst of lighted candles because of fear of one kind or the other or because of any other type of misfortune. The question is whether this is enough to expose the faithful to this type of danger and torture because of just ordinary fear. The activity so involved may be psychologically vital in relieving the fear but whether it

---

660 T.Onoyinma, Attention Please, Op. Cit., p.13

661 L. Madubuko, Healing and Liturgy, Seminar Paper on Healing Ministry, Emene, Enugu, 11th – 14th February 1992, p.19

662 Ibid., p.19

663 K.Chigo, Healing Ministry on fire, Op.Cit., p.81

has an overt value remains a question. The torture and the danger involved are enormously great and grave. While prescribing this type of healing prayer to our Christians, one should consider the danger of the fire from the candle burning the client or even setting the whole house on fire where twelve candles are lighted at the same time with the client immersed in meditative prayer or slumber. Again what type of liturgy prescribes the indecent and unhealthy rubric of going to prayers in nudity with the supplicant lying on bare cement floor? This practice reminds me of one of the popular priest–healers who asks his clients to bath in the middle of their compounds while performing some rituals prescribed by the priest in question. Information gathered shows that majority of these clients are working class ladies who have some pride to protect, so most of them perform the bathing rituals in the nights. What a ritual!

Building an edifice on the cross of Christ buried on the ground according to Madubuko can be an eloquent way of building on the victory of Christ over all forces, including the evil spirits. But the question remains whether the ministers of healing who bury crucifixes on the ground have the same intelligent thought pattern with the Liturgy Scholar. We have earlier remarked in this work that the problem with the healing ministry in lgboland is not in the healing ministry itself but in the mode of operation.

Most of the ministers, who bury crucifixes and bottles of holy water at the four corners of people's houses, give the impression that the buried items serve as prevention of the evil spirits and evil men or any type of enemies, including sickness from entering people's houses.[664] This therefore gives the impression that the crucifixes and the other items buried on the ground are meant to serve the place of Igbo traditional Charms and Amulets. The traditional Igbo invite the traditional medicine man "dibia" to his compound when he has problems of life. And most of the times, the dibia buries some charms somewhere in the compound especially at the spots where he believes are the entrance routes of the evil spirits into the compound. Do we understand this practice of the healers of burying the crucifixes as a replacement of the practice of burying of charms of the dibia? If

664 cf. T. Onoyinma, Attention Please, No 1, Op. Cit., p.12: Sometimes some people bring more than one crucifix to a Catholic priest to bless. If you ask the owner of these sacramentals what he does with more than one of them, he/she replies that after the consultation with one prophet or prophetess, an order has been given that these sacramentals should be buried at the four corners of the house to block or prevent the entrance of any devil or bad spirit. Any enemy crossing those places or any of these points shall have his or her bad plans or charm destroyed. This obtains with those who may be sick or have an attack of the evil spirit which many people emphasise and believe. This means that any type of sickness has some devils responsible for it. This is really misleading because there will be as many devils as there are sicknesses and this is strange. This makes the devil countable and numerical.

we so understand, do we then believe the evil spirits have pathways from where they come into people's houses? And if we believe this too, do the buried crucifixes actually prevent the evil spirits from gaining access into the said compounds?

Supposing the evil spirits avoid the spots at which the sacramentals are positioned what happens? Can these evil spirits, we feel shall not cross those points, not pass unnoticed since they are spirits and invisible? Does the faith of the people grow stronger, weaker or do some of them find out by themselves that their faith and God's presence can help them more than thinking of check–points for the evil spirits? Of course the sacramentals remind us of God, Jesus, Mary and the Saints and we have to venerate these sacramentals but is burying them any veneration?[665]

Or is this taken as inculturation? If this is taken as inculturation of the practice of the dibia, we must know that inculturation has to take its proper course. We have to be careful "not only of a wild accretion of ritual formulae, but even serious aberrations justified by some as inculturation"[666]

If the building of an edifice on the crucifix is seen as a way of building on the victory of Christ over all forces, a thorough Catechesis on the theology of the cross (suffering), should have been the most comfortable or adequate companion to the practice of the burying on the crucifix, in which case the Christians concerned may not hold the impression that no enemy including sickness may have entrance into their compounds. Instead that will mean that the Christians will be ready to handle every problem that come their way on the strength of the cross of Christ buried in their houses. The victory of Christ on the cross was built on His suffering, death on the wood of the cross and the glorious resurrection from the dead.

Here, it may even be necessary to remind ourselves also, that the Roman Catholic Rubrics state that to drive away evil spirits or the devil, the priest "ought to have the crucifix at hand or somewhere in sight,"[667] and not to have it hidden or buried to be destroyed by termites or exposed to rusting. "One will see to it too that the sacred objects are not treated improperly or that no injury is done them by the evil Spirit."[668] Moreover, the use of the sacraments and sacramentals must be according to the Sacred Canon, which states that,

665 Ibid., p.14–15

666 S.C.., No 59

667 Roman Catholic Rubrics on Exorcisms, No. 13., cf also T.Onoyinma, Attention Please, p.14, Shall the devil not be more afraid to see a hanging crucifix than the one buried and gradually destroyed by the sand?

668 Ibid., No. 13

only the Apostolic See can establish them and approve their rites and formulae, which should be accurately observed at their celebrations and use. (C. 1167)

And for any priest to introduce a new or revise the use of the sacramental,

account must be taken of the primary principle of enabling the faithful to participate intelligently, actively and easily. The circumstances of our times must also be considered.[669]

And this provision must be at the discretion and approval of the Ordinary of the place and the Episcopal conference of the region.

5.3.6 Outlandish testimonies and self advertisement of the ministers

Giving of testimonies have been part and parcel of the mode of operation of the healing ministry. This is how it was done at the first organised prayer/healing ministry in the Catholic Church in Igbo society of Nigeria.

Participants who are convinced that God has answered their prayers and wish to make it public do so at the appropriate time. This helps to encourage others and to break monotony. They usually bring offering of different kinds, ranging from animals and money to brooms. They are instructed not to go over reach themselves to get what to offer, and to come out to testify even if one has nothing to offer. But they always have something to offer even if it is only 50 kobo in envelope.[670]

There are many other genuine reasons to allow the giving of testimonies to serve as a part of the format of operation for the healing ministry. Testimonies are "meant to teach them gratitude to God and to fortify the faith of those yet waiting on God's own good time for their own healing."[671] 1t is also known that some people who attend the prayer–healing ministry hold that,

listening to the testimonies of other sufferers has a therapeutic value: through listening to the sufferings of others, they create enough courage to help them endure their own problems.[672]

Giving of open testimonies to God during prayer/healing ministry by those who received one Messing or the other from God is encouraged as a sign of gratitude to God and to encourage the people's faith and belief in the healing work of

669 S.C. No. 79
670 G.Ikeobi, Catholic Response to the Challenge of 'Prayer Houses' Op. Cit., p.273
671 U. Igboaja, Healing Ministry at the Pastoral Centre Ugwu di nso, Eke, Op. Cit., p.3
672 L.Mbefo, Priests and Healing Ministry in the Nigerian Church, Op. Cit., p.2

Jesus Christ. There is nothing wrong in giving thanks to God and acknowledging that God has wrought wonders in one's life. But just like some other aspects of the healing service, the issue of giving testimony is being exaggerated. Unlike Christ the divine healer who never encouraged those he healed to go about advertising him, some healing ministers use the place of testimonies to sound their personal trumpet and give outlandish testimonies on miraculous activities attributed to themselves, genuine or not. Some are even said to stage–manage the practice of giving testimony. Any wonder E. Uzukwu says that,

there is a fascination with the gift or Charism of healing. Gifted priests and Charismatics show little restraint in publicizing their "miracle rain" through "testimonies" in imitation of the fundamentalist (American style) Christian groups[673]

Writing on the areas where problems exist in the healing ministry in Nigeria, M.C. Asuzu says,

Self advertisement of the "faith healer's ministry", which any blind man can see even when they try to camouflage this self–advertisement in all. A kind of way; Jesus' healing apostolate is a full anti– thesis of this abuse.[674]

Jesus Christ never advertised his own healing works. He even warned his disciples not to rejoice that the devils obey them. They should instead be happy that their names are written in heaven. Is the same admonition not relevant for the healing ministers of today? Why should the disciples of today turn deaf ears to the admonition of the master and go about singing their own praises, seeking for fame and honour and canvassing for larger crowds of clients?

The researcher has personally listened to some of the priest–healers really advertising themselves not only during the testimonies but also during homilies by broadcasting some of the wonders that are said to have been accomplished through their healing ministries. Some occasionally make some uncomplimentary and damaging remarks about other priest–healers that perhaps they found as rivalries.

Some healers even pronounce curses on some other healers and their clients. This sounds unimaginable but it is true. Some of the ministers too, encourage their clients to give superfluous testimonies on wonder works they claimed to have performed. Such clients are normally called up by the ministers themselves or by their lieutenants to come forward and testify.

The miracles or healing works granted by Jesus Christ through the prayer sessions should not be advertised at all. Testimonies can be given but,

---

673 E.Uzukwu, A listening Church, Op. Cit., pp.122–123

674 M.C. Asuzu, Healing Apostolate of the Church, Op. Cit., p.5

great discipline is to be observed to discourage testimonies, which aim at exciting admiration or adulation of the minister for the Charism is not for the good of the individual minister but for the good of the Church and it is not even a proof that the individual minister is holier or more powerful than the others, for the gift is gratuitously given and not as a result of merit on the part of the individual minister of healing.[675]

Christ abhors that and always discourages that.

In the New Testament, healing accounts (i.e. testimonies) are simple, straightforward and humble. They were never aimed at glorifying or admiring any person as a wonder worker. They were never aimed at making any one's fame to glow and spread to attract others' attention. Christ himself even hid away from the people who wanted to make him a king or make him popular. When will our priests begin hiding away as Christ did, from the sycophants who come to fan their fame of popularity but with underlying selfish interests which most of the times are unknown to the priests concerned.

May our priests who are gifted with this gift of healing try to avoid any testimonies or things invented to boost their prestige and ego. The authentic healer after Christ must be humble and wise. And to Our Lord Jesus Christ should all glory and honour be given for any healing works of whatever type. God is jealous with his glory and will share it with no one.

5.4 Pastoral Challenges

Having identified and examined the emergence and operation of the prayer/healing ministry in Igbo society of Nigeria, we tried to uncover some of the importance and the contribution of the ministry to the entire mission of Jesus Christ in the area. We discovered that among other things, the healing ministry has done a lot in strengthening the faith of the Christians of that part of Nigeria. A good number of the Christians who are cold have woken up from their slumber and many others who abandoned the Catholic faith are trooping back into the Church in great numbers. It has also helped in the process of inculturation which is being nurtured and encouraged today by the universal Church. Such practices as the indigenisation of the Church music by use of local musical instruments in singing and prayers during Eucharistic and other celebrations are the handiwork of the Charismatic Renewal and the Prayer/healing ministry. On the other hand, we have noticed that the healing ministry has generated a lot of tensions and prob-

675 A.K.Obiefuna, Directives on Prayer and healing ministry in the Archdiocese of Onitsha, MAS founders Publications, Nkpor, 1996,p.10; Catholic Bishops Conference of Nigeria, Guidelines on Healing Ministry, Lagos, 1997, p.19

lems for the young Church in Igbo land. There are abuses here and there, which are most often caused by over enthusiasm on the part of some Christians and some members of the Clergy.

The healing ministry has in one way or the other exaggerated some aspects of the life and teaching of the Church. In an attempt to inculturate some practices of the Church, the ministry in some way is drifting back to some of the traditional beliefs and practices of Igbo traditional religion, which the Church has considered contrary to the gospel of Christ. We have seen some of these in the previous pages. The healing ministry is an integral part of the mission of Jesus Christ on earth, and it has a lot of good things to offer to the Church and to the people of God. Consequently the Church in her attempt to control the excesses in the ministry is also trying her possible best not to extinguish the spirit blowing in the Church. Instead she is doing all within her capacity to face the challenges posed by the mode of operation of this loved ministry for a better execution of the mission of Jesus Christ, which He entrusted to his disciples some two thousand years ago.

The Catholic Church in Igbo society is very much aware of the challenges resulting from the healing ministry. She has intervened particularly in controlling some of the abuses introduced into the Church by the prayer–healing ministry. This she has done through the efforts of the Hierarchy of the Church, individual persons and Institutions of Theology. The First Missiology Symposium on Healing and Exorcism organised by the Spiritan International School of Theology (SIST), Atakwu, Enugu, from May 18–20, 1989 was a case to reckon with. Individual bishops were also known to have called to order and dialogue some of the priests and attendants of healing and prayer sessions, who are known to have introduced some practices that are foreign to the Church's traditions and teachings. There are also combined efforts by the Bishops to face the Challenge. The National Theological Conference on the Healing ministry, organised under the auspices of the Catholic Bishops Conference of Nigeria at Emene, Enugu in 1992 was another step forward. The aim of the Seminar was to allow the "true image of the Church and her healing ministry to remain intact and according to the mind of Christ in keeping with the apostolic Tradition."[676]

Nigerian theologians, priests and laymen presented various papers at the Seminar. The priest–healers were also invited to be present to make their own observations and contributions towards the success of the Seminar. They gave their own side of the story and tried to clarify certain issues and questions that arose since it is obviously clear that the problem with the healing ministry is not

676 A.K.Obiefuna, National Theological/Pastoral Seminar on healing ministry, Seminar Paper on healing Ministry, February 11th–14th 1992, Emene, Enugu, p.2

with the phenomenon of healing and prayer but with the manner of the operation of the ministry. Some of the topics raised and discussed include:

Priests and healing ministry in the Nigerian Church.
The healing apostolate of the Church in the light of modern day faith healing.
Healing and Liturgy.
Scripture and healing.
Healing care ministry in the Church.
Modern ministry and healing apostolate.

Another joint step already taken to curb some of the abuses found in the healing ministry was the drawing of the Guidelines for the healing ministry in the Catholic Church all over Nigeria issued by the Catholic Bishops Conference of Nigeria in 1997. The aim of the guidelines was to direct the practices of the ministry and allow the healing ministry to operate freely in Nigeria.

But in spite of the efforts of the hierarchy of the Church to curb the abuses of the healing ministry, the abuses continued to persist. Some new ones rear up their ugly heads in different ways, especially with many more priest–healers and ministers emerging all over the place on daily basis. A good number of the new healers come up with many new ideas and practices since they know that "many of our people are mad for new manifestations of God's presence forgetting that they are already living in and with God's presence."[677]

Many of the ministers of healing are ready to do anything provided they sell through the society their own style of healing, not minding the type of dangerous teachings and doctrines they mete out to our not yet well–informed Christians to swallow. There are some of the ministers, who preach,

that aborted babies have not arrived in heaven because they were not yet baptised, before they were killed in the wombs. So to baptise them, some people during a public prayer crusade or a private interview with these "prophets" to pray for the sins of those children, then a general prayer that can be called a general Absolution is held. Then water is sprinkled in the same crowd that has prayed for these children. Then, these children are so baptised and can then see God. Most rejoice at this especially those who might have been involved in the abortion or those worried about the fact of heaven in reference to a non baptised child.[678]

677 T.Onoyinma, Attention Please No.1 Op. Cit., p.9

678 T. Onoyinma, Attention Please *No.* 1, p.1 7: The Catholic Church has never taught that you can baptise people who died many years or months or even days ago. We are not taught that you baptise an unborn baby in the womb either so that the child if aborted can have the seal of baptism. The Catholic Church does not teach that we baptise invisible objects or people in the air, Baptism too is not retroactive so that

What a theological aberration and a misdirection of the faithful!

The Catholic Church never in any way or manner teaches that medically certified dead people can be baptised to give them the seal of baptism, which they never received before. Baptising an aborted child is not the same with giving a conditional baptism or anointing to somebody in danger of death or in occasions of doubt where death of the person is not yet certified, as in the case of an accident. Let this type of ministers stop deceiving the faithful who have some problems of life, all in the name of the healing ministry.

Our suggestion to this brand of ministers is, to allow Christ to heal these brothers and sisters by praying for them and teaching them how to pray when they are in one problem or the other. They are also advised to celebrate the Eucharist with them and give them the normal authentic Catholic instructions on Suffering and the cross without confusing the people. They should also instruct them on the healing effects and the healing power of the sacrament of penance. We assure such ministers that their charisma (if they have any) will continue to be there and still be effective without their trying to be abnormal and teach inauthentic doctrines. Having identified the efforts being made by the Church to confront these abuses and implied challenges of the healing ministry, we note that the Catholic Church in Igbo Society has still a big job to accomplish if the healing ministry is to exist in the area with minimal problems.

Before concluding this chapter I would like to mention that the aborted–children belong also to the group that attracts the sympathy and care of the church. It is also maintained that they (the aborted children) through the merciful act of God are united with Christ in his suffering, death and resurrection. The last chapter takes care of the general conclusion.

---

the gap between the past and the present be closed...Some people who are not babies die after an accident and nobody talks of baptising them after they have been buried.

6. Chapter Six – Conclusion

6.0 Preliminary Remark

The Church of Nigeria is intensively involved in the area of medical care. This aspect has already been treated in section 4.4.2 of this work under the "Medical Service of the Church/Congregations of Hospitals in Nigeria" Healing and Caring of the Sick is an indispensable and innate vocation of the Church. Without this aspect, the existence and worth of the church in Nigeria will be questionable. The Church should therefore concern herself with the continuation of this duty and its spread to every ambient of the society, for example, in social stations of all human endeavour. The Church should not limit herself only to liturgy and law.

6.1 General Conclusion

Days are gone when the Catholic Church was thought of as a Church of Liturgy and law, centred on Tradition, Hierarchy and Sacraments. The missionary task is no more considered the prerogative of the Clergy and Religious who worked in close union with the princes and governors of the colonial powers whose "objects of new missionary thrusts were not so much on spreading the gospel as on extending the Churches of the mother countries".[679] Today the Church always talks of and insists on the proclamation of the Gospel and evangelisation and new evangelisation of the people. When the Vatican spoke of Evangelisation, she generally meant "the proclamation of the basic Christian Message of Salvation through Jesus Christ."[680] Pope Paul VI wishing to engage the entire Church in the dissemination of the Gospel "described evangelisation as the deepest identity of the Church, which exists in order to evangelise."[681]

And he added that, "there can be no evangelisation without explicit proclamation of Jesus as Lord."[682]

679 A.Dulles, John Paul II and the New Evangelisation: What does it mean?, in R. Martin & P. Williamson, John Paul II & the New Evangelisation, Ignatius Press, S. Francisco, 1995, p.26

680 Ibid., p.26

681 Evangelii Nuntiandi, (hereafter as E N), No.14

682 E N, No.22

Carrying the evangelical shift a stage further, John Paul II issued repeated calls for a new evangelisation of the world. He insists that,

new evangelisation cannot be new in its content, since its theme is always the one Gospel given in Jesus Christ. If it arose from ourselves and our situation, there would be no salvation in it.[683]

"Evangelisation however, can and should be new in its ardour, its methods, and its expression."[684] It must be heralded with new energy and in a style and language adapted to the people of our day."[685]

Having declared that the Universal Church today talks of the new evangelisation of the Gospel of Jesus in its method and expression without destroying the content of the Gospel, we call for the Healing Ministry in Igbo society of Nigeria to toe this new line of evangelisation. Jesus Christ is the healer of his people who instituted his healing ministry and set up the pattern of operation for the Christian healers of all ages. He called his ministers to follow the footstep laid down by him who is their Lord and Master.

The healing ministry of Jesus Christ is one of the most attractive and loved areas of his mission on earth, yet one of the most controversial and reactional. Jesus came to give sight to the blind, to make the cripples walk, the lepers cleansed, the deaf began to hear and even the dead raised to life and the gospel was above all preached to the poor (Mtt 11:2–6). This mission he entrusted to his Church through his first apostles and disciples, who carried it through places and centuries and today, it has reached the Igbo land of Nigeria.

The emergence of the healing ministry in Igbo society of Nigeria has a double dimensional effect on the life of the people and on Christianity in the area. We know that the healing ministry has generated some tensions and anxieties for the yet growing Church of Igboland to contend with. On the other hand, it has gone a long way to elevate the faith in many Christians and has helped in the evangelising of the culture of the Igbo people and the Igbo culture and life trying to make its own impact on the gospel message. The healing ministry has made some other positive contributions towards evangelising and fortifying the Christian faith in the area, the negative aspects of the ministry not withstanding.

---

683 Opening Address, Santo Domingo, Oct. 12, 1992, No.6, in A.T. Hennelly, ed., Santo Domingo and Beyond, Maryknoll, N.Y., 1993, pp.44–45, in A. Dulles John Paul II and the New Evangelisation in R.Martin and P.Williamson, Op. Cit., p.28

684 "The task of the Latin American Bishops, Address to CELAM, March 9, 1983, p.661 in A.Dulles, John Paul II and the new Evangelisation, in R. Martin & P. Williamson, Op. Cit., p.28

685 A.Dulles, John Paul II and the new Evangelisation, in R. Martin & P. Williamson, Op. Cit., p.28

There is therefore the need for the Local Church in Igboland, including the hierarchy and the faithful, to adopt a more positive attitude towards the healing ministry and the healing ministers. The Local Church should see the healing ministry according to the spirit of New Evangelisation as the ministry of Jesus Christ and that of entire member of the Christ's faithful and not as that of the ministers of healing and their adherents. This will very much help in looking at the abuses in the ministry with more constructive mind with the view of correcting, reorganising and establishing firmly the ministry without giving room for possible extinction of the ministry. This therefore calls for regular organisation of conferences and workshops on prayer and healing ministry for the healing ministers and the entire presbyterium on the diocesan level and occasionally on the regional and national levels.

Pastors of souls should also see the prayer/healing ministry as part of their vocation to the priesthood, a responsibility, which every pastor should embrace to give life to their flock. If the shepherds do not take care of the flocks, the thief can break in and scatter the flocks. At the same time, the lay faithful should try to see the prayer and healing sessions as part of the normal Christian life and not as anything extra–ordinary. This calls for introduction of in the sense of the church organised prayer sessions in more parishes in the dioceses. Here the faithful should be taught what it means to pray and how to pray well and do it themselves and not waiting for the pastors to always pray for them. This should also be accompanied by an intensified Catechesis on the theology and the saving power of the cross. The importance of the healing power of the sacrament of penance should also be strongly emphasised.

With regard to the issue of some of the phenomena and forces believed to harass people and cause sickness in the society, we propose that more research should be taken up in the area. Scientifically speaking, and theology taken its place as the science of God, the belief in most of these forces like the "Ogbanje" syndrome, "Muo mmili" and other such forces is basically superstitious, since there are not yet enough and clear data to meaningfully interpret the validity of their existence. But since many of the faithful believe very much on the existence of these forces, the Church cannot pretend to overlook the development. There is therefore need for a thorough study of these phenomena or forces. There is also a need for intensified process of evangelisation of the culture of the people and intensified Catechesis by the pastors of the people. Adequate support needs to be given to the Igbo expression of the gospel in all ramifications. It is therefore, our task to seek to translate the Gospel into forms suited to our culture, so as to make it well understood and well lived by our people, and also be able to guide and defend it. Hence writing on inculturation for the African Synod, A. Shorter remarks,

The inculturation of African marriage institutions and traditions of integral healing must not be side stepped by the Synod. Explicit encouragement should be given to valid experimentation, and the idea of a moratorium on inculturation in the Church must be vigorously repudiated. There must be no hesitation whatever in describing inculturation as both urgent and necessary for Africa and for the Church as a whole.[686]

On intensifying the process of inculturation in the Church, in Igbo Society, particularly in the area of healing, we have to take a look at some of the practices already inherent in the healing ministry in the area. We have noticed within the course of our research that there are certain practices, which the Ministers of healing apply that seem to be working for them and their clients but which are not quite conversant with the traditional teaching of the Church. Some of such practices tend to stem from the traditional religion and culture of the people. That means that some of the healing ministers are going bach to the traditional world–view of the people to minister to the Igbo Catholics of this time. This move by some of these ministers should not be neglected completely and condemned. This is so because as the gospel Christianises the Igbo culture, the culture has to give some expressions to the gospel. The Ibos accepted the gospels brought by the missionaries, rejecting some part of their cultures but there are still many aspects of the culture of the Ibos that are good and need to be revered. The Igbo Christians therefore still tend towards some of these cultures. A good number of them rear up their heads in the prayer/healing ministry. This therefore calls for the attention of the Church in Igbo land. The Church has to take a proper examination and study of these practices, expose their theological contents morally, liturgically and pastorally. Then after the studies, comes a need for a proper Catechesis and inculturation of the practices. According to John Paul 11, "A faith which does not become culture is a faith which has not been fully received, not thoroughly thought through, not fully lived out."[687]

This process of evangelising the culture with special reference to the operation of the healing ministry can begin with the manner of the use of the sacramentals by some of the ministers. Such practices as the burying of the crucifixes on the ground and the various practices of praying with the candles can be studied, be better evaluated and evangelised. One of the Igbo prominent Liturgy Scholars and a deep thinker, L. Madubuko had already taken a step on persuading the Church into taking a move in this direction of inculturating some of the practices

686 A.Shorter, The African Synod, A personal response to the Outline document, St. Paul's Publication, Africa, 1991, p.145

687 John Paul II, in L'Osservatore Romano, 28 June 1982, pp.1–8, in A. Sorter, The African Synod, Op.Cit., p.52

of the healing ministry. Talking generally on liturgical symbols, during the National Seminar in Emene in 1992, he said,

The use of the symbols, which are under the general law of the sacramental era, is to be in accordance with the nature of the symbolic material except where there is a clear direction from the Lord. And precisely on the issue of the buried crucifix which is one single practice of the healing ministry that attracts a near unanimous outcry, he says that the triumph of Resurrection which is the principal message of the crucifix has nothing to fear from the dirt of the earth; and building an edifice on the top of the crucifix would be an eloquent way of building on the victory of Christ over all forces since as a religious symbol we understand the crucifix as the embodiment of the reality of Christians victory over the last enemy of man i.e. death and devil.[688]

Madubuko also talked of evangelising the practice of praying with lighted Candles in form of a cross, and lying to sleep within such a cross. We have made our little contributions towards a better understanding of these two practices which are already wide spread in the healing ministry in Igbo society of Nigeria. The Church in Igbo land can introduce an organised study of these two and similar practices found in the healing ministry in Igbo Society and from there continue the process of inculturation of the practices of the healing ministry in Igboland. These practices, I believe with proper study and Catechesis, removing the aspects that are aberrations or contrary to the traditional theology of the Church, will form a good basis for proper inculturation of Igbo culture and religion. Our calls towards inculturation of some of these practices, I believe is not in haste.

While it is perfectly true that one should not be hasty or superficial in carrying out inculturation, it is a necessary and normal activity of the Church, and one which requires reflection, analysis and planning, like any other activity. John Paul 11 has described it as "particularly urgent" (Redemptoris Missio 52), and there are many in Africa who will agree with him."[689]

This is in order since the Universal Church allows anything good in the Tradition and religion of any group of people. It is not too early neither is it too fast for the Church in Igbo land and in Nigeria in general to continue to appreciate things beautiful enough in the culture of the people. These are to be examined and put into use in such a way that they can bring about a successful implementation of the aspirations of the people.

One of the major reasons for the Lineamenta during the African Synod was to reflect the Synod's African character and to stress the contribution of Africa to the universal

---

688 Cf. L.Madubuko, Healing and liturgy, Seminar Paper on healing Ministry, Op.Cit., pp.18–19

689 Cf. A Shorter, The African Synod, St. Paul's Publication, Op. Cit., p.64

Communion of the Church. It was meant to draw lesson from history particularly with regards to past failures of Christianity in African Continent. Among the reasons listed for the disappearance of the once flourishing North African Church was its failure to inculturate. It remained an essentially Latin Church, and no attempt was made to translate the Bible and liturgy into local indigenous languages, or to use elements of local indigenous cultures to create a deeply rooted national Church which could survive the onslaught of Islam. On the other hand the Church survived in Egypt and Ethiopia precisely because it adopted Coptic and Ethiopian languages and cultures.[690]

The Church continues to evangelise the cultures of her people in order to bring the faithful closer to Christ the incarnate Son of God and to give the Church in particular area strong rooted foundation to move ahead and avoid extinction by external forces.

On the part of the priest–healers and other healing ministers, we call on them to work in understanding with the Authorities of the Church. Priest–healers should not see their Superiors and Local Ordinaries as threats or enemies working against their special gifts of God. They should try to avoid laying unnecessary emphasis on personal charisma as if these are the most important aspects of their life as priests. They should bear it in mind that these charismas are for the building and edification of the Community of Christ's faithful and not for self–fascination and aggrandisement. Priests–healers are also called to avoid any moves that give the impression that the healing ministry is a quick means of acquiring any material wealth. They should therefore pray for humility to avoid unnecessary and undue emphasis on public testimony and allow praise to God who is the ultimate source of all healings. Finally, we recommend the study of Pastoral Theology of Health and Healing in our Senior Seminaries to help nip in the bud, the problem of the excesses and abuses in the healing ministry.

690 A. Shorter, The African Synod: A personal response to the outline document , St. Paul's Africa, 1991, p.26

Anhang

Abbreviations

Vatican II Documents and Papal Magisterium

A G	Ad Gentes
D H	Dignitatis Humanae
D V	Dei Verbum
E A	Ecclesia in Africa
E N	Evangelium Nuntiandi
E S	Ecclesiam Suam
G S	Gaudium e Spes
H P D	Humanae Personae Dignitatem
L G	Lumen Gentium
M E	Mysterium Ecclesiae
M S	Misericordiam Suam
N A	Nostrae Aetate
O P	Optatum Totius
P O	Presbyterorum Ordinis
R M	Redemtoris Missio
S C	Sacrosantum Concilium
S D	Salvifici Dolores
S R S	Sollicitudo Rei Socialis
U R	Unitatis Redintegratio

Abbreviations from other works

A D	Anno Domino (Year of the Lord)
A T R	African Traditional Religion
AAS	Acta Apostolicae Sedis
Afer	African Ecclesiastical Review (Kenya)
AIDS	Acquired Immune Deficiency Syndrome
B T S	Bigard Theological Studies
C C M	Catholic Charismatic Movement

C C R	Catholic Charismatic Renewal
C C	Catechismo della Chiesa
C E P	Congregation for the Evangelisation of peoples
C I W A	Catholic Institute of West Africa (Port–Harcourt, Nigeria)
C U E A	Catholic University of East Africa (Kenya)
Cf	Confer
CMS	Church Missionary Society
Co	Companions
Dec.	December
ed, eds	Editor, Editors
etc	Etcetera (and others)
Feb.	February
Ff	And following
HIV	Human Immunodeficiency Virus
I T R	Igbo Traditional Religion
Ibid.	Ibidem
Jan.	January
N J	New Jersey
N Y	New York
NGO	Non Governmental Organisations
No	Number
Op. Cit.	Opus Citatum (Works already cited)
P C 1 D	Pontifical Council for Inter Religious Dialogue
p. (pp)	Page (pages)
Rev.	Reverend
S 1 S T	Spiritan International School of Theology (Attakwu, Nigeria)
S E C A M	Symposium of Episcopal Conference of Africa and
Vol.	Volume
W A T R	West African Traditional Religion

Selected Bibliography

Dictionaries and Encyclopaedias

A New Dictionary of Christian Theology, Edited by Richardson, A. & Bowfrn, J., SCM Press, 1991.

Calwer Bibellexikon, Herausgegeben von Otto Betz, Beate Ego und Werner Grimm in Verbindung mit Wolfgang Zwickel, Stuttgart 2003

Lexikon für Theologie und Kirche Walter Kasper mit Konrad Baumgartner, Horst Bürkle, Klaus Ganzer, Karl Kertelge, Wilhelm Korff, Peter Walter, Zehnter Band, Thomaschristen bis Zytomyr, Herder, Freiburg. Basel. Rom. Wien, 2001

The Concise Oxford Dictionary of Current English, Allen, R.E., (ed.) (8 edition), New York, 1990.

Encyclopaedia of Biblical Theology Bauer, J.B., , Sheed and Ward, London, 1 977.

Dictionary of Comparative Religion, Brandon, S.G.F., (ed.), New York, 1 970,Theological Dictionary of the New Testament Bromley, G.M., Eerdmans Publishers, 1985.

International Dictionary of the New Testament Theology, Brown, C., Volume 1 1, Michigan, 1986.

Dictionary of Pentecostal and Charismatic Movements, Burgess, S. M., & McGee G. B., (eds.), Grand Rapids, Michigan, 1988.

The Interpreters Dictionary of the Bible Buttrick, G. A., (ed.), an illustrated Encyclopaedia, Vol. 2, Nashville, 1985.

A Dictionary of Pastoral care, London Cambell, A.V., (ed.), London, 1977. The Collegeville Pastoral Dictionary of Biblical Theology, Carrol, S & co (eds.), Liturgical Press, Minnesota, 1996.

Dizionario di Teologia Pastorale Sanitaria, Cina, G., Locci, E., Rocchetta, C., Sandrin, L., (eds.), Edizione Camilliane, Torino, 1997.

Dictionary of Medical Ethics, Duncan, A.S., Dunstan, G.R., Melbourn, R.B., (eds.), Darton, Longmans, London, 1981.

Encyclopaedia of Theology: Sacramentum Mundi, Vol. 3, Burns and Oates,VV. Germany, 1987.

Foreman, J.B., Collins English Gem Dictionary, London, 1974.

The Interpreters Dictionary of the Bible George, A. B., (ed.), Abigdon Press, Nashville, 1985.
The Advanced Learners Dictionary of current English, Hornby, A.S., Gatenway, E.V., Wakefield, H., Oxford University Press, London, 1965.
The Encyclopaedia of Religion, Vol. 3, Mircea, E., Macmillan, New York, 1987.
The Encyclopaedia of Religion, Vol. 6, Mircea, E., Macmillan, NewYork, 1 987.
New Catholic Encyclopaedia, Washington, 1981.
Encyclopaedia of Theology: a concise Sacramentum Mundi, Rhahner, K., (ed.), Burns and Oates, London, 1977.
The Catholic Encyclopaedia, revised and updated Robert, B., (ed.), Thomas Nelson Publishers, New York, 1987.
Encyclopaedia Britanica, Vol. 13, University of Chicago Staff, (ed.), Chicago Toronto, 1984.
Dictionary of Biblical Theology, Xavier Leon–Duffour, (ed.), London, 1970.

Works

Aguaowo, M.G.U., Health in Traditional Nigeria Society, Leuven,1985.
Ashley, B.N., Rourke, K.D., Ethics of healthcare, CHA, St. Louis, 1986.
Baldwin, R., The Healers, Huntington, Indiana, 1986.
Barclay, W., Prayers for heip and healing, Glasgow, 1976.
Brown, C., Miracie and the critical mind, Eerdmanns Publication, Michigan,1984.
Buckley, M., His Healing Touch: Freedom through good relationships, Harper Collins, London, 1987.
Byrant, C., Depth psychology and religious belief, Darton, Longman, and Todd, London, 1987.
Chigbo, K. , Catholic Healing ministry on fire, Abakiliki, 1997.
Cobb E. H., Christ Heafing, London, Washington, Capetown 1933.
Coyle, T., (ed.), Christian ministry to the sick, London, 1986.
Davies S. L., Jesus the healer, Possession, Trance and Origins of Christianity, S.C.M. Press, London, 1995.
De Grandis, R and Schubbert, L., Healing through the Mass, Resurrection Press, New York, 1992.
De Grandis, R., Lay person's manual for the healing ministry, St.Paul's publication, Makati, Philipines, 1988.
Edgar, N.J., Understanding health: An introduction to the holistic approach to health, London, 1972.

Emiliano Tardif & Philippe Madre, Das Charisma der Heilung und Gebete um Heilung, Vier–Türme–Verlag, Münsterschwarzach, 1995.
Ezeanya, S.N., Healing in Traditional African society, West African Religion, 17, Nsukka, 1976.
Fitchter, J.H., Healing ministries, St. Paul's, New Jersey, 1986.
Galipeau, S.A., Transforming Body and Soul: Therapeutic wisdom in the gospel healing stories, New Jersey, 1990.
Geisler, N.L., Miracies and modern thought, Michigan, 1982.
Glenon, C. J., Your healing is within you, Houdder and Stoughton, London, Sydney, 1978.
Graham, H., Time, Energy, and Psychology of healing, London, 1990.
Gumede, M. V., Traditional healers, Capetown, 1990.
Gunstone, J., Healing Power, Servant books, Michigan, 1987.
Hacker, G., The Healing Stream: Catholic Insight into the ministry of healing, Dalton, Longman and Todd, London, 1998.
Haring, B., Healing and revealing, Slough, London, 1984.
Haring, B., Medical Ethics, St. Paul's Publication, London, 1977.
Haring, B., The healing power of peace and non–violence, Slough, England, 1986.
Haron, F., Burnside, J., Health and human values, New Haven, London,1983.
Harrie, C.W., Resist the Devil: a pastoral guide to deliverance prayer, Green Lawn, 1988.
Hayes, H., Von de Poel, C.J., (eds.), Healthcare ministry: a handbookforchaplains, NewJersey, 1990.
Heijkoop, H.L., Faith healing, speaking in tongues, signs and miracles in the light of the scriptures, Kaduna, 1994.
Henri J.M. Nouwen, Seelsorge, die aus dem Herzen kommt, Herder, Freiburg, Basel, Wein, 1989.
Ikeobi, G., Effective prayer and Christian basis for spiritual healing, Okeke Charity Press, Nnewi, 1975.
Kane, T., The healing touch of Affirmation, Affirmation books, Massachusetts, 1976.
Keller, A. Schmerz–Leid–Tod: Verlag Butzon & Berecker Kevelaer, 1980.
Kelsey, M. Healing and Christianity, S.C. M. Press, London, 1973.
Kelsey, M.T., Psychology, Medicine and Christian healing, San Francisco 1988.
Keneth, M., Healing the family tree, Sheldon press, London, 1992.
Krippner, S., & Villoldo, A., The realms of healing, California, 1976.
Levine, S., Healing into life and death, London, 1987.
Lenz, H., Das Feuer neu entfachen – Lachen, Verl., BE –Team, 2004
Linn, D., Linn, M., Healing Life's hutis, New York, 1977.

Leuninger, E., Die Entwicklung der Gemeindeleitung – St. Ottilien: EOS–Verl., 1996
Leuninger, E., Dialog in der Kirche – Limburg: Lahn–Verl., 1992.
Leuninger, E., Wir sind das Volk Gottes, Frankfurt am Main: Knecht, 1992, 1.Aufl.
Leuninger, E., Die missionarische Pfarrei, Limburg: Lahn–Verl., 1981
Mackrell, G., The Healing Miracles in Marks Gospel, Slough England,1987.
Ifeanyi, V., The Catholic Church and the Challenges of the Traditional System of Healthcare in Nigeria, Rome, 1989.
MacNutt, F., Healing,Ave Maria Press, U.S.A., 1974.
Manus, C., Mbefo, L., Uzukwu, E., Healing and Exorcism. – The Nigerian experience, Snaap Press, Enugu, 1992.
Marsch, M., Healing through the Sacraments, Liturgical Press, Collegeville, Minesota, 1989.
Maslow, A.W., Motivation and Personality, Harper and Row, New York, 1970.
Mayeroff, M., On Caring, Harper and Row Publishers, London, 1972.
McCoy, K. C., Genetic Counselling and the Catholic Healthcare Institutional response in the United States, Rome, 1986.
McGuire, A., Handerson, J., Mooney, G., The economics of healthcare, London, New York , 1988.
McManus, J., Healing in the Spirit. – Inner healing and deliverance in today's Church, London, 1994.
Meehan, B.M., The Healing Power of Prayer, Ligouri Publications, U.S. A., 1988.
Milingo, E., The World in between.– The Christian Healing and struggle for spiritual survival, Ibadan, 1986.
Monge, M. A., Ethical practices in health and diseases, Manilla, Philippines, 1994.
Niederschlag, H., Prophetischer Protest – Vallendar–Schönstatt: Patris–Verl., 2003
Njoku, S., Curses, Effects and Reiease, Christian Living Publication, Enugu,1993.
Nwankwo, D.O., Healing: Challenges of African Traditional and Christian Religions, Tropical Fish Paradise, Festac town, Lagos, no date.
O'Neill, A., Charismatic healing in every day life, Ireland, 1991.
Onyemenagam, J.O., Pastoral Care of the Sick in lgbo Community of Nigeria, Rome, 1985.
Probst, M., Plock, H., Richter, K., Kommunionfeier mit Kranken. Eine Handreichung für Priester und Laien, Essen: Driewer 2 – 4. Aufl. 1973

Richter, K., Plock, Probst, M., Liturgie mit Kranken, Krankensalbung – Hausmessen – Stärkung im Tod; Essen, Driewer 1973
Richter, K., Probst, M., H. Plock, Zeichen der Hoffnung in Tod und Trauer. Ein Werkbuch für die Pastoralliturgische Praxis, Freiburg–Einsiedeln: Herder – Benziger 2 Aufl. 1978
Rhymer, J., The Miracles of Jesus, Slough, United Kingdom, 1991.
Richards, J., The question of healing services, London, 1989.
Sandford, J. A., Healing and Wholeness, St. Paul's, New York, 1977.
Sandford, J.A., Healing body and Soul. – The meaning of illness in the New Testament and in Psychotherapy, Louiseville, Kenturchy, 1992.
Scalan, M., lnnerhealing, Dublin, 1979.
Schmiedel, J., Das Konzil und die Orden – Vallendar–Schönstatt, Patris–Verl., 1999
Schmiedel, J., In seinem Herzen ein Feuer – Vallendar, Patris–Verl., 1999
Shorter, A., Jesus and the Witch doctor.' An approach to healing and wholeness. London, New York, 1985.
Sofoluwe, G.O., Benneth, F.J., Principles and Practice of Community Health in Africa, University Press, Ibadan, 1985.
Thomas, L. & Alkire, J., Healing as a parish ministry: mending body, mind and spart, Ave Maria Press, lndiana, 1992.
Thomas, L., The healing team: a pastoral guide for effective ministry, New York, 1987.
Turner, J., The Healing Church, Christian Journals, Beifast–Dublin Ottawa, 1978.
Unger, M.F., Demons in the world today, Tyndale house publishers, Wheaton, Illinois, 1974.
Uzorma, N.M., Occult grand master now in Christ, Osasu publication, Benin, 1993.
Weil, A., Health and Healing, Houghton, Boston, 1983.
Weiser, A., Jesu Wunder – damals und heute Katholisches Bibelwerk GmbH, Stuttgart, 1976.
Wilkinson, J., Christian Ethics in healthcare, Handsel Press, Edinburgh, 1988.
Wright, G., Our Quest for Healing, Green Hurst Press, Cheltenham Glos, U.K., 1981.

Works on Igbo and African Traditional Life

Achebe, C., Morning Yet on Creation, Day Essays, Heinemann, London, 1982.
Achebe, C., Things fall Apart, Heinemann, London, 1978.

Achebe, Chinwe., The World of Ogbanje, Forth Dimension, Enugu, 1986.
Adegbola, E.E.A., (ed.), Traditional Religion in West Africa, Ibadan, 1983.
Amadi, E., The Concubine, London, 1978.
Amponsah, K., Topics on West African Traditional Religion, Vol.II, Cape Coast, 1975.
Anigbo, 0.A.C., Commensality and Human relationship among the Igbos, Enugu, 1987.
Arinze, F. A., Answering God's call, London, 1983.
Arinze, F. A., Sacrifice in Ibo Religion, lbadan, 1970.
Arthur, G. L., The Lower Niger and it's Tribes, London, 1968.
Bascon, W. R., (ed.) Continuity and Change in African Culture, University Press, Chicago, 1975.
Basden, G. T., Among the Ibos, London, 1966.
Basden, G.T., Niger lbos, London, 1966.
Blakely, T. D., and co. (ed.), Religion in African experience and expression, London, 1994.
Bohannan, P., African Outline, Penguin Books Harmondsworth, 1964.
Edeh, E., Towards an Igbo Metaphysics, U.S.A., 1985.
Egudu, R & Nwoga, D., lgbo traditional verses.
Ejizu, C., lgbo Ritual Symbols, Enugu, 1986.
Eliade, M., From Primitive to Zen: A thematic source book of the history Religion, London, 1967.
Esomonu, L.E., Respect for Human Life in lgbo Religion and Morality,
Rome, 1981.
Forde, D. & Jones G.I., The lbo and lbibio – speaking peoples of South–Eastem Nigeria, 1962.
Gelfand, M., The African Witch, E & S Livingston Ltd, 1967.
Glyn, L. A., The Lower Niger and it's tribes, London 1968.
Green, M.M. , lgbo Village Affairs, London, 1964.
Green, M. M., Land Tenure in Igbo Village, London, 1941.
Gumede, M. V., Traditional Healers, Capetown, 1990.
Henderson, R. N., The king in every man: Evolutionary Trends in Onitsha Ibo Society and Culture, New Haven, Yale University Press,Chicago,1975.
Idowu, E.B., African Traditional Religion, London, 1973.
lfemesia, C., Traditional Humane Living among the lgbos, Enugu, 1979.
Igwegbe, 1., Newmann's Sacramental theological thinking: it's relevance to Africans, Rome, 1994.
Ilogu, E., Christianity and Igbo Culture, New York, 1974.
Isichei, E., A history of the lgbo peopie, London, 1960.
lwu, M., African Ethnomedicine, Snaap Press, Enugu, 1986.

Jordan, J., Bishop Shanahan of Southem Nigeria, London, 1949.
Kato, B.H., African Cultural Revolution and Christian Faith, Jos, 1976.
Kirwan, M.C., The Missionary and the Diviner, Mary Knoll, New York, 1 988.
Leonard, A.G., The Lower Niger and it's Tribes, London, 1906.
Lucas, J. 0., Religion in West Africa and Ancient Egypt, Lagos, 1970.
Madu, R.O., Studies in Africa and Africa American Culture: African Symbols, Proverbs, and Myths, New York, Paris, 1992.
Mbefo, L., Re–shaping of African Tradition, Enugu, 1988.
Mbiti J. S., The Prayers of African Religion, London, 1975.
Mbiti, J. S., Bible and Theology in African Christianity, Nairobi, 1986.
Mbiti, J. S., Concept of God in Africa, London, 1970.
Mbiti, J. S., The lntroduction to African Religion, London, 1975.
Mbiti, J.S., African Religion and Philosophy, London, 1977.
Meek, C., Law and Authority in a Nigerian tribe, London, 1937.
Metuh, 1. E., African Religions in Westem Conceptual schemes: The problem of Interpretation, Jos, 1991.
Metuh, 1. E., and Ojoade, 0., Nigerian Cultural Heritage, Jos, 1990.
Metuh, 1. E., God and Man in African Religion, London, 1981.
Metuh, 1.E., Comparative Studies of African Traditional Religions, Imico Press, Jos, 1987.
Moinoukin, M., Akan and Ga–Adangme peopie of the Gold Coast, London,1975.
Mozia, M., Solidarity in the Church and Solidarity among the lgbos of Nigeria, Rome, 1982.
Nkwo, M., lgbo Cultural Heritage, Vol. 1, University Publication Onitsha.
Nwabara, S.N., lboland: a century contact with Britain, 1860–1960, London,1977.
Nwogugu, Family Law in Nigeria, Ibadan, Hienemann, 1974.
Nwosu, V. A., (ed.), The Catholic Church in Onitsha: people, places and events (1885 – 1985), Onitsha, 1985.
Nzeako, J. U.T., Omenala ndi lgbo, London, 1977.
Nzekwu, 0., Ward of Noble Wood, London, 1961.
Obuna E., African Priests and celibacy, Rome, 1986.
O'Donohue, J., New wine, old botties: A study of the concepts of African Traditional Religion and their continuing influence today,Sweden,1994.
Obi, C. A., (ed.), Hundred Years of the Catholic Church in Nigeria, Onitsha, 1985.
Obiagwu, M.C., Our Praying Fathers, Rome, 1983.
Obuna, E., The people of God as educators to peace and violence among the lgbos of Nigeria, Rome, 1986.

Odinkemelu, L., Mammy Water in the society: Her influence in lgbo Culture, Ihiala, 1986.
Okafor, F., Africa at Crossroads, New York, 1974.
Okpala, M.M., The lgbo peopie and the search for security, Rome, 1985.
Onyeocha, A. E., Family Apostolate in lgboland, Rome, 1983.
Parrinder, G., Africa's Three Religions, Sheldon Press, London, 1969.
Parrinder, G., African Traditional Religion, London, 1975.
Parrinder, G., West African Traditional religion, London, SPCK, 1962.
Smith E., African ldeas of God, London, 1961.
Talbolt, P. A., Some Nigeria Fertility Cult, Oxford University Press, London, 1929.
Thorpe, S. A., African Traditional Religion, Pretoria, South Africa, 1992.
Uchendu, V.C., The Igbo of South–Eastem Nigeria, New York, 1965.
Udo, R.K., Nigeria, Area and Population, in Encyclopaedia Britannica, (ed.) University of Chicago, 1984, Vol. 13.
Westermann, D., Africa and Christianity, Oxford London, 1937.

Papal Documents

John Paul II, Apostolic Letter, Salvifici Doloris, 11 February 1984, AAS 66(984).
Apostolic Letter, Dolentium Hominum, 15 February 1985, AAS 77(1985).
Apostolic Exhortation, Familiaris Consortio, 22 November 1981, AAS 74 (1982).
Apostolic Exhortation, Pastores dabo vobis, 25 March 1992.
Apostolic Exhortation, Christi Fidelis laici, 30 December, 1988, AAS 81 (1989).
Apostolic Exhortation, Catechesi Tradendae, 16 October, 1979, AAS 71 (1979).
Apostolic Exhortation, Dominicae Canae, 24 February, 1980.Encyclical Letter, Redemptor Hominis, 4 March 1979, AAS 71 (1979).
Evangelisation in the Modern World, Evangelium Nuntiandi, 8 December, 1975, AAS 68 (1976).
Ecclesiae in Africa, Post Synodal Exhortation, 14 September, 1995, AAS 88 (1996).
Address to Nigerian Bishops, 17 February 1982, AAS 74 (1982).
Paul VI, Encyclical Letter, Humanae Vitae, 25 July,1968, AAS 60 (1968).
Encyclical Letter, Mysterium Fidei, 3 September 1965, AAS 62 (1965).
Encyclical Letter, Ecclesiam Suam, 6 August 1964, AAS 6 (1964).
Apostolic Constitution on Penance, Paenitemini, 17 February, 1966, AAS 63 (1966).

Apostolic Constitution on the Sacrament of Annointing, Sacram Unctionem Infirmorum,30 November, 1972, AAS 65 (1973).
Decree Promulgating the New Order of Penance, Reconciliationi, 2 December, 1973.
Africae Terrarum, Message to the people of Africa, 29 October 1967, AAS 59 (1967).
Leo XIII., Apostolic Letter, Catholicae Ecclesiae, 20 November 1880, Actes de Leon, XIII.

Conciliar Documents

Actio Pastoralis Ecclesiae, Instruction on Masses for Special Gathering, 15 May 1969, AAS 61 (1969).
Apostolicam Actuositatem, Decree on the Apostolate of the Lay People, 18 November, 1965, AAS 58 (1966), 837 – 864.
Dei Verbum, Dogmatic Constitution on Divine Revelation, 18 November, 1965, AAS 58 (1966).
Eucharisticum Mysterium, On the Worship of the Eucharistic Mystery, 25 May 1967, AAS 59 (1967).
Gaudium et Spes, Pastoral Constitution on the Church in the Modern World, 7 December, 1965, AAS 58 (1966).
Hominum Dolores, Introduction to the rite of anointing and to the Pastoral Care of the sick, 7 December, 1972.
Infirmis Cum Ecclesiae, On the new rite of the anointing and the Pastoral Care of the sick, 7 December 1972, AAS 65 (1973).
Lumen Gentium, Dogmatic Constitution on the Church, 21 November, 1964, AAS 57 (1965).
Misericordiam Suam, Introduction to the New Order of Penance, 7 February 1974.
Mysterium Ecclessiae, Declaration in defence of the Catholic Doctrine on the Church against some present day errors, 24 June, 1973, AAS 65 (1973).
Nostrae Aetate, Declaration on the Relation of the Church to Non –Christian Religions, 28 October, 1965, AAS 58 (1966).
Optatam Totius, Decree on the training of the Priests, 28 October, 1965, AAS 58 (1966).
Presbyterium Ordinis, Decree on the ministry and life of Priests, 7 December 1965.
Sacrosanctum Concilium, Constitution on the Liturgy, 4 December, 1963, AAS 56 (1964).

Other Church and Episcopal Documents

Congregation for Divine Worship and the Discipline of the sacraments – The Roman Liturgy and Inculturation, Vatican Press, Vatican City, 1994.
Coriden, J.A., & co (eds), The Canon Law; text and Commentary, St Paul's Publication, New York, 1985.
International Theological Commission, Christianity and the world Religions, Vatican City, 1997.
Obiefuna, A. K., Directives on Prayer Ministry and Healing Ministry in the Archdiocese of Onitsha, MAS Founders Publications Ltd, Nkpor, 16 October, 1996.
Pontifical Commission for the Apostolate of Healthcare Workers: Religious in the world of suffering and health, Rome, 1987.
Pontifical Commission for the Apostolate of Healthcare Workers: The Laity in the world of suffering and health, Rome, 1987.
Pontifical Commission for the Apostolate of Healthcare Workers: The Training of the priests and the pastoral care of the sick, Vatican City, 1990.
Pontifical Council for Inter Religious Dialogue and Congregation for Evangelisation of the Peoples, Dialogue and Proclamation, 19 May 1991, Vatican City, 1991.
Pontifical Council for pastoral Assistance, Charter for healthcare workers, Vatican Translation, St. Paul's Books and Media, Boston, 1995.
The Catechism of the Catholic Church, St Paul's Publication African/Libreria Editrice, Vatican, Vatican City, 1994.
The Catholic Bishops' Conference of Nigeria, Guidelines for the healing ministry in the Catholic Church in Nigeria, 14 September 1996, Lagos, 1997.
The Code of Canon Law, Vatican City, 1983.

Pastoral and other Theological Works

Aixala, J., Searching the scriptures, St. Paul's Publication, Allahabad,1982.
Akukwe, F.N., Towards a New society, Enugu, 1988.
Apostoli, A., The Gift of God: The Holy Spirit, New York, 1997.
Arinze, S., Increase your wisdom, Snaap Press, Enugu, 1993.
Ayandale, E.A., The missionary impact on modem Nigeria, 1842 1914, Ibadan,1966.
Bertsch, L., Leitideen Künftiger Sakramentenpastoral, in: Wiener, J./Erharter, H. (Hg.), Zeichen des Heils, Vien 1975

Bertsch, L., Tendenzen der Veränderung und Erneuerung der Sakramentenpastoral, in: Pastroaltheologische Informationen 1976

Betz, J., Art.:Krankensalbung, in: Handbuch theologischer Grundbegriffe Bd. I (hg.Von H.Fries), Münschen 1962

Bührer, M., Anregungen für die Krankenpastoral. Auf der Suche nach neuen Wegen, Müunschen/Luzern 1977

Bowers, M.K. u.a., Wie können wir Sterbenden beistehen? München/Mainz 1971, 1973

Brown, R., New Testament Essays, Chapman, London, 1965.

Browne, M., & African Faith and Justice net work, (eds), The African Synod, Documents, Reflections, Perspectives, Orbis Books, Mary Knoll, New York, 1 996.

Collins, G.O., Interpreting Jesus, Chapman, London, 1985.

Dhavamony, M., Christian Theology of Inculturation, Editrice Pontificia Università Gregoriana, Roma, 1997.

Domeris, W, The portraits of Jesus,– Mark, Collins Publications, London,1987.

Ekechi, F.K., Missionary enterprises and rivalry in Igboland, 1857–1914, London,1972.

Ekwunife, A.N.O., Nwosu, V.A., Nzomiwu J.P.C., (eds) Renewal of priestly life and ministry: The Nigerian experience, Snaap press, Enugu, 1995.

Gula, R.M., Ethics in Pastoral Ministry, Paulist press, New York, Mahwah, New Jersey, 1996.

Gusmer, C.W., And you visited me: Sacramental ministry to the sick and the dying, Pueblo Publishing Company, New York, 1989.

Guttler, M., The portraits of Jesus: Mark, Collins publication, London, 1 987.

Guy, H. A., The life of Christ, Macmillan, London, 1974

Guy, H. A., The synoptic gospels, Macmillan, London, 1974.

Heiler, F., Prayer –. A study in the history and psychology of Religion, London,1932.

Latourelle, R., The miracles of Jesus and the theology of miracles, New York, 1988.

Martin, R., and Williamson, P., John Paul 11 and the New Evangelisation, Ignatius Press, San Francisco, 1995.

Martinez, L.M., The Sanctifier, St Paul's Publication Boston, 1985.

Martins, R.P., New Testament Foundations: A Guide for Students, Vol 2, Acts Revelation, Pater Noster Press, Australia, 1978.

Mgbobukwa, J., Inculturation: A positive approach in the Nigerian Church, Pacific Publishers, Obosi, 1994.

Moody, R.A., Life after life: The investigation of a phenomenon, survival of bodily death, Bantan books, London, New York, Sydney,1976.

Ndiokwere, N., Africa Today, and Tomorrow, Vol. 1, Onitsha, 1994.
Ndiokwere, N., Prophecy and Revolution.– The role of Prophets in the independent African Churches and in the Biblical Tradition, SPCK, London, 1981.
Nleanya, 0., A., Critical Introduction to the Traditions of Jesus, Enugu 1991.
Nouwen, H., Creative Ministry, Image book, New York, 1978.
O'Grady, J.F., The four Gospels and the Jesus traditions, New Jersey, 1989.
Okolo, C., The Igbo Church and the quest for God, Pacific Press, Obosi, 1985.
Okure, T., Paul van Thiel et alii, 32 Atticies evaluating Inculturation of Christianity in Africa, AMECEA Gaba Publications, Kenya, 1990.
Onoyinma, T., Aitention Please No. 1, Snaap press, Enugu, 1996.
Palmer, B., (ed) Medicine and the Bible, Pater Noster Press, Australia, 1986.
Perkins, P., New Testament introduction, St. Paul's, Bombay, 1992.
Publication Department, CUEA, Nairobi, (ed), The Gospel as Good News for African Cultures, A Symposium on the Dialogue between Faith and Culture, CUEA Publications, 1999.
Sabourin, L., The divine miracles discussed and defended, Rome, 1987.
Saldanha, J., Inculturation, St Paul's Publication, Bandra, Mumbai, 1997.
Schineller, P., A handbook on Inculturation, New York, 1990.
Shorter, A., The African Synod: A personal response to the Outline document, St. Paul's Publication, Africa, 1991.
Sigo, J., Miracie age, Kaduna, Nigeria, 1990.
Sullender, R.S., Grief and Growth, New Jersey 1985.
Theissen, G., The miracie stories of the early Christians, T and T Clark, Edinburgh, 1983.
Touhey, J.F., Caring for persons with Cancer and Aids, CHA, St. Louis, 1985.
Uzukwu, E.E., A listening Church.– Autonomy and Communion in African Churches, Orbis Book, Mary Knoll, New York, 1996.
Vaughan, R.P., Basic skills for Christian counseilors: an introduction for pastoral ministers, St. Paul's publication, New York, 1987.

Articles and Journals

Achebe, Chinwe, The Ogbanje Phenomenon: An Interpretation, in C.U.Manus et al., "Healing and Exorcism: The Nigeria Experience", Enugu, 1992, pp. 24 – 43.
Agnew, M.B., Charismatic Movement, in "New Catholic Encyclopaedia", Washington, 1981, pp.157–159.

Akpunonu, P.D., Healing in the Bible and in the Church.' The Nigerian experience, in "Bigard theological studies", July – December, 1995, vol. 15, No. 2, pp. 5 – 17.
Anike, O., Miracie or Magic?, Misunderstanding and Aberration in the healing ministries, in "Touch Magazine", Enugu, April – June, 1993.
Asuzu, M.C., Healing Apostolate of the Church, Seminar paper, Emene, Enugu, February, 1992.
Bibel und Kirche – Wunder – Geschichten von Gottes Kraft 61. Jahrgang 2.Quartal Stuttgart, 2/2006
Boyle, J., The concept of health and the right to healthcare, "On Moral Medicine", (ed), Lammers, S.E:, and Allen V., Michigan, 1987.
Boylon, A. The rite of Anointing and Viaticum, in Tom Coyle, (ed.), "Christian Ministry to the sick", London, 1986, pp. 20 – 38.
Bradley, P.B., Healing in the Charismatic Movement, "The Catholics in Nigeria, Religions, Nsukka, Vol. 2, No. 2, Dec. 1977.
Bundesministerium für Familie, Senioren, Frauen und Jugend: Fünfter Bericht zur Lage der älteren Generation in der Bundesrepublik Deutschland, Berlin, August, 2005.
Cahallan, D., The WHO definition of health, in "On Moral Medicine", (ed), Lammers, S.E., and Allen, V., Michigan, 1987.
Chappell, P.G., Healing Movements, in Burgess S.M., & McGee G.B., (eds), "The dictionary of Pentecostal and Charismatic Movement", Grand Rapids, 1988.
Constantelos, Charity, in Mircea E., (ed.) "Encyclopaedia of Religion, Vol.3", London, 1987.
Dulles, A., John Paul 11 and the New Evangelisation – What does it mean?, in R. Martin and P. Williamson, John Paul 11 and the New Evangelisation, Ignatius Press, San Francisco, 1995, pp.25 – 39.
Ejizu, C., Cosn?oiogical Perspective on Exorcism and Prayer–Healing in Contemporary Nigeria, in C. U. Manus &co (eds), "Healing and Exorcism: The Nigerian Experience", Enugu, 1992.
Eneja, M.U., Goodwill Message, in C,U.Manus &co, "Healing and Exorcism: The Nigerian Experience", Enugu, 1992.
Enusani, G., Healing and Deliverance ministry: What is really happening? Seminar Paper on Healing ministry, Emene–Enugu, 1 llh _ 14 Ih February, 1992.
Ezeokeke, P.E., A layman's reflection on some Pastoral problems, in B.T.S., Vol. 1, No.2, July – Dec., 1994.
Faniran,J., Charism and Authority: A case study of the Charismatic Renewal in Nigerian Church, "Nigerian Journal of Theology", Vol. 7, No.1, June 1993.

Gillman, J., Charism, in Stuhllmueller (ed.), "The Collegeville Pastoral Dictionary of Biblical Theology", Minnesota, 1996.
Gomez J. A., The Care of the sick in the history of the Church, in "Dolentium Hominum", No. 31, 1996..
Graber, F., and Mutter D., Heal, in Brown C, "International Dictionary of the New Testament Theology", Vol. 2, Michigan, 1986.
Green, S.E., Religion, History and the Supreme Gods in Africa, in "The Journal of Religion in Africa", Vol. XXVI, Fasc. 2, May, 1992.
Greenberg, J.H., Africa as linquistic area, in W.R. Bascom, (ed) "Continuity and Change in African Culture", Chicago, 1975.
Hellberg, J.H., The Makumira consultation on the healing ministry of the Church, in "African theological journal", NO. 1, 1968.
Heron, B., Praying for Healing, in Tom Coyle, (ed), "Christian Ministry to the Sick", London, 1986, pp. 91 – 103.
Hetson, J., VVanjobi, R., Annointing and Healing in Africa, in "Spearhead Magazine", No. 71, Gaba publication, 1982.
Hinnebusch, P., The Bible in the Charismatic Movement, in W.R. Farmer et al. (eds), "The International Bible Commentary", Liturgical Press, Collegeville, Minnesota, 1998, p. 1 56.
Ibekwem, D.D., Testimony, Seminar Paper on Healing Ministry, Emene, Enugu, 1 lth _ 14 th February 1992.
Igboaja, U., Healing Ministry at the Pastoral Centre Ugwu di nso, Eke, Seminar paper, Emene–Enugu, February, 1992.
Ikeobi, G., Sickness, Prayer and Healing, in "Mulumba magazine", Vol. 3, No.1, Enugu, Dec. – June 1989.
Ikeobi,G., Healing and Exorcism.– The Nigerian Pastoral Experience, in C.U.Manus et al., (eds), "Healing and Exorcism – The Nigerian Experience", Enugu, 1992.
Ilkeobi, G., Catholic Response to the Challenge of Prayer Houses: The origin of Tuesday Prayer in Onitsha, in Nwosu, V.A., "TheCatholic Church in Onitsha: people, places and events (1885–1985)", Onitsha, 1985.
Ikeobi, G., Priests, Healing and Healing ministry, in A.N.0. Ekwunife et al., (eds), "The Renewal of Christian Life and Ministry: The Nigerian experience", Snaap press, Enugu, pp. 212–237.
Ikeobi, G., What 1 think God is doing in and through me, Seminar paper, Emene – Enugu, February, 1992.
Kamugisha, J.M., African proverbs as sources of wisdom, in "African Christian Studies", (ed), Namwera, L., Catholic University of East Africa, (CUEA), Nairobi, Kenya, Vol. 12, No. 4, Dec. 1996.
Madubuko, L., Igbo Worid View, in B.T.S., Vol. 14, No. 2, July–Dec., 1994.

Madubuko, L., Healing and Liturgy, Seminar paper on Healing ministry, Emene–Enugu, 1992.

L'Osservatore Romano, English edition, 18 th October 1973.

Maimela, S.S., Religion and Culture: Biessings or Curse?, in "The journal of Black Theology in South Africa", Vol. 5 No 1, Mäy 1991.

Manus, C.U., Miracle Workers1Healers as divine men: their role in Nigeria Church and society, "Asian Journal of Theology", Vol. 3, No. 2..

Mbefo, L., Priests and Healing ministry in the Nigerian Church – A Theological reflection, Seminar Paper, Emene–Enugu, 1992.

Meier, J., Jesus, in "The New Jerome Biblical Commentary", London, 1992.

Metuh, 1. E., African Traditional Medicine and Healing: a theological and pastoral reappraisal, in Lucerna, Bigard Memorial Seminary, Enugu, Jan. – June 1985,Vol. 6, No. 1

Metuh, 1. E., Theological status of African Traditional Religion, in the Journal of Inculturation theology, Vol. 1, No. 2, Catholic Institute of West Africa, (CIWA), Port–har–court, Nigeria, 1994.

Monge, M.A., Integral Care of the Sick.– The rolle of spiritual help, in "Dolentium Hominum", No. 12, 1989.

Musopole, H.C., Witchcraft Terminology, The Bible, and African Christian theology.– An exercise in Hermeneutics, in African Christian Studies, (CUEA), Nairobi, Vol. 8, No. 4, Dec. 1992.

Norbert, M., Environmental Condition to promote and defend health, in "Dolentium Hominum" No. 7, Yr 3, No. 1, 1988.

Nwankwo, L.C., Nigerian priests and Catholic Charismatic Renewal of Nigeria, in Ekwunife, A.N.O., & co (eds), "Renewal of priestly life and ministry: The Nigerian experience", Snaap press, Enugu, 1995.

Nyamiti , C., African Tradition and the Christian God, in "Spearhead", No 49, p. 48.

Nyamiti, C., African Ancestral Veneration, in "African Christian Studies", (CUEA), Nairobi, Vol. 9, No. 3, Sept. 1993..

Nyamiti, C., The problem of evil in African cultures and today's African Inculturation and Liberation Theologies, in ACS, (CUEA), Nairobi, Vol. 1 1, No. 1, March, 1995.

Nyamiti, C., The Trinity from an African Ancestral perspective, in ACS, (CUEA), Nairobi, Vol. 12, No. 4, Dec., 1996.

Obiagwu, M.C., MorallSpiritual care of the terminally sick, Conference Paper, Onitsha, 1995.

Obiefuna, A.K., National Theological/Pastoral Seminar on Healing Ministry, Seminar Paper, Emene–Enugu, February 1992.

Okolo, B.C., Healing ministry in the Nigerian Church: Dangers next door, in "Bigard Theological Studies", Vol. 14, No. 2.

Onaiyekan, J., The Priesthood in Owe traditional Religion, in Adegbola A.E., "Traditional Religion in W. Africa", lbadan, 1983.

Onwuka, S. C., 1 was a juju priest, in Adegbola A, "Traditional Religion in W. Africa", Ibadan, 1983.

Pellegrino, Edmund., Every sick person is my brother or sister, in Dolentium Hominum, Year 111, No 7, 1988, pp. 65 – 70.

Pilch J.J., Healing, in Stullmueller (ed.), The Collegeville Pastoral Dictionary of Biblical Theology, Minnesota, 1996.

Ramsey P., The Indignity of Death with dignity, in Lammers, S.E. & Allen V, (eds.), "On Moral Medicine", Michigan, 1987.

Redford J., The Healing Word: Scripture and the Pastoral Ministry to the Sick, in T. Coyle, (ed.), "Christian Ministry to the sick", London, 1986.

Romain, W., C.M.S. Archives, Niger Mission, CA31034, "Journal of a visit to Ossomare", 1869.

Ryan, R., Healing and the mission of the Church, in C. Stuhlmueller, (ed), "The Collegeville Pastoral Dictionary of Biblical Theology", Minnesota, 1996.

Taylor, E.B., Primitive Culture, 1, London, 1913, p. 1, in M. Dhavamony, Christian Theology of Inculturation, Rome, 1997, p. 41.

Turner, H.W., History of an Independent Church. – The Church of the Lord (Aladura), Vol. 1, London, 1967, pp.6–8.

Ukpong, J., Christology and lnculturation: A New Testament Perspective, in R. Gibelini,(ed), "Paths of African Theology", SCM Press, London, 1994.

Umeagudosu, M. A., The primacy of prayer in African spirituality, (Traditional and Christian), in ACS, CUEA, Nairobi, Vol. 9, No. 1, March, 1993..

Umeagudosu, M.A., The healing of the Gerasene demoniac from a specifically African perspective, in ACS, CUEA, Nairobi, Vol. 12, No.4, Dec. 1996..

Uzukwu, E.E., lnculturation and Liturgy (Eucharist), in R. Gibelini (ed), "Paths of African Theology", SCM Press, London, 1994.

Viviano, B.T., The gospel of Matthew, in "The New Jerome Biblical Commentary", London, 1992.

Walsh, J.C., The History of the rites, in T. Coyle (ed.), "Christian Ministry to the sick", London, 1986, pp. 4 – 19.

Wilkinson, P., A Theology of sickness, in T. Coyle (ed), "Christian Ministry to the Sick", London, 1986.

Wiseman, D.J., Medicine in the Old Testament Worid, in Palmer B., (ed), "Medicine and the Bible", Pater Noster, Australia, 1986.

World Health Oraganisation, Guide to Planning Health Promotion for AIDS Prevention and Control, Geneva, 2000.

World Health Organisation, Global Health Agenda, 11th General Programme of Work, Geneva, 2006.
Zuese, E. M., African Traditional Religion, in "Abingdon Dictionary of Living Religions",

Vincent Chijioke Onunkwo

Peace in the Social Teachings of Pope John Paul II: Its Relevance to the Igbo of Southeastern Nigeria

Frankfurt am Main, Berlin, Bern, Bruxelles, New York, Oxford, Wien, 2006.
324 pp.
European University Studies: Series 23, Theology. Vol. 834
ISBN 978-3-631-55217-9 · pb. € 56.50*

This study aims at re-evaluating the traditional Igbo conception and practice of peace and the doctrines of Pope John Paul II. By using an expository and evaluative approach, the author concludes that the Pope's teachings and pronouncements remain relevant in the life and experiences of Igbo Christians. This is a work which Western audiences will find informative and which will provide hope and inspiration for African readers whose lives are touched daily by the havoc of violence and war. The human need for peace, wholeness, love, and an encounter with the Sacred are characteristics that transcend individual cultures. Thus, all readers from all lands can recognize for themselves a role in the cause for peace and harmony for humankind.

Contents: Igbo traditional and religious attitudes to war and peace · Western context of the social teachings of Pope John Paul II.

FSC
www.fsc.org
MIX
Papier | Fördert
gute Waldnutzung
FSC® C083411

Kolibri 360 GmbH
Ferdinand-Jühlke-Straße 7
99095 Erfurt, Deutschland
produktsicherheit@kolibri360.de

Druck:
CPI Druckdienstleistungen GmbH
im Auftrag der
Kolibri 360 GmbH
Ferdinand-Jühlke-Str. 7
99095 Erfurt